Clinical Neurodynamics

This book is dedicated to:
My mother and father, Reta and Frank Shacklock
My children, Lucy and Oliver

For Elsevier

Commissioning Editor: Heidi Harrison
Development Editor: Siobhan Campbell
Production Manager: Morven Dean
Design: George Ajayi

Clinical Neurodynamics

A new system of musculoskeletal treatment

Michael Shacklock M.App.Sc, Dip. Physio.
Director
Neurodynamic Solutions
City Physiotherapy and Sports Injury Clinic
Adelaide, Australia

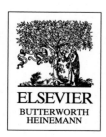

ELSEVIER
BUTTERWORTH
HEINEMANN

EDINBURGH LONDON NEW YORK OXFORD PHILADELPHIA ST LOUIS SYDNEY TORONTO 2005

ELSEVIER
BUTTERWORTH
HEINEMANN

First published 2005

ISBN 0 7506 5456 2

British Library Cataloguing in Publication Data
A catalogue record for this book is available from the British Library

Library of Congress Cataloging in Publication Data
A catalog record for this book is available from the Library of Congress

Notice
Medical knowledge is constantly changing. Standard safety precautions must be followed, but as new
research and clinical experience broaden our knowledge, changes in treatment and drug therapy may
become necessary or appropriate. Readers are advised to check the most current product information
provided by the manufacturer of each drug to be administered to verify the recommended dose, the
method and duration of administration, and contraindications. It is the responsibility of the
practitioner, relying on experience and knowledge of the patient, to determine dosages and the best
treatment for each individual patient. Neither the Publisher nor the author assumes any liability for
any injury and/or damage to persons or property arising from this publication.

    Neither the publishers nor the author will be liable for any loss or damage of any nature occasioned
to or suffered by any person acting or refraining from acting as a result of reliance on the material
contained in this publication.

          The Publisher

your source for books,
journals and multimedia
in the health sciences
www.elsevierhealth.com

The
Publisher's
policy is to use
**paper manufactured
from sustainable forests**

Printed in China

Contents

About the author   vii

Preface   ix

Acknowledgements   xiii

Chapter 1: General neurodynamics   1

Chapter 2: Specific neurodynamics   31

Chapter 3: General neuropathodynamics   49

Chapter 4: Diagnosis of specific dysfunctions   77

Chapter 5: Diagnosis with neurodynamic tests   97

Chapter 6: Planning the physical examination   105

Chapter 7: Standard neurodynamic testing   117

Chapter 8: Method of treatment: systematic progression   153

Chapter 9: Cervical spine   159

Chapter 10: Upper limb   175

Chapter 11: Lumbar spine   195

Chapter 12: Lower limb   217

Glossary   239

Index   243

About the author

Michael Shacklock graduated as a physiotherapist from the Auckland School of Health Sciences in 1980. During his undergraduate training, he quickly developed an interest in manual therapy and has pursued this interest throughout his career. He worked in public hospitals and private practices for several years in New Zealand before travelling to Adelaide, South Australia, to take part in postgraduate study. In 1989, he completed a Graduate Diploma in Advanced Manipulative Therapy at the University of South Australia and converted this to a Master of Applied Science in 1993. He has taught internationally for over 15 years and has given numerous keynote and invited presentations throughout the western world. His Masters thesis was on the effect of order of movement on the peroneal neurodynamic test, in which he discovered the concept of neurodynamic sequencing. Since then he has studied mechanics and physiology of the nervous system, performing research and writing publications on the subject. Michael edited the extremely successful book Moving in on Pain and has published in Physiotherapy, Manual Therapy, the Australian Journal of Physiotherapy and New Zealand Journal of Physiotherapy.

Michael's recent area of research has been the *in vivo* imaging of mechanical function of the nervous system and he teaches clinical neurodynamics internationally. He owns and directs a city based sports physiotherapy practice and is an associate of Specialised Physiotherapy Services. Most recently he founded Neurodynamic Solutions with the express purpose of disseminating the practical application of clinical neurodynamics.

NEURODYNAMIC SOLUTIONS COURSES

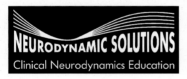

Courses in clinical neurodynamics as presented in this book are available world wide. If you are interested in holding or attending a course, workshop or seminar in this area or would like more information, please contact Neurodynamic Solutions.

Contact details:
Neurodynamic Solutions
6th floor, 118 King William Street
Adelaide SA 5000
Australia

Ph: +61 8 8212 4886
Fax: +61 8 8212 8028
E-mail: admin@neurodynamicsolutions.com
Web: www.neurodynamicsolutions.com

Preface

Neurogenic disorders are common and their incidence is probably underestimated (Bennett 1997). With many recent developments in their management, it is merciful that they can now be treated with non-invasive physical methods. The notion of adverse neural mechanics has been present for many years and probably longer than we know. Wittingly or unwittingly, the first known description of a neurodynamic test was on the Edwin Smith Papyrus by Imhotep in 2800 BC, in which a leg straightening manoeuvre was performed in the diagnosis of low back pain in workers injured whilst building the Egyptian pyramids (Beasley 1982; Dyck 1984). However, between then and now, much has happened and it is fascinating to note that, in addition to the neurodynamic tests for the lower quarter, the three major tests for the upper limb nerves (median, radial and ulnar) had been documented and illustrated pictorially by the 1920s and 1950s (Bragard 1929; Von Lanz & Wachsmuth 1959). Their anti-tension counterpart postures were also illustrated next to these neurodynamic tests (Figs i, ii and iii).

In the context of therapy, neural mobilization has undergone massive development, particularly in the last thirty-five years since Gregory Grieve, Geoffrey Maitland, Robert Elvey and David Butler published their work. Such an awareness of mechanical function of the nervous system has developed to the point where, for therapists dealing with pain and the musculoskeletal system, proficiency in neurodynamics has

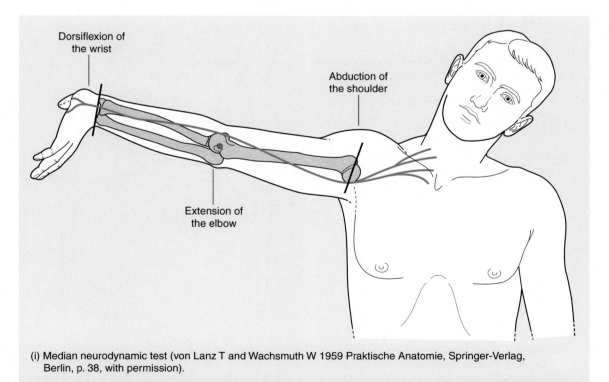

Dorsiflexion of the wrist

Abduction of the shoulder

Extension of the elbow

(i) Median neurodynamic test (von Lanz T and Wachsmuth W 1959 Praktische Anatomie, Springer-Verlag, Berlin, p. 38, with permission).

Figure P.1   The three main neurodynamic tests as described by Lanz and Wachsmuth in 1959.

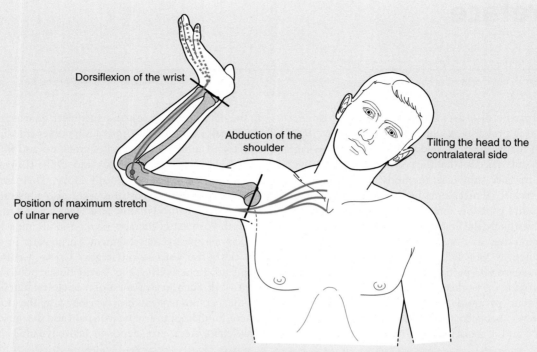

(ii) Ulnar neurodynamic test (von Lanz T and Wachsmuth W 1959 Praktische Anatomie, Springer-Verlag, Berlin, p. 41, with permission).

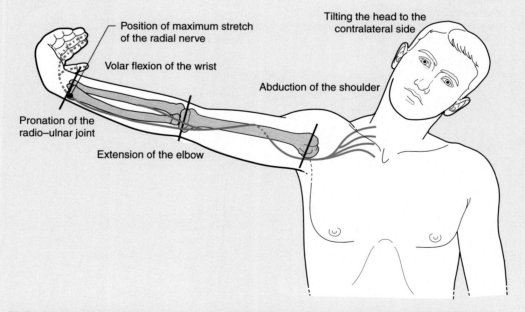

(iii) Radial neurodynamic test (von Lanz T and Wachsmuth W 1959 Praktische Anatomie, Springer-Verlag, Berlin, p. 47, with permission).

Figure P.1(*Continued*)

become a standard requirement. Nevertheless, an author whose work passed relatively unnoticed was Grieve (1970). The reason this paper is important is that in it Grieve commented on, for the first time that I am aware of in the physiotherapy literature, the notion of sensitivity of neural tissues being a key factor in whether they produce symptoms. He remarked on the possibility that inflamed neural tissues may well be more likely to produce abnormal neurodynamic tests as opposed to those on which pressure was exerted by pathologies such as disc bulges. He also alluded to the possibility that nervous system processing could be a means by which neurodynamic tests might change with spinal manual therapy. These aspects have undergone somewhat of a renaissance and they turn out to be key facets of current thinking in clinical neurodynamics.

Publications on neural problems are often complex, making it difficult for the clinician to apply neurodynamic techniques safely and effectively. My experience in teaching the approach around the world has led me to the conclusion that there is a gap in clinical expertise and resources. My intention with this book therefore is not to provide a detailed review of the literature but to quench the thirst in the clinician for a practical book that is balanced with enough theory to make sense of the practical application, with emphasis on selection and application of manual techniques that attack the causative mechanisms. For that reason, I have written this for the clinician who requires an understanding of the fundamentals of, and advances in, neurodynamics in relation to the musculoskeletal system. Emphasis in the early parts is on theoretical neurodynamics. What then follows is a system of how to work out patient problems; including classifications of dysfunctions; how to plan a safe and appropriate physical examination; how *not* to provoke pain, yet still have a beneficial effect; how to establish whether the nervous system is abnormal and how to construct a treatment regimen using a progressive system of mobilization techniques.

Functional neuroanatomy has been presented in numerous peer reviewed journals and is summarized well in other monographs (Breig 1960, 1978; Sunderland 1978, 1991; Butler 1991), so this aspect is not presented, other than some of the key points relevant to neurodynamics. New aspects that have not been presented elsewhere are proposed, such as a practical and systematic method of working through neurodynamic problems, with the final outcome being that the therapist understands, and can practise, this exciting subject more proficiently. This book is also intended to be an update so as to provide new options for treatment that the clinician may never have previously considered. One of the key aspects is the treatment of neurodynamic problems in conjunction with the musculoskeletal system. After all, many neural problems have their causes in the musculoskeletal system and, unfortunately, the emphasis in the past has been on mobilizing the nervous system per se, at the expense of integrating treatment of the musculoskeletal system. Neural mobilizations, particularly stretches, have at times been the mainstay of treatment, rather than being applied in a way that addresses how the body really moves, that is, in an integrated fashion that includes the relational dynamics between both the neural and musculoskeletal systems.

The general format of this book follows the process of clinical neurodynamics from beginning to end, from the perspective of the therapist. Even so, much of what therapists generate in treatment comes from our patients which makes it tempting to start this book from the patient's presentation, work backwards into the theory of what might be wrong, then finish with the anatomy and biomechanics. This is actually the way I do most of my learning, because many of the best questions come from the clinic. However, this can not easily be achieved in a book because learning is a circular process that involves constant revisiting and reorganizing knowledge so that it eventually grows into a flexible construct on which to base treatment. Some knowledge of the basic framework is required to start with. Hence, the first few chapters consist of theoretical neurodynamics and pathodynamics (general and specific) and the basis for diagnosis and treatment and are referred to in the later chapters.

One of the key principles in this book is that mechanics and physiology of the nervous system must be linked in the clinician's mind so that safe and effective decisions can be made. For too long now, the terms 'neural tension', 'neural stretch' and 'neural provocation' have been dominant and, even though the situation is improving, more change is necessary. Hence, the concept of neurodynamics, as I originally conceived it (Shacklock 1995a, b), is the mainstay of this book.

With the above in mind, I felt the need to produce an approach that is in some ways uniquely useful to the clinician. The approach is therefore characterized by the following:

1. links between mechanics and physiology of the nervous system
2. integration of neurodynamics with musculoskeletal functions
3. a new movement diagram that enables the clinician integrate musculoskeletal and neural mechanisms
4. a new system for determining the kind and extensiveness of examination and treatment based on neurodynamics and neuropathodynamics
5. the concept of neurodynamic sequencing and various options in assessment and treatment
6. new diagnostic categories of specific dysfunctions based on neuropathodynamics
7. treatment progressions derived from the above.

This text is about a particular modality in the treatment of neuromusculoskeletal disorders. As such, the approach is peripheralist and will have limitations that the reader should bear in mind. I am not a peripheralist (I am actually a biopsychosocialist), but I still believe that afferent mechanisms play a great role in producing pain and suffering. Nevertheless, it is common for therapists to diagnose more frequently the problems they have recently learned about, which raises the possibility of false diagnosis due to raw enthusiasm. At all times, the reader will realize that clinical neurodynamics is only one aspect of management of the person in pain and all other relevant information should be included in clinical decision making. For instance, the existence of a neural problem does not necessarily mean that a treatment with a neurodynamic technique is warranted. This could be because other treatments may attack the causative mechanisms more effectively or neurodynamic application may be contraindicated. Clearly, the biopsychosocial approach to neural problems will place this book in its rightful place as just a modality of treatment that will be effective in some patients and not in others.

Clinical neurodynamics is for clinicians dealing with musculoskeletal disorders with peripheral neurogenic pain mechanisms, including those of the nerve root and peripheral nerve. There is no assumption that all problems are as such, or that the treatments presented in this book act only on peripheral mechanisms. The clinician will naturally and responsibly establish that it is appropriate to treat patients with clinical neurodynamics before doing so.

References

Beasley A 1982 The origin of orthopaedics. Journal of the Royal Society of Medicine 75: 648–655, cited by Dyck P 1984 The lumbar nerve root: enigmatic eponyms. Spine 9(1): 3–5

Bennett G 1997 Neuropathic pain: an overview. In: Borsook D (ed), Molecular Neurobiology of Pain, Progress in Pain Research and Management, vol 9. IASP Press, Seattle: 109–113

Bragard K 1929 Die Nervendehnung als diagnostisches Prinzip ergipt eine Reihe neuer Nervenphänomene. Münchener Medizinische Wochenschrift 48(29): 1999–2000

Breig A 1960 Biomechanics of the Central Nervous System. Almqvist and Wiksell, Stockholm

Breig A 1978 Adverse Mechanical Tension in the Central Nervous System. Almqvist and Wiksell, Stockholm

Butler D 1991 Mobilisation of the Nervous System. Churchill Livingstone, Melbourne

Dyck P 1984 Lumbar nerve root: the enigmatic eponyms. Spine 9(1): 3–5

Elvey 1979 Brachial plexus tension tests and the pathoanatomical origin of arm pain. In: Idczak R (ed) Aspects of Manipulative Therapy. Lincoln Institute of Health Sciences, Melbourne: 105–110

Grieve G 1970 Sciatica and the straight-leg raising test in manipulative treatment. Physiotherapy 56: 337–346

Shacklock M 1995a Neurodynamics. Physiotherapy 81: 9–16

Shacklock M 1995b Clinical application of neurodynamics. In: Shacklock M (ed) Moving in on Pain, Butterworth-Heinemann, Sydney: 123–131

Sunderland S 1978 Nerves and Nerve Injuries. Churchill Livingstone, Edinburgh

Sunderland S 1991 Nerves Injuries and Their Repair: A Critical Appraisal. Churchill Livingstone, Edinburgh

Von Lanz T, Wachsmuth W 1959 Praktische Anatomie. Ein lehr und Hilfsbuch der Anatomischen Grundlagen Ärztlichen Handelns. Springer-Verlag, Berlin

Acknowledgements

Not all authors who have performed work in the area of physical treatment of neurogenic pain have been quoted for each of their single contributions. There comes a time when facts and figures mature into common knowledge and it is cumbersome to acknowledge everything and everyone. If this offends, I apologize in advance, for no offence is intended. However, I thank some of these authors for their contributions; Allison Bell, Dr Alf Breig, Dr Michel Coppieters, Louis Gifford, Dr Jane Greening, Toby Hall, Helen Jones, Dr Gerrit Jan Kleinrensink, Paul Lew, Dr Peter Selvaratnam, Brigitte van der Heide and Max Zusman. I also thank Kurt Lehermayr, Kelly Filmer and Cory Banks for their contribution to the artwork.

Because of their substantial and osmotic contribution to the way this book has materialized, several key people resoundingly deserve acknowledgement. Robert Elvey is the first. For it was in 1984, whilst practising in Nelson, New Zealand, at Michael and Sita Monaghan's Physical Medicine Centre and Nelson Public Hospital that I came across a dilapidated copy of his pioneering paper on the pathoanatomical origin of arm pain (Elvey 1979). Its battered appearance was on account of it having been used so much. It aroused in me a fervent interest in things neural and, from then on, I was transfixed by the possibility that nerves might hurt and could be treated with our hands. The second person who has had a substantial effect on this book is David Butler. Without him, I doubt if this book would have ever come about. His own book, Mobilisation of the Nervous System, was such an innovative icon for clinicians and it brought into our profession a whole new world – the notion that the entire nervous system was a mechanical organ that could be treated. In being involved with him since the late 1980s through the 1990s, I learned a freedom of thought and an inspiration that is always welcome in the clinical professions. Helen Slater also deserves thanks because it was from her that I learned such disciplined and critical thought which I can only partly emulate in this book. I also wish to thank Geoffrey Maitland and Associate Professor Patricia Trott who, directly or indirectly, mentored me through the process of logical analysis of clinical problems, without which this book would have little to offer. Dr Sheila Scutter and Ms Maureen Wilkinson (School of Medical Radiation, University of South Australia) are to be thanked for their valuable contributions and support during our work on cadavers and imaging of nerves.

I wish also to acknowledge the late Professor Emeritus Patrick Wall, whose steadfast and deadly honest dialogue on pain and the neurosciences, unfaltering humanitarianism and open-mindedness helped me conceptualize the systematic approach in this book. When it comes to logical thought, there is no leeway when conversing with such a man, who had an exceptional ability to pinpoint the key issues right from the start.

I also wish to thank my students and colleagues, who have provided me with the stimulus to fashion the contents of this book into what it is now. They have offered me criticism and support without which this book would not have taken its current form. The clinic and classroom are the garden from which this book has grown and my students are to be thanked for this.

A special thanks is extended to my senior commissioning editor at Elsevier Science, Mrs Heidi Harrison. It was she who helped me gain the confidence to write this book with her positive feedback, support, flexibility and exquisite knowledge of how to write a book for the health professional. Authors are often high maintenance clients and, after hundreds of late night e-mails from me, I am sure she had to bite her tongue more than a few times in order to smooth out the wrinkles during the making of this book.

Lastly, the person who deserves the most thanks is my wife, Linda, who, for several years, has contended with the vissicitudes of an errant husband, and who still supported me to the end. During lengthy periods of absence due to international teaching commitments, she diligently cared for our two children and parenting on your own is much more difficult than writing a book. To her I am eternally grateful and, to some extent, a significant part of this book is hers. I only wish that it could reward her as it has me.

M.S.

Reference

Elvey R 1979 Brachial plexus tension tests and the pathoanatomical origin of arm pain. In: Idczak R (ed) Aspects of Manipulative Therapy. Lincoln Institute of Health Sciences, Melbourne 105–110

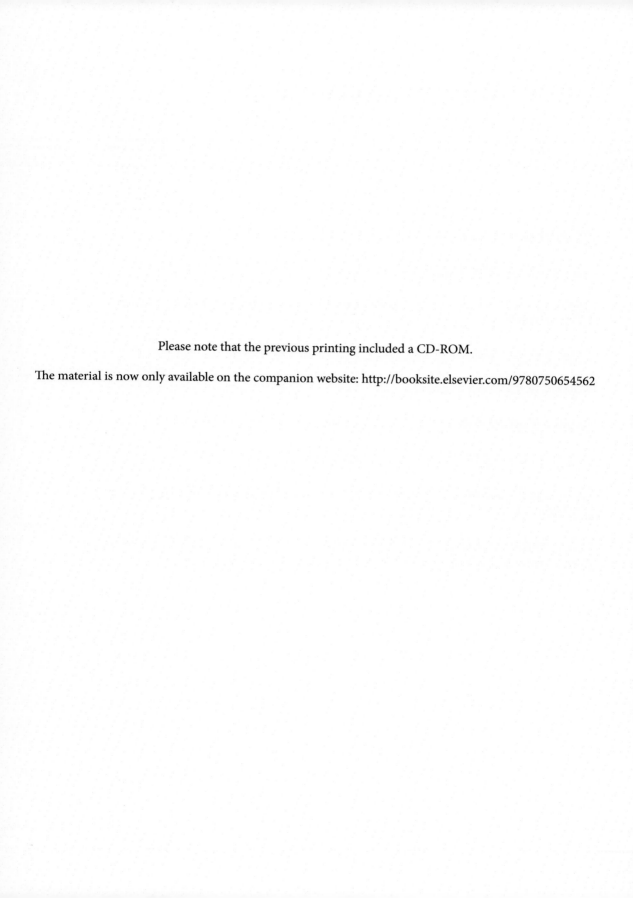

Please note that the previous printing included a CD-ROM.

The material is now only available on the companion website: http://booksite.elsevier.com/9780750654562

General neurodynamics

1

The concept of neurodynamics

General layout of the system

Primary mechanical functions of the nervous system – tension, sliding, compression

How nerves move

A new movement diagram

Nervous system responses to movement

Links between mechanics and physiology

Nervous system physiology and the innervated tissues – neurogenic inflammation

Neurodynamic sequencing – how the concept began, definition, sliders and tensioners, accuracy in testing, personalizing the sequence

THE CONCEPT OF NEURODYNAMICS

As the concept of 'neural tension' emerged, and as my understanding of it developed, I became increasingly uncomfortable with the word 'tension'. This was because, for therapists, the corollary of 'tension' is 'stretch', which they did. Neural stretching then became a mainstay of neural mobilization, placing patients at risk, because stretching may irritate nerves and provoke pain. Consequently, therapists who were not confident in the approach were, at best, flummoxed by the occurrence of a positive test and tentatively fiddled in the hope that something good would come out of their exploits. At worst, they gave up on neural mobilization for fear of provoking the patient's symptoms. Sometimes, they revisited neural problems more gently but not very effectively. Hence, I came to the belief that aspects of nervous system function, such as movement, pressure, viscoelasticity and physiology were equally important and were at that time being omitted from the analysis. These thoughts prompted me to write the paper 'Neurodynamics' (Shacklock 1995a) with the purpose of stimulating serious integration of mechanics and physiology of the nervous system in the manual treatment of neuromusculoskeletal disorders. In his book Adverse Mechanical Tension in the Central Nervous System, Breig (1978) had already discussed physiology of the nervous system being affected by mechanics. However, tension was the focus, it was from a surgical perspective, and links between mechanics and physiology were not comprehensively or specifically brought into physical treatments. Now that so many improvements have made it possible and justifiable to treat nerves with much more science and safety, neurodynamics has thankfully become a standard aspect of treatment of neuromusculoskeletal disorders.

As I originally conceived it, the concept of neurodynamics has essentially remained the same in terms of the fundamental points but, in addition, it has evolved further to integrate mechanical and physiological mechanisms in a way that makes it easier and safer to apply neurodynamic techniques. Also, in this book, neurodynamics is integrated with musculoskeletal function and neurodynamic sequencing is developed on. The following is an update and breakdown of neurodynamics into its essential aspects, ready for clinical application. For clarity, I have divided the subject into two main sections, general neurodynamics (this chapter) and specific neurodynamics (Chapter 2). General neurodynamics is concerned with fundamental mechanisms that apply to the whole body, no matter what region. Specific neurodynamics applies to particular regions of the body to cater for local anatomical and biomechanical idiosyncrasies that the therapist must take into account to make examination and treatment more specific to the patient's needs.

Definition
Clinical neurodynamics is essentially the clinical application of mechanics and physiology of the nervous system as they relate to each other and are integrated with musculoskeletal function.

GENERAL LAYOUT OF THE SYSTEM

A three part system

The following conceptual model is a framework on which to base neurodynamic techniques. The concept is presented in this manner because of its accuracy and the fact that it provides the foundation on which the application of neurodynamics can be made systematic. A three part system is used in which the tissues of the body are categorized with respect to the nervous system. This is not to say that the nervous system is necessarily the most important component, but if we intend to analyse events with respect to it, then this approach serves our purpose. Another reason for considering the nervous system as follows is that it enables us to categorize its dynamics according to the relevant components so that diagnosis and treatment can be derived from the causal mechanisms (Fig. 1.1).

Mechanical interface

The body is the container of the nervous system in which the musculoskeletal system presents a mechanical interface to the nervous system (Shacklock 1995a). The mechanical interface can also be called the nerve bed and consists of anything that resides next to the nervous system, such as tendon, muscle, bone, intervertebral discs, ligaments, fascia and blood vessels. The interface behaves like a flexible telescope in which the

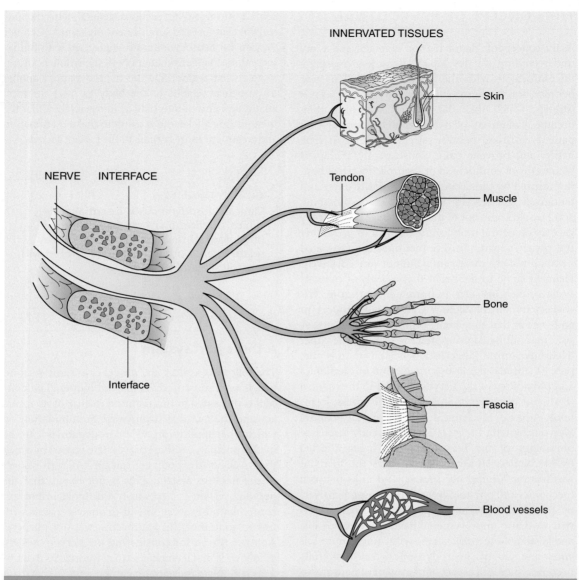

INNERVATED TISSUES

NERVE   INTERFACE

Skin

Tendon

Muscle

Bone

Interface

Fascia

Blood vessels

Figure 1.1   General layout of the nervous system in relation to the musculoskeletal system.

nervous system is contained and whose movements the nervous system must follow. During daily movements, the telescope elongates and shortens, bends, twists and turns, resulting in simultaneous changes in the neural structures. In doing so, the complexity of interactions between the nervous and musculoskeletal systems is a natural part of body movement. A good knowledge of these events is a key part of clinical practice, so that assessment and treatment can be directed specifically toward them.

Neural structures

The neural structures are simply those that constitute the nervous system. Included are the brain, cranial nerves and spinal cord, nerve rootlets, nerve roots and peripheral nerves (including the sympathetic trunks) and all their related connective tissues. The connective tissues of the nervous system are formed in the central nervous system by the meninges (pia, arachnoid and dura maters) and in the peripheral nervous system by the mesoneurium, epineurium, perineurium and endoneurium. In terms of pain mechanisms, the dorsal root ganglion, nerve roots and peripheral nerves are considered to create peripheral neurogenic mechanisms. Even so, and paradoxically, the connective tissues of the nervous system produce a form of nociceptive mechanism. This is because they are also innervated tissues and act through the nociceptors.

Although they are interdependent, functions that are located in the neural structures can be divided into mechanical and physiological types. The primary mechanical functions in the nerves are tension, movement and compression and the key physiological functions are intraneural blood flow, impulse conduction, axonal transport, inflammation and mechanosensitivity.

Innervated tissues

Innervated tissues are simply any tissues that are innervated by the nervous system. Virtually all tissues are likely to be innervated, whether directly by nerve endings or by the psychoneuroimmune connection. However, this book is concerned with the direct neuronal connections of the nervous system with its innervated tissues for three reasons. The first is that they provide the basis for some causal mechanisms that therapists should pay particular attention to. Such an example would be injury to the innervated tissues by way of overstraining them. This could in some cases produce excessive stretching of a peripheral nerve or nerve root and clinical sequelae. Also, in terms of physiology, the nervous system interacts in both afferent and efferent directions with the innervated tissues and these actions can be clinically important. More detail on this aspect is presented at various stages throughout this book.

The second reason for making specific reference to the innervated tissues is that they provide the therapist with the opportunity to move nerves. For instance, a mechanism by which therapists can use the innervated tissues to test the femoral nerve and its associated nerve roots is by movement of the quadriceps muscle. Stretching the muscle applies tension to the nerve and therefore yields techniques for testing and treatment. Another example is the median nerve stress test as it applies tension to the median nerve with extension of the middle finger (Laban et al 1989). Many other examples exist and they are used later in this book.

The third reason for presenting the importance of the innervated tissues is that, surprisingly, sometimes treatment of the innervated tissues is the best way to treat what seems to be a neural problem. For instance, a nerve root disorder may produce trigger points in the muscles innervated by the related nerve root. In the absence of a thorough examination of the innervated tissues, pain in these muscles would typically be termed referred pain and the muscles would often be ignored. However, with the knowledge that neurogenic inflammation and Kingery's effects may occur in these muscles in the presence of a mechanosensitive nerve root, it may be essential to treat the muscles as part of treatment of what started as a nerve root disorder and ends as a multifactorial problem.

PRIMARY MECHANICAL FUNCTIONS OF THE NERVOUS SYSTEM

General points

The nervous system possesses a natural ability to move and withstand mechanical forces that are generated by daily movements. This capacity is essential in the prevention of injury and malfunction. For the reader to progress to the clinical application stages of this book, it is important that the key mechanical functions of the nervous system are understood clearly because they form the basis for much of the systematic approach presented.

For the nervous system to move normally, it must successfully execute three primary mechanical functions; withstand tension, slide in its container, and be compressible. Ultimately, all mechanical events in the nervous system stem from these three functions, such that the more complex mechanical events that occur during human movement are merely combinations of tension, sliding and compression. These three primary events occur in both peripheral and central nervous systems. However, they are often achieved in different ways because of the existence of regional differences in anatomy and biomechanics. Always, each of the component mechanical events will interact with the others. However, in some cases, it is possible to ascertain that a particular component dominates the clinical problem. Present is the opportunity for the clinician to deliberately bias examination and treatment techniques to the specific neurodynamic components.

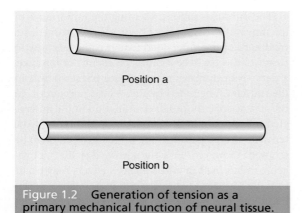

Figure 1.2   Generation of tension as a primary mechanical function of neural tissue.

Position a

Position b

a. Tension

The first of the primary mechanical events in the nervous system is the generation of tension. Since the nerves are attached to each end of their container, the nerves are lengthened by elongation of the container, which, as mentioned, behaves like a telescope. The joints are a key site at which the nerves are elongated. The mechanisms by which forces are transmitted between the container and the nerves are complex and are described in more detail later in this chapter. Stronger parts of the nervous system, e.g. the sciatic nerve, can withstand well over 50 kg of tension (Symington 1882) (Fig. 1.2).

Perineurium

The perineurium is the primary guardian against excessive tension and is effectively the cabling in the peripheral nerve (for review, see Sunderland 1991). Densely packed connective tissue and forming each fascicle, the perineurium possesses considerable longitudinal strength and elasticity. It allows peripheral nerves to withstand approximately 18–22% strain before failure (Sunderland & Bradley 1961; reviewed in Sunderland 1991).

b. Sliding of nerves

The second primary mechanical event in the nervous system is the movement of the neural structures relative to their adjacent tissues (McLellan & Swash 1976; Wilgis & Murphy 1986). This is also called excursion, or sliding, and occurs in the nerves longitudinally and transversely. Excursion is an essential aspect of neural function because it serves to dissipate tension in the nervous system. Just as gaseous molecules move down the pressure gradient from regions of high to low density producing equalization of pressure, so do nerves slide down the tension gradient by displacing toward the point of highest tension to produce an equalization of tension throughout the neural tract.

Longitudinal sliding

The sliding of nerves down the tension gradient enables them to lend their tissue toward the part at which elongation is initiated. This way, tension is distributed along the nervous system more evenly, rather than it building up too much at one particular location. An illustration of the protective effect of neural sliding is the following. Blood flow in peripheral nerves is blocked at 8–15% elongation (Lundborg & Rydevik 1973; Ogata & Naito 1986), yet the nerve bed that contains the median nerve elongates by 20% between full elbow flexion and extension (Millesi 1986). If the sliding of the nerve from its proximal and distal ends toward the site at which tension is applied (the elbow) did not occur, neural ischaemia would result. However, the median nerve continues to function normally even if we hold our elbow straight for a sustained period. This is because the actual strain in the nerve is probably only 4–6% (Millesi et al 1995) and is due to the nerve sliding toward the elbow from the wrist and shoulder. Another example of the protective effects of longitudinal sliding is the straight leg raise, in which the sciatic/tibial nerve bed elongates by up to 124 mm (Beith et al 1995). Calculated in a person 1.75 m tall, this would amount to approximately 14% elongation of the nerve bed. It is not normal to produce nerve failure with the straight leg raise and means that the nerve is protected from excessive elongation by an intrinsic mechanism, that is, sliding. In contrast, nerves are more likely to malfunction if additional movements are performed that prevent sliding by creating a simultaneous increase in neural tension from both ends. Such examples in the case of the median nerve are contralateral lateral flexion of the neck, glenohumeral abduction and wrist and finger extension. The addition of elbow extension would now produce neural symptoms even in the normal subject. This introduces the phenomenon of convergence and is discussed later (Fig. 1.3).

Transverse sliding

Like longitudinal movement, transverse sliding is also essential because it helps to dissipate tension and pressure in the nerves. Transverse excursion occurs in

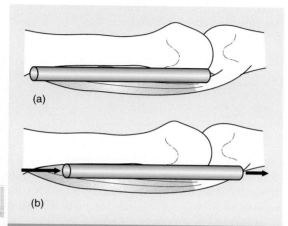

(a)

(b)

Figure 1.3   Longitudinal sliding capacity of peripheral nerve.

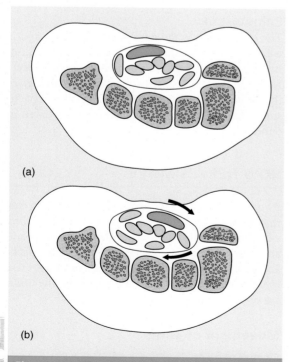

(a)

(b)

Figure 1.4   Transverse sliding of the median nerve at the wrist.

two ways. The first is to enable the nerves to take the shortest course between two points when tension is applied. This is particularly important in locations where transverse movement is a key part of the nerve's local biomechanics, for example, the superficial peroneal nerve over the ankle. The second means by which transverse movement occurs is when nerves are subjected to sideways pressure by neighbouring structures, such as tendons and muscles. Sideways pressure induced by movement of the flexor tendons causes the median nerve at the wrist to slide transversely out of its resting position (Nachamichi & Tachibana 1992; Greening et al 1999). In certain positions, neck movement can be seen to move this nerve out of its original position in the nerve's attempt to take the shortest course between the hand and neck (Shacklock & Wilkinson 2000, unpublished recordings, School of Medical Radiation, University of South Australia). Also, we have observed significant transversus movement in the median and posterior interosseous nerves at the elbow during supination and pronation movements (Shacklock et al 2002, unpublished recordings, School of Medical Radiation, University of South Australia). Specific combinations of upper limb and spinal movements can be used to deliberately produce transverse sliding of nerves (Shacklock & Wilkinson 2001). Various combinations of sliding movements that can be produced by limb and spinal movement are illustrated in the CD that accompanies this text (Fig. 1.4).

Mesoneurium and internal sliding of fascicles

Sliding of peripheral nerves in their bed is provided by specific connective tissues (Lang 1962; Millesi 1986). At surgery, and in cadavers, the mesoneurium has been observed to be a thin multilayered membrane made of loose connective tissue that has distinct boundaries and behaves in a fashion similar to the synovial membrane around tendons (Rath & Millesi 1990). Another dimension of neural sliding is the movement of particular fascicles on their neighbouring bundles. This interfascicular sliding is permitted by interfascicular epineurium which also consists of soft and loose connective tissues (Millesi et al 1990). The capacity of nerves to function in this way means that they can respond internally as well as externally to the forces to which they are subjected.

3. Compression

Compression is the third primary mechanical function of the nervous system. Neural structures can distort in many ways, including the changing of shape according to the pressure exerted on them. A clinical example of compression exerted by the mechanical interface is wrist flexion pressing on the median nerve at the wrist in Phalen's sign (Phalen 1951). Another is elbow flexion applying pressure on the ulnar nerve at the elbow (Gelberman et al 1998). In these cases, bone and tendon combined with muscle and fascia are what press on the nerve. The spinal equivalent of these manoeuvres is extension ipsilateral lateral flexion, which closes the spinal canal and intervertebral foraminae around the nerve roots. In this way, the mechanical interface transmits forces to the nervous system which then responds to these demands by altering its own dimensions and position. The nervous system effectively moves down the pressure gradient (Fig. 1.5).

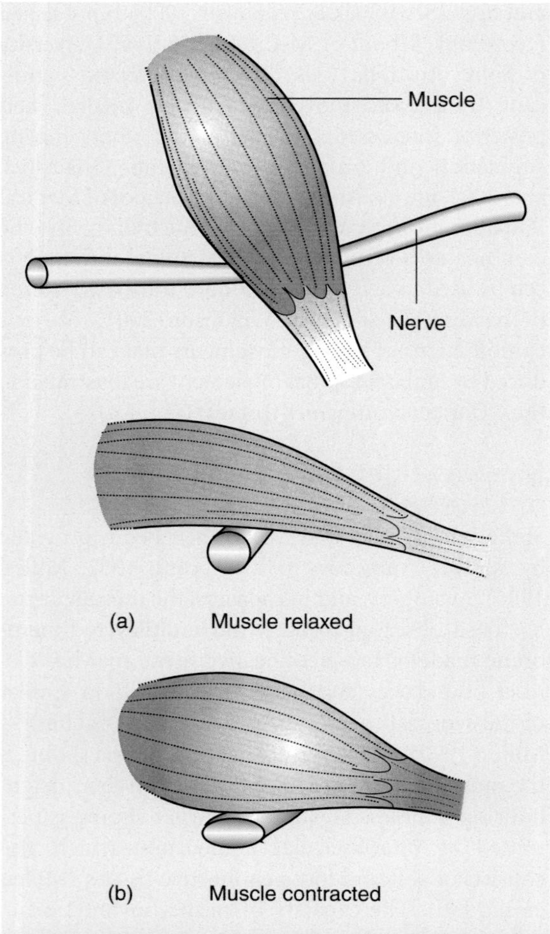

> Illustration of real-time imaging of compression and distortion of nerve tissue with movement of the neighbouring tendons.

Of particular clinical value in the above context are movements of the mechanical interface. This is because sometimes it is necessary to deliberately adjust the position of the interface so as to alter the amount of pressure on neural structures in making diagnosis and treatment specific to the existing problem. Pressure on the nervous system can be increased or decreased, depending on whether a closing or opening movement is performed.

Epineurium

The epineurium is the padding of the nerve and is what protects the axons from excessive compression. It consists of finer and less densely packed connective tissue than the perineurium, a feature that gives the nerve spongy qualities and enables the nerve to spring back when pressure is removed (reviewed in Sunderland 1978, 1991).

HOW NERVES MOVE

As mentioned, the three primary mechanical events that the nervous system relies on are tension, sliding and compression. They occur interdependently and are caused by a complex series of events. The mechanisms by which body movements produce these events, and how they can be used by the therapist, are presented below.

Movement of joints

Convergence

Movement of joints is the first way that movement-inducing forces are applied to the nervous system. An

(a)   Muscle relaxed

(b)   Muscle contracted

Figure 1.5   Compression of nerve tissue with contraction of adjacent muscle.

increase in length of the neural container occurs on the convex side of joints and this dimension decreases on the concave side. The neural events that follow joint movement are therefore influenced by where the nerve is situated relative to the joint axis. If the nerve lies on the convex side, it will be subjected to elongation forces, whereas, if the nerve is located on the concave side, it will be subjected to shortening forces.

Even though the container elongates around the nerves on the convex side of the joint, the nerves do not follow this movement entirely. This is because neural tissue is 'lent' from each end of the nerve tract toward the point where interface movement occurs. This partly offsets increases in neural tension as the nerves slide down the tension gradient, mentioned earlier. Relative displacement of the nerves toward the joint then occurs. The nerves slide in the direction of the joint because that is where elongation is initiated. The effects at the two ends of the system summate to produce little or no movement of nerves relative to the joint roughly at its midpoint. This phenomenon is called 'convergence' and is provided by the capacity of the nerves to 'lend' their tissue and slide in the direction of the joint from both ends of the nerve tract. The overall reason for convergence occurring is that tension is effectively applied at the joint that is moved.

Having said the above, it depends on the observer's point of reference. A component of convergence is actually an illusion created by displacement of nerves relative to bone in which the interface telescopes outward from the joint further than the nerves do. Because the nerves do not telescope as far as the interface does, to avoid excessive increase in tension, they must be lent tissue from either end and consequently slide toward the joint. This occurs at the same time as the nerve tissue undergoing a small amount of true internal elongation and is indeed a paradox (Fig. 1.6).

Convergence occurs in the limbs (Smith 1956; McLellan & Swash 1976) and spine at the most mobile of spinal segments (C5–6, C4–5) during sagittal movements (Adams & Logue 1971; Louis 1981). The point of convergence is a site where displacement of nerve tissue relative to bone reaches zero. Convergence appears to be a universal neurodynamic event and occurs opposite joints that are moved or, if several joints are moved, convergence will be most evident adjacent the joint that moves the most.

Generally, movement of a single joint will not evoke much tension in neural structures because

nerves can slide toward the joint from other areas, keeping the tension low. However, elongation of the nerves at several points along their course, such as at contiguous joints, reduces the amount that the nerves can slide, or 'lend' neural tissue, toward any particular joint. For this reason, movements of several joints in series produces greater elongation of the neural tissues than when only one joint is moved. A neurodynamic test utilises this principle by combining movements of several connected joints and the related innervated tissues and results in the summation of the above events.

Nerve bending

The bending of a neural structure around its interface is a good example of the combining of fundamental events to produce a more complex action. The ulnar nerve at the elbow is a case in point. As the elbow flexes, the nerve, being on the convex side of the joint, is elongated. Simultaneously, the nerve must bend around the bony trochlea, at which point the nerve is also compressed by three mechanisms. The first is the need for the nerve to take the shortest course between its two ends, which results in the nerve being pushed against the trochlea, undergoing increased internal pressure. The second compression mechanism is produced by the structures over the nerve, particularly fascia that forms the roof over the cubital tunnel pushing on the top of the nerve. The third is by an increase in tension in the nerve producing approximation of its fascicles. Tension is produced in the nerve by a further two mechanisms: a. the nerve being on the convex side of the joint makes it take a longer course around the joint than if it were on the concave side; b. the bending of the nerve produces more tension in the part of the nerve that is furthest from the joint axis. Hence, even within the nerve, different parts undergo different events, depending on the local intricacies (Fig. 1.7).

Movement of the innervated tissues

In addition to longitudinal forces being applied to the nervous system from the joint adjacent to the nerve, the innervated tissues can be used to produce such events. For instance, in the lower limb, dorsiflexion of the foot and toes can be used to apply tension to the sciatic nerve as this movement is combined with the straight leg raise or slump tests. The slump test is an example of using the points of nervous system fixation at each end of the nerve tract to

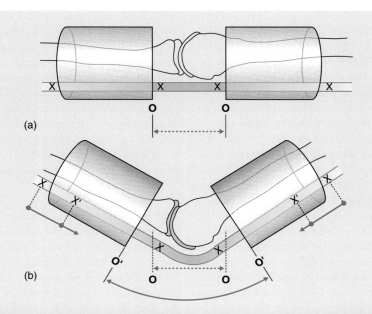

Figure 1.6   Convergence of the nerve tissue toward the joint that is moved. (a) neutral position. The position O marks the interface as if O represents a point adjacent the nerve. X marks points on the nerve. (b) flexed position. O' shows the new position of the interface produced by flexion of the joint. Note that it appears that X has moved inward toward the joint line but in fact it is the movement of O to the position of O' (outward from the joint) that produces the phenomenon of covergence. The dotted arrow line represents the position of the interface in the neutral position (O) (Fig. a). X' indicates the new position of the nerve tissue in the flexed position relative to the interface, but again, this effect is produced by the outward movement of the interface.

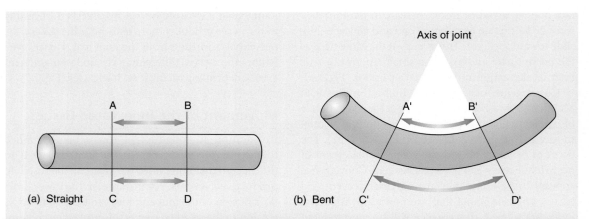

Figure 1.7   Internal effects of nerve bending. Different parts of the nerve undergo different events. The parts further from the joint axis will undergo more change in tension than those closer to the joint axis.

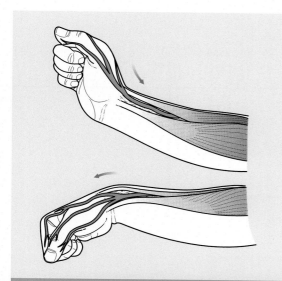

Figure 1.8   Application of tension to the radial sensory nerve with the use of flexion/adduction of the thumb and ulnar deviation of the wrist. The neurodynamic test for false diagnosis of de Quervain's disease is effectively Finkelstein's test combined with the radial neurodynamic test (for technique see Chapter 7).

apply elongation forces to the nervous system. The nervous system is attached to its container at the top end by the dura inserting into the cranium and at its bottom end by the digital nerves terminating in the toes. Hence, movements that increase the distance between the two end points in the nervous system (at the head and feet) will increase tension in the nerves and evoke neural movement. Knowledge of the innervated tissue sites for the nervous system is an integral part of clinical neurodynamics and can be particularly useful in the diagnosis of which components are relevant to the patient's problem. An example of this is the application of a modified radial neurodynamic test for the radial sensory nerve in the case of de Quervain's disease (Fig. 1.8).

Movement of the mechanical interface

Defining opening and closing around the nervous system

A new movement diagram

It is important at this point that the reader be acquainted with the exact definitions of opening and closing. In a diagrammatic representation, each event occupies its unique direction in the movement complex in which the movement is considered relative to the nervous system. An axis passes through the diagram and illustrates the neutral position as it divides the opening and closing sides. The movement of closing reduces the distance between the neural tissues and movement complex and therefore causes pressure to be exerted on the nervous system. Opening occurs in the direction away from the nervous system and therefore produces a reduction in the pressure on the neural elements.

The reason for creating this type of movement diagram is that the nervous system must at times be analysed in terms of what occurs in its mechanical neighbour. The position and mechanical function of the musculoskeletal tissues relative to the nervous system can be illustrated on this diagram which extends Maitland's movement diagram to incorporate the two-way dynamics (opening and closing) of the mechanical interface in relation to the nervous system (Maitland 1986) (Fig. 1.9).

The reason for placing both opening and closing movements in the same conceptual framework is that the dynamic relationships between the two are important in their effects on the nervous system. For instance, the movement complex might show an increase in both opening and closing, placing altered forces on the nervous system. This would constitute multi-directional instability with expansion of the neutral zone and would require motor control exercises to reduce forces on the nervous system. Alternatively, a reduction in opening can occur whilst, at the same time, closing can be normal. In this case, even though the nervous system is not pressed on directly by the interface, the nervous system may never be sufficiently relieved of pressure. This constitutes a distinct kind of mechanical dysfunction that is often missed and requires a technique that opens the interface without closing it and is perfectly suited to specific passive movements, especially in the spine. Yet another kind of dysfunction would be excessive closing with reduced opening. This would produce migration of the neutral zone toward the neural structure and may need correction. Different types of interface dysfunctions exist and these are covered in more detail in Chapter 4 on diagnosis of specific dysfunctions.

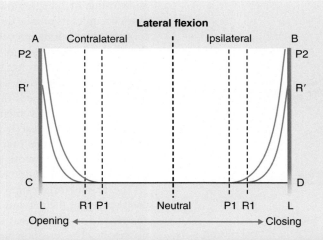

Figure 1.9 A new movement diagram to illustrate the interactions of the musculoskeletal and nervous systems in physical examination of neurodynamic disorders. Modelled from Maitland's diagram, it includes the essential aspects of his creation, however in addition, it takes into account opening and closing movements in relation to the relevant neural structure. Typically, this would include movements such as ipsilateral and contralateral lateral flexion in closing or opening the intervertebral foramen respectively. Similar analysis can be applied to peripheral joints and nerves.

Application of the movement diagram

The proposed movement diagram can be used by the clinician to document and analyse the movement-related events in the mechanical interface in relation to the nervous system. It assists in mechanical diagnosis, clinical reasoning and the development of the best treatment. In using the diagram, the therapist comes to specific conclusions about the relational dynamics between opening and closing and how they may be treated. Naturally, production of the diagram requires proficiency in manual examination of the musculoskeletal and nervous systems and the ability to document accurately the physical and subjective findings.

Closing mechanisms

Definition

Closing mechanisms are those that produce increased pressure on a neural structure by way of reducing the space around it.

A clinical example of using a closing mechanism is Phalen's test (Phalen 1951, 1970), which closes the carpal tunnel structures around the median nerve and compresses the nerve. Since closing is universal, it can be applied to many areas of the body. A spinal example is the performance of extension/lateral flexion which exerts pressure on the ipsilateral nerve roots in their intervertebral foraminae. Closing manoeuvres such as this are particularly useful in diagnosis of an interface component to neural problems.

Closing mechanisms can be relatively independent of longitudinal effects in nerves. Again with Phalen's test, even though the median nerve is compressed by flexion, tension in the nerve is reduced because the nerve is located on the concave side of the joint. This is in contrast with the ulnar nerve at the elbow, which, in the process of being compressed by elbow flexion (Pechan & Julis 1975), is also tensioned by this movement (Tsai 1995; Grewel et al 2000). The nerve passing over different sides of the joints is what causes such regional differences and is an important aspect of modifying neurodynamic tests to suit the patient's needs.

As mentioned, compression of neural structures occurs by virtue of the nerve container closing around the nerves. Given the right conditions, in addition to tunnel and joint structures pressing on nerves, so can muscles. Compression of nerves by muscles during their contraction is a normal phenomenon. However, an example of excessive muscle contraction with resultant neuropathy is the posterior interosseous nerve being compressed by the supinator muscle in cases of supinator tunnel syndrome (Werner et al 1980). Stretching this muscle also applies pressure to the nerve and this kind of event can also occur in other nerves (Werner et al 1985a, 1985b).

In relation to causes of neural problems, it is possible that excessive contraction of a muscle that is situated adjacent to a peripheral nerve could irritate or compress the nerve. This may not cause changes in nerve conduction, particularly if the compression is not severe and is only intermittent. However, this could be quite painful.

On the subject of diagnosis, it is possible with physical testing to ascertain whether an interface component has primarily a contractile or stretch component. In addition, it may be necessary to perform an examination that is more sensitive than the standard one, taking into account the subtleties in interface dynamics. This is achieved by combining a mechanical test for the relevant nerve with active contraction or passive stretch of the interfacing muscle and would test the interplay between the two. In the examination of interactions between joint, muscle and nerve, clinical tests can be combined with other closing or opening mechanisms, for instance, joint position. Clearly, systematic examination of all the relevant components is necessary to ascertain the pertinent aspects.

Opening mechanisms

Definition
Opening mechanisms are those that produce reduced pressure on a neural structure. The reduced pressure occurs when the space around the neural structure is increased by a particular manoeuvre.

Like closing mechanisms, opening ones are also universal. In the extremities, opening mechanisms would consist of elevating the scapula for thoracic outlet syndrome, straightening the elbow for ulnar

neuritis and releasing the piriformis muscle to reduce pressure on the sciatic nerve. In the spine, flexion and contralateral lateral flexion would reduce pressure on the contralateral nerve roots.

Intervertebral foramen opening and closing differ from joint opening and closing

It is important at this stage to emphasize the point that intervertebral foramen opening and closing are not the same as joint opening and closing. For instance, in the cervical spine, the posterior intervertebral joints are opened by contralateral lateral flexion and ipsilateral rotation. However, if one observes on a skeleton the effect of these movements on the dynamics of the intervertebral foramen, it can be seen that this combination actually produces a degree of closing of the foramen because the posteroinferior corner of the upper vertebral body at the foramen moves backward into the foramen. The movement produces approximation of this part of the vertebral body toward the superior facet of the segment below, closing down the anteroposterior dimension in the foramen. Instead, the best movements to open the foramen are flexion, contralateral lateral flexion, and contralateral rotation. These movements are used extensively in the treatment of dysfunctions of the mechanical interface for various types of radiculopathy, as presented later.

The importance of specificity in mechanical diagnosis

The above section illustrates the importance of separating different mechanical events in examination so that diagnosis and treatment can be directed at the specific pathodynamic mechanisms. For instance, a patient might have an interface closing problem rather than a neural tension problem and it would be important to bias physical tests and treatment to the relevant component. Also important is the point that clues about which component dominates the problem can be obtained clinically because the signs and symptoms will frequently reflect the neurodynamic mechanisms. The patient whose provoking movement is a squeezing action, triggering pins and needles in the first three digits of the hand, may have an interface problem such as excessive contraction of the pronator teres muscle. In which case, the physical examination may include a neurodynamic test that incorporates contraction and/or stretch of the muscle to ascertain if a disorder of this closing mechanism is present, given appropriate circumstances. However, this is quite an extensive technique for which specific guidelines on selection are presented in Chapter 6.

THE NERVOUS SYSTEM IS A CONTINUUM

Transmission of forces along the system

The nervous system is a very long organ. As such, it provides unique features that explain many clinical problems that are not attributable to other systems and can be utilized by clinicians who treat neuromusculoskeletal problems. The following illustrates the value in making clinical use of the length of the system.

Neck movements, particularly flexion and extension, produce changes in position and tension in the lumbar spinal cord and nerve roots (Breig & Marions 1963). Macnab (1988, personal communication) has stated that, at surgery, the lumbosacral nerve roots can be seen to move with dorsiflexion of the foot whilst the lower limb is held in the straight leg raise position. Another example of this mechanical continuum is the inward movement of the eyes with a bilateral straight leg raise. It is possible that the eye movement is induced by tension that passes along the spinal cord and brain to the optic nerves.

During body movement, tension is applied to the nervous system at the site at which the force is first initiated. As the force increases, the ensuing tension takes a short time to be transmitted further along the system (Tani et al 1987). This slight delay is caused by the nervous system being viscoelastic and slightly wrinkled and loose whilst at rest (Zöch et al 1989, 1991; Millesi et al 1995). Forces pass along the system as the slack in the system is taken up.

For a movement of one motion segment, gentle forces are transmitted only a short distance along the nervous system and will be dissipated easily. As the applied force increases in magnitude, its effects spread further along the nervous system from the site of force application (Tani et al 1987). This has important implications for the clinician because force and range of joint movement are significant variables in neurodynamic testing. When the nervous system is in a relaxed state, gentle forces will produce mainly local effects. However, in the tensioned state, even

small forces can be used to move neural tissue that is located far remote from the site of force application. If the elbow and shoulder joints are positioned so as to offer relaxation of the median nerve, wrist movements will not greatly influence the brachial plexus. Conversely, if the shoulder is positioned in abduction and the elbow in extension, forces will be transmitted to the plexus with only small movements of the wrist.

Structural differentiation

Through its continuous nature, the nervous system provides the capacity for manual differentiation of symptoms as important aspects of diagnosis and treatment. In certain situations, nerves can be moved with good specificity, simply because of the continuous nature of the nervous system. A good example of this is the production of symptoms in the wrist and forearm with the median neurodynamic test 1 (Butler 1991). Contralateral lateral flexion of the neck produces proximal movement of the nerves in the forearm and wrist without producing longitudinal movement in adjacent fascia, muscles or tendons (McLellan & Swash 1976; Shacklock & Wilkinson 2001).

> Dynamic illustration of structural differentiation i.e. specific movement of the median nerve at the wrist.

> **! Key point**
> Structural differentiation is performed with all neurodynamic tests in order to gain information on whether neurodynamic events participate in the mechanism of symptoms. Differentiation is achieved when the therapist moves the neural structures in the area in question without moving the musculoskeletal tissues in the same region. Any change in symptoms with the differentiating manoeuvre may indicate a neural mechanism.

The question of whether structural differentiation selectively moves the neural structures arises when it is possible that fascia and tendons pass long distances in a similar fashion to nerves. The complete validity of structural differentiation is not yet proven. However, it appears that differentiation may be mechanically valid in some circumstances. Our research group has shown that the median nerve at the wrist can be moved in a highly specific manner. The nerve can be moved in specific directions relative to its interfacing tissues, such as bone and tendon according to the neurodynamic sequence (Shacklock & Wilkinson 2001).

Spread of mechanical changes

Mechanical events at one site in the nervous system can produce a cascade of related events along the system. Passive neck flexion produces tension in the lumbosacral nerve roots, wrist extension can produce tension in the brachial plexus and dorsiflexion of the ankle moves the sciatic nerve. The mechanism by which mechanical forces spread along the nervous system paves the way for pathomechanical changes at one location in the nerve tract to produce secondary pathological effects in other parts of the system. Tethering of the spinal cord so that it can not move effectively produces greater elongation of distant spinal cord and dural tissue than normally (Adams & Logue 1971; Yamada et al 1981). This is important because patients frequently report that pain in one area has developed only since the development of a prior mechanical problem in another area. A classical example of this is acute low back pain resulting in a subsequent stiff neck, especially when the slump test is abnormal. Another is the adolescent who gradually develops low back pain which is later accompanied by hamstring tightness with bending over, and this later spreads up the system to produce neck pain and headaches. These people frequently have a tight nervous system in which the problems can spread along the tract. Neurodynamic solutions exist for these patients.

NERVOUS SYSTEM RESPONSES TO MOVEMENT

Dynamics between neural tension and neural movement

Biomechanics

The following is a brief analysis of the timing of tension and movement of the nervous system during body movement. As forces are applied to the relaxed nervous system with a particular joint movement, the nerves at the site of force application move first then, as tension passes along the system, the more remote contiguous nerves commence movement. Hence, a delay exists between movement of the nerves at locations remote from the site of force application. In this early part of joint movement, the primary event in the nervous system is the taking up of slack.

In the mid-range, the slack is absorbed and the rate of neural sliding increases. Then, later in the joint movement, the slack and capacity of the nerves to slide have been consumed, causing the tension in the nerves to rise. These points are useful clinically because the therapist can visualize what occurs during neurodynamic techniques and make use of subtle variations in technique.

In summary, events occur in the following order during a joint movement; taking up slack early in the range, rapid neural sliding in the mid-range; then finally tension builds in the nervous system as nerve movement diminishes at the end range. These points are illustrated in Charnley's (1951) and Smith's (1956) classic studies on the movements and tension changes in the lumbosacral nerve roots during the straight leg raise. From 0°–35°, the slack in the sciatic nerve is taken up and little movement on the neural structures takes place. Movement in the nerve roots is most rapid between 35° and 70° and ceases between 70°–90°. Because the movement capacity is now consumed, a rapid increase in tension occurs from approximately 60° onward. These events will naturally vary between individuals and region in the body. However, the principles of load transmission in relation to neural movement are fundamental and it is important to appreciate them in the application of neurodynamic tests.

Application to treatment techniques

The above illustrates some key points for the application of different techniques. A slider technique will need to be a large amplitude movement through the mid-range. A tensioner will need to be performed more toward the end range of joint movement. Combinations of techniques can be performed in which large amplitude movements can be performed in the same mobilization as an end range aspect to the technique. This would produce sliding and tension in the nerve. Alternatively, if the intention is to do something minimal to a nerve, a technique that simply takes up the slack can be used.

Force application and viscoelasticity

The nervous system is a viscoelastic organ. This feature provides great opportunities for the therapist because it may be possible to influence the intrinsic mechanical function of nerves through movement.

Most of the safe viscoelastic effects that occur during the application of forces to neural structures are likely to occur within a few seconds of force application (Tani et al 1987; Millesi et al 1995). Clearly this has important implications. Most of the mechanical benefits of mobilization will occur in this time and to hold a neurodynamic technique longer may place the neural structure at risk because of a possible build-up of intraneural ischaemia with time. It appears that, generally, because of the risks associated with stretching, neural *movement* is better than *stretch* because it is safer and is likely to be at least as effective. Movement techniques and exercises will also be tolerated better by patients than potentially uncomfortable stretching.

LINKS BETWEEN MECHANICS AND PHYSIOLOGY

The proposal that mechanics and physiology of the nervous system are interdependent forms the basis for the concept of neurodynamics (Shacklock 1995a). Acceptance of this idea enables the clinician to take into account, not just the effects of mechanical changes on neurological function, but also pain mechanisms. In doing so, the clinician then has access to the central nervous system and biopsychosocial aspects of pain and disability which, although not covered in this book, are essential in the management of the person in pain.

Examples of the links between mechanics and physiology of the nervous system are pressure and tension in neural structures producing ischaemia and reducing axonal transport (Lundborg & Dahlin 1996). Improving physiology through treatment of mechanical function is also an integral part of the concept of neurodynamics and can be highly effective in both diagnosis (Coveney et al 1997; Selvaratnam et al 1997) and treatment (Shacklock 1995b; Sweeney & Harms 1996; Rozmaryn et al 1998). Releasing pressure or tension in a nerve could improve its physiology and clinical correlates. Furthermore, offering the patient a

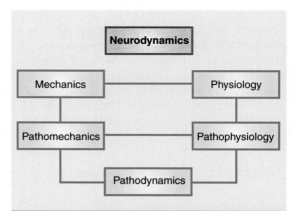

Figure 1.10 The concept of neurodynamics includes links between mechanics and physiology of the nervous system in which interactions occur both ways and can be capitalized on therapeutically. Mechanical treatment may therefore be used to improve physiology in the nervous system and the clinical correlates (from Shacklock M 1995a, Physiotherapy, with permission).

new way to move may reduce irritation of a neural structure, providing relief of pain and disability.

Not only do mechanical events influence physiological functions, but these interactions also occur the other way around. Diabetes, a problem that causes pathophysiology in nerves, results in increased susceptibility of nerves to compression (Dellon et al 1988, reviewed in Mackinnon & Dellon 1988; Mackinnon 1992). Hence, it is important that the clinician take into account the physiology of nerves as part of making decisions on clinical neurodynamics (Fig. 1.10).

PHYSIOLOGICAL EVENTS

Intraneural blood flow

Regulation of intraneural blood flow – a balancing act

Blood flow in nerves is regulated by a fascinating system that intertwines the efferent and afferent systems with amazing interplay and subtlety. The reason for including this in clinical neurodynamics is that changes in intraneural blood flow, particularly through the inflammatory process, are a way in which nerves may cause pain without producing changes in conduction velocity. Furthermore, inflammation of nerves can be a way for daily movements and mechanical tests to become abnormally painful. Intraneural blood flow is regulated by a mechanism that constantly balances vasoconstriction, vasodilation and secretion.

Vasodilation and constriction

In an extraordinary twist, the blood flow of peripheral nerves is actually regulated by nerves (nervi vasa nervorum) (Bove & Light 1995b, 1997a, 1997b). Nociceptors and sympathetic fibres are the relevant types of nerve fibre because they are what do the controlling. When stimulated, in addition to potentially producing pain (Zochodne 1993), the nociceptors (C fibres) in the connective tissues of the nerve exert a vasodilator effect on the local blood vessels. They achieve this by releasing substance P and calcitonin gene-related peptide from their terminals onto the walls of the blood vessels in the nerve (Zochodne & Ho 1991a; Zochodne et al 1995; Zochodne et al 1997; Schaafsma et al 1997). The release of these vasoactive and pro-inflammatory substances from the nerve's nociceptors is tonic and subject to change, depending on whether they are stimulated or sedate. Stimulation of the nerve's nociceptors triggers increases in intraneural blood flow at the site of stimulation (Zochodne & Ho 1991b). This is particularly important because repetitive mechanical stimulation is likely to increase intraneural blood flow and, if excessive, create an inflammatory or oedematous response in the nerve (Fig. 1.11).

At the same time that the nerve's nociceptors produce vasodilation in the nerve, the sympathetic nerve terminals that enter the nerve with blood vessels exert a counterbalance with vasoconstriction and reduced intraneural blood flow (Zochodne & Low 1990; Zochodne et al 1990). This function is similar to what occurs in musculoskeletal tissues.

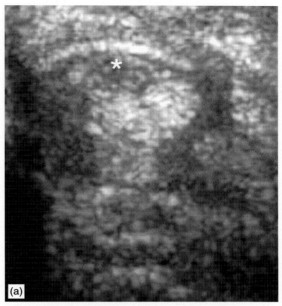

(a)

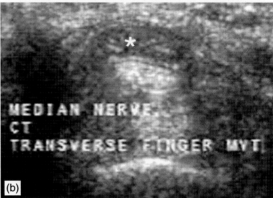

(b)

Figure 1.11   Median nerve in the carpal tunnel. (a) Normal . The nerve* adopts the shape of the neighbouring tendons and appears reasonably light in appearance. (b) Abnormal – swollen and pressurized median nerve* at the carpal tunnel in a case of carpal tunnel syndrome. The nerve is also darker indicating increased fluid in the nerve. Even though not to scale, the nerve is larger compared with the size of the adjacent tendons and it is more round than its normal counterpart. Thickened epineurium can be seen as a silvery line on the under surface of the nerve.

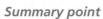

Summary point

A complex balancing act occurs between the vasodilatory effects of the nerve's nociceptors and constricting effect of the nerve's sympathetic supply. The balance may be upset by adverse changes in mechanics or physiology, as with friction irritation, excessive pressure or stretch or altered physiology in the nerve.

Maintenance of blood flow during movement

The flow of blood through the nervous system is highly relevant to the treating practitioner because of the effects of mechanical stresses on blood flow and their potential for danger when performing neural mobilization. Nerves need a continuous supply of blood because they are particularly sensitive to oxygen deprivation and fail quickly in such circumstances. During normal movement, nerve blood flow is preserved through an intricate system of vessels that distort with the nerve. At rest, the vessels are coiled so that, when the nerve is elongated, the blood vessels become uncoiled rather than stretched (illustrated in detail in Sunderland 1978, 1991; Lundborg 1988). This natural flexibility in the vessels provides for some distortion of the nerve to occur without compromising blood flow. However, even though these protective features support ongoing blood flow, limits exist, whereby nerves can fail in the presence of excessive forces, particularly compression and tension.

Effects of tension

Tension in nerves produces a reduction in intraneural blood flow. At 8% elongation, the flow of venous blood from nerves starts to diminish and at 15%, all circulation in and out of the nerve is obstructed (Lundborg & Rydevik 1973; Ogata & Naito 1986). The blockage is caused by stretching and strangulation of the intraneural vessels (Denny-Brown & Doherty 1945) and is of primary interest to the therapist for safety reasons. Tension also reduces blood flow in the spinal cord (Fujita et al 1988) and is an important safety consideration in spinal neurodynamic testing, for instance, with the slump, passive neck flexion and straight leg raise tests.

Time is also an important factor in intraneural tension. If nerves are held at only 6% strain for one hour, nerve conduction reduces by 70%. If the duration of the stretch is increased, greater ischaemia and a longer recovery time will eventuate. Clearly, the longer the nervous system is held in an elongated position, the greater is the likelihood of producing adverse effects. One of my patients told me that, whilst at work, he fell between two large rollers which forced him into the full slump position. He was a printer by trade and, due to a large amount of noise at the factory, his screams for help were not heard for approximately 15 minutes. Cauda equina symptoms developed and remained for many months afterwards.

Effects of compression

As discussed earlier, the mechanisms to maintain continuous blood flow in the nerves during mechanical

stress have their limits. The failure threshold for compression is approximately 30–50 mmHg. In cases where pressure exceeds this value, hypoxia and impairment of nerve blood flow, conduction and axonal transport occur (Gelberman et al 1983; Ogata & Naito 1986; reviewed in Lundborg & Dahlin 1996; Rempel et al 1999). Failure of this kind also occurs in nerve roots (Olmarker et al 1991; Cornefjord et al 1996, 1997; reviewed in Rydevik 1993). Compression of nerves is a normal part of human movement. Therefore, it is clear that normal movement does not usually produce sufficient compression to impair physiological functions. However, in a nerve with prior compromise, changes in pressure of a magnitude smaller than that in normal nerves could be sufficient to produce neuropathic symptoms with normal neurodynamic forces.

Tension and compression have cumulative effects

As mentioned above, both tension and compression of nerves influence intraneural blood flow. Tension and compression on neural tissues can also have cumulative effects, such that compressed neural structures are more likely to fail in the presence of mild tightness (Fujita et al 1988). Hence, in the patient, compression and tension may interact to produce symptoms and it will be important to take into account both components.

Relevance of intraneural blood flow to neurodynamic techniques

As far as the application of manual techniques is concerned, the therapist must take into account the fact that intraneural blood flow will fluctuate with many of the movements performed on the patient. In patients with a nerve problem (e.g. the nerve may be swollen, compressed, inflamed or scarred), the failure threshold to mechanical stress could be lower than normal, so extra care must be taken. This point relates to the idea that decisions on the extent of manual techniques to be applied can be based on neurodynamics and be made systematic. For instance, in the case of an ischaemic and mechanically hypersensitive nerve, it will be necessary to limit the extent of manual techniques so as not to provoke the problem. Conversely, a nerve that is not ischaemic will safely tolerate, and may need, a less restricted approach.

The above reinforces the concept of neurodynamics (Shacklock 1995a), where physiology must be included in management of mechanical problems in the nervous system.

Pain and stretch from the nervous system

Peripheral nervous system

Sensory nerves exist in the connective tissues of peripheral nerves (Hromada 1963) and, in terms of sensation, it appears that they provide nociception and proprioception.

C-type nerve fibres exist in the epineurium of peripheral nerves and evidence for their role as nociceptors comes in several forms. The first line of evidence is through their chemical structure in which they house substance P and calcitonin gene-related peptide (Zochodne & Ho 1993; Bove & Light 1995a), which is a characteristic feature of C nociceptors. The second piece of evidence is that a hallmark of C nociceptors is that they are activated by the application of capsaicin, the active ingredient in chilli peppers. When stimulated by capsaicin, C fibres in epineurium indicate their presence and nociceptive functions by secretion of substance P and CGRP (calcitonin gene-related peptide), producing vasodilation and inflammation in the nerve (Zochodne & Ho 1993) through the nervi vasa nervorum. The third line of evidence for nociceptors being present in the connective tissue of nerves comes from neurophysiological studies. Strong stretch of the connective tissues around the nerve roots activates sensory fibres in the related dorsal root (Bove & Light 1995a). Hence, nociception and stretch through application of forces may arise directly from the nervous system.

It is logical that stretch receptors with high thresholds should exist in the nervous system because this would provide an ideal means of protecting the nervous system against excessive mechanical stress.

Central nervous system

Many of the nerve fibres located in the dura (cerebral and spinal) also show the features of nociceptors. They contain and release substance P, produce inflammation when stimulated and are sensitive to capsaicin (Fricke et al 2001; Moskowitz et al 1983, 1989; Peitl et al 1999; Yamada et al 2001). The sensory innervation for the spinal dura spreads and overlaps several levels cephalad and caudad (Groen et al 1988) and even passes through the sympathetic trunk in a distinctly non-segmental fashion (Konnai et al 2000). This explains the clinical observation that dural pain is not segmental because it does not follow expected dermatomes, myotomes and scleratomes (Cyriax 1978).

Although, technically, dural pain is neurogenic, it may also be classified as nociceptive because this kind of pain is activated through nociceptors that are located in connective tissues. In terms of pain presentation, dural pain will have features similar to nociceptive pain. Dural pain will be provoked by movements that mechanically stress the dura and may also show an inflammatory pattern.

Clearly, many similarities between nociceptive innervation of the central and peripheral nervous systems exist. The above may help explain pain and stretch sensations from manoeuvres that stretch or compress the nervous system, also the development of abnormal pain with neurodynamic tests.

NERVOUS SYSTEM PHYSIOLOGY AND THE INNERVATED TISSUES

Inflammation and the peripheral nervous system

Overview – neurogenic inflammation

Neurogenic inflammation is inflammation in the tissues produced by efferent actions of the peripheral nervous system. The mechanism is located in the C fibres of the peripheral nerve, dorsal root ganglion and nerve root.

The nervous system exerts powerful influences on inflammatory mechanisms in the musculoskeletal tissues (Chahl & Ladd 1976). In the dorsal root ganglion, the cell bodies of C fibres in peripheral nerves and dorsal nerve roots produce calcitonin gene-related peptide and substance P. When stimulated at the nerve root, peripheral nerve or nociceptor, the C fibres release these chemicals into their innervated musculoskeletal tissues. This results in vasodilation and can lead to inflammation (Bayliss 1901; Lembeck & Holzer 1979; Kenins 1981; Levine et al 1984; Ferrell & Russell 1986; Pintér & Szolcsànyi 1988; O'Halloran & Bloom 1991; Levine et al 1993). Changes in blood flow and inflammation are the result of activity in the nociceptors and their axons in which impulses pass antidromically toward the periphery, in addition to the usual passing of impulses orthodromically to the central nervous system for sensory processing (Fig. 1.12).

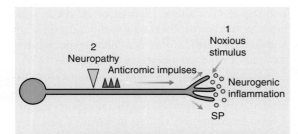

Figure 1.12   Peripheral sites at which inflammation of innervated tissues can be triggered – peripheral nerve and nerve root. The impulses initiated at the neuropathy site pass antidromically to produce the release of substance P (SP) and calcitonin gene-related peptide into the tissues, a process called neurogenic inflammation.

Summary points

Inflammation in both the neural and musculoskeletal tissues is regulated by the nervous system.

Changes in peripheral nervous system physiology, such as in cases of peripheral neuropathy and nerve root disorders, can cause changes in the inflammatory response in the musculoskeletal tissues.

In some patients, neuropathy produces changes in inflammatory mechanisms in the tissues supplied by the damaged nerves (Helme & Andrews 1985; Cline et al 1989; Xavier et al 1990; Shacklock 1995b) by either increasing or decreasing the delivery of inflammatory chemicals to the innervated tissues. The inflammatory changes can at times be a product of certain kinds of neuropathy, as discussed in more detail in Chapter 4 (neuropathodynamics).

Implications for the clinician

In some cases, it is important to pay close attention to physiology in the innervated tissue as a means of understanding the function of the nervous system. We must also be prepared to accept that there are instances where the musculoskeletal system expresses neural events through changes in physiology in its tissues. It can be necessary to assess and treat the innervated tissues as part of managing neural disorders.

Assessment of the inflammatory response

Testing of the inflammatory response can be performed by the clinician in the form of stimulating the nociceptors mechanically in the skin over the musculoskeletal structure in question (Lynn & Cotsell 1992). A change in the amount of reactive vasodilation in the skin compared with the contralateral side can suggest a particular type of neuropathic problem. Reduced vasodilation may correlate with a denervation problem whereas increased redness may correlate with a hypersensitive neural tract. Variations in neurogenic inflammation can occur in the presence of neuropathy (Parkhouse & Le Quesne 1988; Goadsby & Burke 1994).

Another implication in relation to testing the innervated tissues relates to the nerve root problem that produces pain in the related innervated area (e.g. skin, muscle and fascia). Patients, in whom the proximal symptoms have improved, can continue to experience pain and swelling in the distal innervated tissues due to pathophysiology in the related nerve root. In these cases, palpation of the innervated tissues is often painful and can show trigger point-like tenderness. Consequently, direct local treatment of the hypersensitive tissues may form part of the management of the nerve root problem, an aspect that is often overlooked.

NEURODYNAMIC SEQUENCING

How the concept began

The first time I thought of neurodynamic sequencing was in observation of responses to neurodynamic testing in asymptomatic subjects. I noticed that, for the same test, different sequences of movements produced symptoms in different locations. The resistance patterns and ranges of motion at specific joints evoked by neurodynamic testing consistently depended on the sequence used. Theoretically, if the same test had been performed, the responses should also be the same, unless each sequence produced its own specific effects. Following this, I analysed the responses of the straight leg raise test in a normal population between three different studies in which the test was performed in different sequences. The selection of subjects and the method of controlling and performing the relevant movements were the same between the studies (Slater 1988; Mauhart 1989). I found that neurogenic symptoms occurred more frequently in the site at which the first movement was performed and performed most strongly (Shacklock 1989). Since then, the subject of neurodynamic sequencing has developed considerably, such that it is now a regular variant in neurodynamic testing.

Overview

Neurodynamic sequencing relies on the principle that the nervous system does not behave uniformly. Instead, areas of high and low tension, movement and pressure exist and these depend on local variations in anatomy, biomechanics and the particular manoeuvres under consideration. The sequence of movements influences the localization of particular mechanical stresses in the nervous system and the directions and order in which the nerves move. Of particular value in this connection is the fact that the clinician can use different movement sequences in diagnosis and treatment. More or less strain can be applied to a particular neural structure, depending on the technique. Also, techniques that reduce neural tension or pressure, or produce a sliding action in a nerve can be applied (see Shacklock & Wilkinson 2001). Neurodynamic sequencing opens up many new avenues in diagnosis and treatment, above and beyond standard testing.

Definition

Neurodynamic sequencing is the performance of a set of particular component body movements so as to produce specific mechanical events in the nervous system, according to that sequence (or order) of component movements.

Many possible sequences exist in which the interface or innervated tissue can be emphasized. It is important that the therapist is proficient in the selection and performance of the key sequences for each part of the body.

Key facts about neurodynamic sequencing

1. The sequence of movements affects the distribution of symptoms in response to neurodynamic testing (Shacklock 1989; Zorn et al 1995).

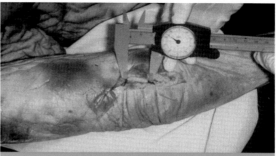

Figure 1.13   Yung-Yuh Tsai's research on the effect of neurodynamic sequencing on the strain in the ulnar nerve at the elbow. Thread markers were placed in the nerve and their separation was measured with different sequences of movement.

2. There is a greater likelihood of producing a response that is localized to the region that is moved first or more strongly (Shacklock 1989; Zorn et al 1995).
3. Greater strain in the nerves occurs at the site that is moved first. Tsai (1995) performed a cadaver study in which strain in the ulnar nerve at the elbow was measured when the ulnar neurodynamic test was performed in three different sequences; proximal-to-distal, distal-to-proximal and an elbow-first sequence. The elbow-first sequence consistently produced 20% greater strain in the ulnar nerve at the elbow than the other two sequences (Fig. 1.13).
4. The direction of neural sliding is influenced by the order in which the component body movements are performed (Lew et al 1994).
5. The principles of neurodynamic sequencing are universal.

These points provide part of the basis for a systematic analysis of the key variables in neurodynamic sequencing and can be applied clinically in making clinical neurodynamics safer and more effective. Tests can be performed with the following variables in mind.

Force

General force application

General force application is simply how hard the therapist pushes or pulls in the performance of a neurodynamic test. The use of too much force provokes symptoms unnecessarily and has caused therapists to avoid neurodynamics. It is preferable for only minimal force to be used in order to gain the necessary information and treat effectively. Instead of magnitude of force being a key part of neurodynamic testing, the emphasis is on specificity of technique and clinical decision making.

Localization of force

The localization of forces with each component movement is important in the performance of neurodynamic tests, for two reasons. First, usually, the pressure applied to the contact points during a standard neurodynamic test should be reasonably even. This ensures that the neural effects are as uniform as possible and prevents inadvertent biasing of stresses to one particular site. Second, forces applied to specific contact points during testing can be varied according to the patient's diagnostic and treatment needs. For instance, if the intention is to involve the ulnar nerve at the elbow, emphasis can be placed on the nerve at this location by applying more force to elbow flexion than to the other components of the ulnar neurodynamic test.

Resistance to movement

Resistance to movement differs from force. Both being important in neurodynamic testing, force relates to what the therapist *does* whereas the perception of resistance is what the therapist *feels*. Frequently, the resistance experienced by the therapist is provided by muscle contraction (Hall et al 1995, 1998; Coppieters et al 1999). However, what causes the contraction is open to speculation. It could be that contraction of the muscles that protect the relevant neural structure is a response to mechanical stimulation of the related neural structure. Howe et al (1977) certainly provided support for this by showing that impulses in the nerve root and dorsal root ganglion are activated by the straight leg raise as the nerve root is stretched and comes into contact with the mechanical interface (vertebral pedicle). Also, in cases of peripheral neuropathy, axons in the median nerve are stimulated during movements that apply tension to the nerve (Nordin et al 1984). In some cases, it is possible that the nerves themselves provide part of the resistance to movement.

Resistance to movement is important for several reasons. It may indicate a protective process that

must be respected, although not always avoided. Resistance is useful in mechanical diagnosis whereby the therapist can decide to avoid resistance or treat into it, depending on the needs of the patient. Generally, therapists are not sufficiently aware of the behaviour of resistance during neurodynamic tests and it is useful to analyse this variable as a routine aspect of learning their application. Movement diagrams are particularly useful for this purpose.

Extent of movement

Whether a neurodynamic test is taken a small or large distance into a movement is a key issue. In my experience, the most common cause of provocation of symptoms with testing is that the therapist has taken the nervous system too far into a provoking movement. Some patients will benefit from an extensive test. However, in others, it will be necessary to limit the test to only performing a couple of key components. In some patients, mere performance of a neurodynamic test will be contraindicated. The basis for planning the extent of examination and treatment, which are a key part of my approach to clinical neurodynamics, are presented in Chapter 6.

Duration of testing

Duration of movement is an important aspect in the application of neurodynamic testing because of the potential for harm with sustained holding. Even though the effects of movement and tension have not been comprehensively researched, it is known that the longer a manoeuvre that increases intraneural tension or compression is held, the greater is the chance of producing neural ischaemia and changes in conduction. The time between elongation to a value such as 12% and the onset of conduction changes is as short as several seconds (Wall et al 1992) and the changes are substantial within one minute in patients with neuropathy (Read 1991). Hence, it is not usually advisable to sustain a neurodynamic test for more than a few seconds. However, in exceptional circumstances, the sustaining of a test may be indicated. Sometimes, patients' muscles protect the nerves so effectively that it may be appropriate to sustain a test so as to increase muscle length in order to make a neurodynamic test more effective. In addition, some patients do not experience symptoms without sustaining a test position. In this situation, a sustained test might also be warranted. Specific evaluation in terms of risk analysis should be performed before application of such a technique and is covered in Chapter 6.

Speed of movement

Speed of neurodynamic testing is another variable that will have distinct effects on the nervous system. Nerves need time to adapt to forces and, in the sensitized state, such needs will be more acute. In this case, a slow technique is less likely to provoke symptoms. Generally, slow techniques are safer than fast ones because the nerves will have the opportunity to adapt to the applied forces and patients will have more time to protect themselves with muscle contraction. Also slow movements are less likely to produce impulses from damaged nerve fibres than fast movements (Howe et al 1977). In the stable and non-irritable state, in which the neural problem is difficult to detect, the nerves might need sensitizing with speed of testing. However, this is rarely advised, and should only be performed by the experienced practitioner and only in appropriate circumstances.

Neurodynamic sliders

Definition
The slider is a neurodynamic manoeuvre whose purpose is to produce a sliding movement of neural structures relative their adjacent tissues.

In some locations, the tissues adjacent to nerves are numerous and the dynamics of these tissues in relation to the nerves vary greatly. Hence, it can be important to distinguish which particular tissues the neural structure must slide relative to. For instance, tendons move differently from bones. In the median nerve at the wrist, the best slider for a nerve on the adjacent tendons is different from a slider for nerve against the transverse carpal ligament and the neurodynamic sequencing for each technique is also different (Shacklock & Wilkinson 2001).

The value of sliders – movement without tension
The value of neural sliders is that they produce significant movement in nerves without generating much tension or compression. Consequently, sliders are generally more useful in the reduction of pain and improving excursion of the nerves. To perform a slider, longitudinal force is applied at one end of the nerve tract whilst tension is released at the other. In an attempt to reduce tension, the nerves slide toward the point where tension is applied, or 'down the tension gradient'. For instance, a slider for the brachial plexus would, in the median neurodynamic test position, incorporate ipsilateral lateral flexion of the cervical spine and elbow extension (distal slider). A proximal slider would make use of contralateral lateral flexion with elbow flexion. Sliders are presented in more detail in the chapters on treatment of specific syndromes.

> Sliders of the median nerve at the carpal tunnel relative to the bones and tendons specifically.

Neurodynamic tensioners

Definition
The tensioner is a neurodynamic test that produces an increase in tension in neural structures. It relies on the natural viscoelasticity of the nervous system and does not pass the elastic limit. Therefore, the technique does not produce damage and, if performed gently, may improve neural viscoelastic and physiological functions.

Uses
Tensioners are used to activate viscoelastic, movement-related and physiological functions in the nervous system. Tension is applied to the neural tissues by increasing the distance between each end of the nerve tract, that is, elongating the telescope in which the nerves are contained and attached at each end.

A key feature of the tensioner is that, in addition to the joints being moved, the innervated tissue is used to apply tension to the nerve. Extension of the fingers with the median neurodynamic test 1, combined with the rest of the test and contralateral lateral flexion of the neck, is an example of a tensioner. Another example is the slump test in which neck flexion, knee extension and dorsiflexion apply tension from both ends of the neural tract. Tensioners are also presented in more detail in the chapters on treatment of specific syndromes.

> **Key point**
>
> A tensioner is *not* a nerve stretch. 'Stretch' implies sudden and permanent elongation in which the elastic limit of the neural structure is passed and results in damage. For obvious reasons, nerve stretching is not recommended and, instead, a tensioner seeks to gently improve the viscoelastic and physiological functions of the neural structure.

Testing for different components – interface, neural and innervated tissue

General

It is possible, and sometimes advisable, to perform neurodynamic tests for each of the different components of a clinical problem. Tests can be biased toward the interface, neural structures or the innervated tissue in any combination. This raises the possibility that, although standard tests (Butler 1991, 2000) are generally useful, they will only be effective in certain situations and frequently need extensive modification.

Mechanical interface

In directing neurodynamic tests toward the dynamic interactions between the musculoskeletal system and nervous system, decisions on which movements to perform will be derived from the mechanics of the interface in relation to the function of the adjacent nerve and needs of the patient. The principle of directing techniques toward the interface is universal, being applicable to all areas of the body. For example, closing manoeuvres are performed to temporarily apply pressure to the nervous system at a specific site. This is to assess how the nervous system tolerates the closing. Also, a closing movement can be used to test whether this movement is involved in the production of symptoms. Being a component of mechanical diagnosis, closing manoeuvres are useful in determining the kind of interface problem. They test the capacity of the interface to execute its normal closing and opening functions and how the nervous system responds to these events.

An example of the above is testing the interface for a brachial plexus problem at the thoracic outlet. Contraction of the pectoralis minor muscle can be performed during the median neurodynamic test 1 in which the effect of pressing of the muscle on the brachial plexus is assessed whilst it is under tension. A standard neurodynamic test in isolation might not be sufficient to detect an interface component to the neuropathodynamics.

Neural

In directing testing toward the neural structures, two types of manoeuvres are employed. Not necessarily in order of importance, the first is the slider, in which the ability of the nerves to perform and respond appropriately to normal gliding movements is assessed, and sometimes treated. The tensioner is the second, in which the ability of the nerves to respond appropriately to mechanical elongation can be a focus (tensioner). The key aspects are whether the neurodynamic movements reproduce the patient's symptoms or show other abnormalities such as reduced range of motion and altered muscle function. More detail on diagnosis with neurodynamic tests is presented in Chapters 4 and 5.

Innervated tissue

Testing of the innervated tissue can be an important aspect of neurodynamic testing and comes in two forms, mechanical and physiological.

In the first instance, mechanical testing of a tendon or muscles that relate to the neural structure can be performed independently of, or in conjunction with, testing of the neural structure. For example, if the calf muscle is painful, it can be tested by contraction or stretch whilst no stresses are placed on the nervous system, that is, the lower limb is in the anatomical position. In the case of combined testing of the nervous system and innervated tissues, contraction or stretch of the calf muscles would be performed whilst the limb is placed in a position that applies force to the neural system. The calf muscles would then be tested in the straight leg raise or slump positions to detect any abnormalities in the interactions between the musculoskeletal and neural systems. Frequently, tests that combine neural and innervated tissue testing are more sensitive than testing each component in isolation and are more advanced than standard testing.

In the second instance, physiological testing of the innervated tissues is discussed later and relates to analysis of the inflammatory response, motor control and neurological examination.

Serial neurodynamic sequences

In order to test the nervous system in a serial fashion, it is at times useful to apply neurodynamic tests in a proximal-to-distal sequence or vice versa. With this technique, the nerves are loaded in a distal direction, starting at the spine and continuing outwards along the extremity. For the median neurodynamic test 1, the movements may therefore be performed in the following order: cervical contralateral lateral flexion, scapular depression, glenohumeral abduction and external rotation, elbow extension and supination, wrist extension, finalized with finger extension.

For the straight leg raise, the movements could be performed in the following order: thoracolumbar contralateral lateral flexion, hip flexion, knee extension, ankle dorsiflexion-eversion and toe dorsiflexion. Naturally, the distal-to-proximal sequence would be performed in the reverse order.

Cephalocaudad sequences can be performed for the spine, in which movements can be executed in the following order; upper cervical flexion, lower cervical flexion, thoracic flexion, lumbar flexion, hip flexion, knee extension, ankle dorsiflexion and toe dorsiflexion and in reverse.

Importance of neurodynamic sequencing

Accuracy in performance of neurodynamic tests

From the above, it is clear that alterations in the performance of neurodynamic tests will produce changes in both the mechanical function of the nerves and the associated symptom responses. It is vitally important that the sequencing between test applications is highly consistent for accuracy reasons. Small changes in sequencing can produce large changes in the response and ranges of motion. Proof of this comes from the straight leg raise test in the following example.

Practical exercise

To test the above points, I recommend that the reader perform the straight leg raise test on a normal subject in two different ways. In the first application, merely rest the hand that controls the knee on the anterior aspect of the knee, immediately below the patella with almost no manual pressure over the joint. Perform the straight leg raise test to the first onset of symptoms and then to 5/10 in severity of symptoms, noting in detail the symptom response, resistance to movement and range of motion at each measured point in the range. The knee can flex a very small amount. Then repeat the test but, this time, apply firm pressure over the knee joint so that the joint can not move at all. The range of motion of straight leg raise will often be smaller and the symptoms will be more easily evoked than in the first application. This illustrates the following point:

Key point

If the neurodynamic sequence is *slightly* different, the test is *completely* different.

Personalizing the sequence for the patient's needs

Protection of the nervous system during a technique – starting remotely

The therapist who is reluctant to perform neurodynamic techniques for fear of provoking symptoms can now learn new sequences that are safer and more effective than before. A neurodynamic sequence can be used in which the mechanical stresses in the relevant nerves are minimal, so that there is little risk of provocation. The nerves that are remote from the site in question can be moved first. This way, the build up of forces at the problem site is gradual and easily controlled. Alternatively, the neurodynamic test can be planned so that a long lever is used to produce small movements in the nerve at a distant site. For instance, elbow flexion/extension for a median nerve problem at the wrist might be used instead of moving the wrist joint, where small movements will produce more intense local neural effects. This is a case of 'starting remotely'.

More localized testing – 'starting locally'

A sequence in which the relevant nerves are moved first can be used to make testing and treatment more specific to the patient problem than a standard approach. The therapist can move the part in question early in testing. An example of this would be a minor tarsal tunnel syndrome or heel pain in which physical signs are difficult to detect and the symptoms are not easily reproduced. The dorsiflexion/eversion straight leg raise could be performed with the first movement at the foot, then the test would be completed by performance of the straight leg raise. This is termed 'starting locally'.

Use of the symptomatic movement or position

Sometimes, a detailed analysis of the movements that provoke the patient's symptoms reveals the likelihood that a refined test is necessary. Hamstring pain serves our purposes here. In the soccer player, who experiences pain in the posterior thigh with kicking a ball, the provoking sequence of movements is early knee extension, followed by late hip flexion. The martial arts practitioner, who also uses a kicking motion, performs an early hip flexion movement, followed by late knee extension. The movements of hip and knee extension are performed in the opposite order between the soccer player and martial artist, which may necessitate personalizing the examination and treatment to each individual. The soccer player may need a standard straight leg raise because it emulates the sequence of kicking a ball. However, the martial artist may need a sequence that starts with hip flexion to approximately 70°, with some additional internal rotation of the hip, followed by knee extension later in the manoeuvre.

NEURODYNAMIC TESTS

Why the name 'neurodynamic tests'?

Since neuromechanical tests evoke changes in neural functions of many domains, it is appropriate to discuss

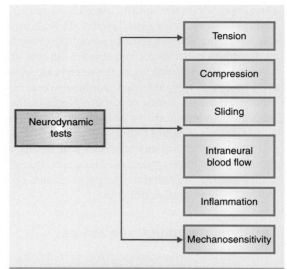

Figure 1.14 Neurodynamic tests and their effects on neural tissues (from Shacklock 1995a, Physiotherapy, with permission).

them in a way that encompasses all their relevant functions. Events that occur with such tests include nerve sliding, changes in cross-sectional area and shape, transverse position, axial rotation, viscoelasticity, intraneural blood flow and mechanosensitivity, to name a few. Hence, the name used to describe the tests should include these aspects and embrace the notion that neurodynamic tests are multidimensional and dynamic in nature. To call them 'tension tests' would be to localize the way we consider them to only two parameters, 'tension' and 'stretch'. This would then encourage diagnosis and treatment to also be restricted to these aspects. Clearly, this would be too narrow a term. The same applies to the term 'neural provocation tests', because, frequently, the intention and actual effect is *not* to provoke symptoms. Therefore, in this book, the tests will be called neurodynamic tests (Shacklock 1995a; Butler 2000) (Fig. 1.14).

Definition

A neurodynamic test is a series of body movements that produces mechanical and physiological events in the nervous system according to the movements of the test.

Use of neurodynamic tests

Neurodynamic tests are used to gain an impression of the mechanical performance and sensitivity of the neural structures and their related interfacing and innervated tissues. These inclusions are necessary because the nervous system must be considered in relation to the musculoskeletal and the central nervous systems (Butler 1998, 2000; Shacklock 1999a, 1999b).

References

Adams C, Logue V 1971 Studies in cervical spondylotic myelopathy: 1 Movement of the cervical roots, dura and cord, and their relation to the course of the extrathecal roots. Brain 94: 557–568

Bayliss W 1901 On the origin from the spinal cord of the vaso-dilator fibres of the hind-limb, and on the nature of these fibres. Journal of Physiology 26, 3: 173–209

Beith I, Robbins E, Richards P 1995 An assessment of the adaptive mechanisms within and surrounding the peripheral nervous system, during changes in nerve bed length resulting from underlying joint movement. In: Shacklock M (ed) Moving in on Pain, Butterworth-Heinemann, Australia

Bove G, Light A 1995a Unmyelinated nociceptors in rat paraspinal tissues. Journal of Neurophysiology 73(5): 1752–1762

Bove G, Light A 1995b Calcitonin gene related peptide and peripherin immunoreactivity in nerve sheaths. Somatosensory and Motor Research 12(1): 49–57

Bove G, Light A 1997a The nervi nervorum. Missing link for neuropathic pain? Pain Forum, Focus 6(3): 181–190

Bove G, Light A 1997b The nerve of these nerves! Pain Forum, Focus 6(3): 199–201

Breig A 1978 Adverse Mechanical Tension in the Central Nervous System. Almqvist and Wiksell, Stockholm

Breig A, Marions O 1963 Biomechanics of the lumbosacral nerve roots. Acta Radiologica. Diagnosis 1: 1141–1160

Butler D 1991 Mobilisation of the Nervous System. Churchill Livingstone, Edinburgh

Butler D 1998 Adverse mechanical tension: a model for assessment and treatment: Commentary: Adverse neural tension reconsidered. Australian Journal of Physiotherapy Monograph 3: 13–17

Butler D 2000 The Sensitive Nervous System. Noigroup Publications, Adelaide

Chahl L, Ladd R 1976 Local oedema and general excitation of cutaneous sensory receptors produced by electrical stimulation of the saphenous nerve in the rat. Pain, 2: 25–34

Charnley J 1951 Orthopaedic signs in the diagnosis of disc protrusion. Lancet 1: 186–192

Cline M, Ochoa J, Torebjork H 1989 Chronic hyperalgesia and skin warming caused by sensitized C nociceptors. Brain 112(3): 621–647

Coveney B, Trott P, Grimmer K, Bell A, Hall R, Shacklock M 1997 The upper limb tension test in a group of subjects with a clinical presentation of carpal tunnel syndrome. In: Proceedings of the 10th Biennial Conference of the Manipulative Physiotherapists' Association of Australia, Melbourne: 31–33

Coppieters M, Stappaerts K, Staes F 1999 A qualitative assessment of shoulder girdle elevation during the upper limb tension test 1. Manual Therapy 4: 33–38

Cornefjord M, Olmarker K, Rydevik R, Nordborg C 1996 Mechanical and biochemical injury of spinal nerve roots: a morphological and neurophysiological study. European Spine Journal 5(3): 187–192

Cornefjord M, Sato K, Olmarker K, Rydevik B, Nordborg C 1997 A model for chronic nerve root compression studies. Presentation of a porcine model for controlled, slow-onset compression with analyses of anatomic aspects, compression onset rate, and morphologic and neurophysiologic effects. Spine 22(9): 946–957

Cyriax J 1978 Dural pain. Lancet 1(8070): 919–921

Dellon A, Mackinnon S, Seiler W 1988 Susceptibility of the diabetic nerve to chronic compression. Annals of Plastic Surgery 20(2): 117–119

Denny-Brown D, Doherty M 1945 Effects of transient stretching of peripheral nerve. Archives of Neurology and Psychiatry 54(1): 116–129

Ferrell W, Russell N 1986 Extravasation in the knee induced by antidromic stimulation of articular C fibre afferents of the anaesthetized cat. Journal of Physiology 379: 407–416

Fricke B, Andres K, Von During M 2001 Nerve fibers innervating the cranial and spinal meninges: Morphology of nerve fiber terminals and their structural integration. Microscope Research and Technology 53(2): 96–105

Fujita Y, Yamamoto H, Tani T 1988 An experimental study of spinal cord traction syndrome. Nippon Seikeigeka Gakkai Zasshi 62(4): 359–368

Gelberman R, Szabo R, Williamson R, Hargens A, Yaru N, Minteer-Convery M 1983 Tissue pressure threshold for peripheral nerve viability. Clinical Orthopaedics and Related Research 187: 285–291

Gelberman R, Yamaguchi K, Hollstien S, Winn S, Heidenreich F, Bindra R, Hsieh P, Silva M 1998 Changes in interstitial pressure and cross-sectional area of the cubital tunnel and of the ulnar nerve with flexion of the elbow. An experimental study in human cadavera. Journal of Bone Joint Surgery 80A(4): 492–501

Goadsby P, Burke D 1994 Deficits in the function of small and large afferent fibers in confirmed cases of carpal tunnel syndrome. Muscle and Nerve 17: 614–622

Greening J, Smart S, Leary R, Hart-Craggs M, O'Higgins B, Lynn B 1999 Reduced movement of the median nerve in carpal tunnel during wrist flexion in patients with non-specific arm pain. Lancet 354: 217–218

Grewal R, Varitimidis S, Vardakas D, Fu F, Sotereanos D 2000 Ulnar nerve elongation and excursion in the cubital tunnel after decompression and anterior transposition. Journal of Hand Surgery 25B(5): 457–460

Groen G, Baljet B, Drukker J 1988 The innervation of the spinal dura mater: anatomy and clinical implications. Acta Neurochirurgica 92, 39–46(Up-to-date description of the innervation of the dura mater)

Hall T, Zusman M, Elvey R 1995 Manually detected impediments during the straight leg raise test. In: Jull G (ed) Clinical Solutions. Ninth Biennial Conference of the Manipulative Physiotherapists Association of Australia, Gold Coast, Queensland: 48–53

Hall T, Zusman M, Elvey R 1998 Adverse mechanical tension in the nervous system? Analysis of the straight leg raise. Manual Therapy 3(3): 140–146

Helme R, Andrews P 1985 The effect of nerve lesions on the inflammatory response to injury. Journal of Neuroscience Research 13: 453–459

Howe J, Loeser J, Calvin W 1977 Mechanosensitivity of dorsal root ganglia and chronically injured axons: a physiological basis for the radicular pain of nerve root compression. Pain 3: 25–41

Hromada J 1963 On the nerve supply of the connective tissue of some peripheral nervous system components. Acta Anatomica 55: 343–351

Kenins P 1981 Identification of the unmyelinated sensory nerves which evoke plasma extravasation in response to antidromic stimulation. Neuroscience Letters 25: 137–141

Konnai Y, Honda T, Sekiguchi Y, Kikuchi S, Sugiura Y 2000 Sensory innervation of the lumbar dura mater passing through the sympathetic trunk in rats. Spine 25(7): 776–782

Laban M, MacKenzie J, Zemenick G 1989 Anatomic observations in carpal tunnel syndrome as they relate to the tethered median nerve stress test. Archives of Physical Medicine and Rehabilitation 70: 44–46

Lang J 1962 Über das Bindegewebe und die Gefäße der Nerven Z. f. Anatomie und Entwicklungsgeschichte 123: 61–79, cited by Millesi M 1986 The nerve gap: theory and clinical practice. Hand Clinics 4: 651–663

Lembeck F, Holzer P 1979 Substance P as neurogenic mediator of antidromic vasodilation and neurogenic plasma extravasation. Naunyn-Schmiedeberg's Archives of Pharmacology, 310: 175–183

Levine J, Fields H, Basbaum A 1993 Peptides and the primary afferent nociceptor. Neuroscience 13(6): 2273–2286

Levine J, Clark R, Devor M, Helms C, Moskowitz M, Basbaum A 1984 Intraneuronal substance P contributes to the severity or experimental arthritis. Science 236(2): 547–549

Lew P, Morrow C, Lew A 1994 The effect of neck and leg flexion and their sequence on the lumbar spinal cord: implications for low back pain and sciatic. Spine 19(21): 2421–2424

Louis R 1981 Vertebroradicular and vertebromedullar dynamics. Anatomia Clinica 3: 1–11

Lundborg G 1988 Nerve Injury and Repair. Churchill Livingstone, Edinburgh

Lundborg G, Dahlin L 1996 Anatomy, function and pathophysiology of peripheral nerves and nerve compression. Hand Clinics 12: 185–193

Lundborg G, Rydevik B 1973 Effects of stretching the tibial nerve of the rabbit: a preliminary study of the intraneural circulation and barrier function of the perineurium. Journal of Bone and Joint Surgery 55B: 390–401

Lynn B, Cotsell B 1992 Blood flow increases in the skin of the anaesthetized rat that follow antidromic sensory nerve stimulation and strong mechanical stimulation. Neuroscience Letters 137: 249–252

Mackinnon S, Dellon A 1988 Surgery of the Peripheral Nerve. Thieme, New York

Mackinnon S 1992 Double and multiple crush syndromes. Hand Clinics 8: 369–390

Maitland G 1986 Vertebral Manipulation, 5th edition. Butterworth Heinemann, London

Mauhart D 1989 The effect of chronic ankle inversion sprain on the plantarflexion/inversion straight leg raise test. Graduate Diploma thesis, University of South Australia

McLellan D, Swash M 1976 Longitudinal sliding of the median nerve during movements of the upper limb. Journal of Neurology, Neurosurgery and Psychiatry 39: 556–570

Millesi H 1986 The nerve gap: theory and clinical practice. Hand Clinics 4: 651–663

Millesi H, Zöch G, Rath T 1990 The gliding apparatus of peripheral nerve and its clinical significance. Annales de Chirurgie de la Main et du Membre Superieur 9(2): 87–97

Millesi H, Zöch G, Reihsner R 1995 Mechanical properties of peripheral nerves. Clinical Orthopaedics and Related Research 314: 76–83

Moskowitz M, Brody M, Liu-Chen L 1983 In vitro release of immunoreactive substance P from putative afferent nerve endings in bovine pia arachnoid. Neuroscience 9(4): 809–814

Nakamichi K, Tachibana S 1992 Transverse sliding of the median nerve beneath the flexor retinaculum. Journal of Hand Surgery 17B: 213–216

Nordin M, Nystrom B, Wallin U, Hagbarth K 1984 Ectopic sensory discharges and paresthesiae in patients with disorder of peripheral nerves, dorsal roots and dorsal columns. Pain 20: 231–245

O'Halloran D, Bloom S 1991 Calcitonin gene-related peptide: a major neuropeptide and the most powerful vasodilator of all. British Medical Journal, 302: 739–740

Ogata K, Naito M 1986 Blood flow of peripheral nerve effects of dissection, stretching and compression. Journal Hand Surgery 11B(1): 10–14

Olmarker K, Holm S, Rosenqvist A, Rydevik B 1991 Experimental nerve root compression. A model of acute, graded compression of the porcine cauda equina and an analysis of neural and vascular anatomy. Spine 16(1): 61–69

Parkhouse N, Le Quesne P 1988 Impaired neurogenic vascular response in patients with diabetes and neuropathic foot lesions. New England Journal of Medicine 318(20): 1306–1309

Pechan J, Julis I 1975 The pressure measurement in the ulnar nerve. A contribution to the pathophysiology of cubital tunnel syndrome. Journal of Biomechanics 8: 75–79

Peitl B, Petho G, Porszasz R, Nemeth J, Szolcsanyi J 1999 Capsaicin-insensitive sensory-efferent meningeal vasodilatation evoked by electrical stimulation of trigeminal nerve fibres in the rat. British Journal of Pharmacology 127(2): 457–467

Phalen G 1951 Spontaneous compression of the median nerve at the wrist. Journal of the American Medical Association 145(15): 1128–1133

Phalen G 1970 Reflections on 21 years' experience with the carpal-tunnel syndrome. Journal of the American Medical Association 212(8): 1365–1367

Pintér E, Szolcsànyi J 1988 Inflammatory and antiinflammatory effects of antidromic stimulation of dorsal roots in the rat. Agents and Actions 25(3/4): 240–242

Rath T, Millesi H 1990 The gliding tissue of the median nerve in the carpal tunnel. Handchirurgie Mikrochirurgie Plastische Chirurgie July 22(4): 203–205

Read R 1991 Stress testing in nerve compression. Hand Clinics 7(3): 521–526

Rempel D, Dahlin L, Lundborg G 1999 Pathophysiology of nerve compression syndromes: response of peripheral nerves to loading. Journal of Bone and Joint Surgery 81A(11): 1600–1610

Rozmaryn L, Dovelle S, Rothman E, Gorman K, Olvey K, Bartko J 1998 Nerve and tendon gliding exercises and the conservative management of carpal tunnel syndrome. Journal of Hand Therapy 11: 171–179

Rydevik B 1993 Neurophysiology of cauda equina compression. Acta Orthopaedica Scandinavica Supplement 251: 52–55

Schaafsma L, Sun H, Zochodne D 1997 Exogenous opioids influence the microcirculation of injured peripheral nerves. American Journal of Physiology 272(1/2): H76–82

Selvaratnam P 1997 Mechanical stimulation to the median nerve at the wrist during the upper limb tension test. In: Proceedings of the 10th Biennial Conference of the Manipulative Physiotherapists' Association of Australia, Melbourne: 182–188

Selvaratnam P, Cook S, Matyas T 1997 Transmission of mechanical stimulation to the median nerve at the wrist during the upper limb test. In: Proceedings of the 10th Biennial Conference of the Manipulative Physiotherapists' Association of Australia 182–188

Shacklock M 1989 The plantarflexion inversion straight leg raise. Master of Applied Science Thesis. University of South Australia, Adelaide

Shacklock M 1995a Neurodynamics. Physiotherapy 81: 9–16

Shacklock M 1995b Clinical application of neurodynamics. In: Shacklock M (ed) Moving in on Pain. Butterworth-Heinemann, Sydney: 123–131

Shacklock M 1999a Central pain mechanisms; a new horizon in manual therapy. Australian Journal of Physiotherapy 45: 83–92

Shacklock M 1999b The clinical application of central pain mechanisms in manual therapy. Australian Journal of Physiotherapy 45: 215–221

Shacklock M, Wilkinson M 2001 Can nerves be moved specifically? In: Proceedings of the 11th Biennial Conference of the Musculoskeletal Physiotherapists' Association of Australia, Adelaide, Australia

Slater H 1988 The effect of foot and ankle position on the 'normal' response to the SLR test, in young, asymptomatic subjects. Master of Applied Science thesis, University of South Australia

Smith C 1956 Changes in length and position of the segments of the spinal cord with changes in posture in the monkey. Radiology 66: 259–265

Sunderland S 1978 Nerves and Nerve Injuries, Churchill Livingstone, Edinburgh

Sunderland S 1991 Nerve Injuries and Their Repair: A Critical Appraisal. Churchill Livingstone, Edinburgh

Sunderland S, Bradley K 1961 Stress-strain phenomena in human peripheral nerve trunks. Brain 84: 102–119

Sweeney J, Harms A 1996 Persistent mechanical allodynia following injury of the hand. Treatment through mobilization of the nervous system. Journal of Hand Therapy 9(4): 328–338

Symington J 1882 The physics of nerve stretching. British Medical Journal May 27: 770–771

Tani S, Yamada S, Knighton R 1987 Extensibility of the lumbar and sacral cord. Pathophysiology of the tethered spinal cord in cats. Journal of Neurosurgery 66(1): 116–123

Tsai Y-Y 1995 Tension change in the ulnar nerve by different order of upper limb tension test. Master of Science Thesis, Northwestern University, Chicago

Wall E, Massie J, Kwan M, Rydevik B, Myers R, Garfin S 1992 Experimental stretch neuropathy: changes in nerve conduction under tension. Journal of Bone and Joint Surgery 74B(1): 126–129

Werner C, Haeffner F, Rosén I 1980 Direct recording of local pressure in the radial tunnel during passive stretch and active contraction of the supinator muscle. Archives of Orthopaedic and Traumatic Surgery 96: 299–301

Werner C, Ohlin P, Elmqvist D 1985a Pressures recorded in ulnar neuropathy. Acta Orthopaedica Scandinavica 56(5): 404–406

Werner C, Rosén I, Thorngren K 1985b Clinical and neurophysiologic characteristics of the pronator syndrome. Clinical Orthopaedics and Related Research 197: 231–237

Wilgis S, Murphy R 1986 The significance of longitudinal excursions in peripheral nerves. Hand Clinics 2: 761–786

Xavier A, Farrell C, McDanal J, Kissin I 1990 Does antidromic activation of nociceptors play a role in sciatic radicular pain? Pain 40: 77–79

Yamada H, Honda T, Yaginuma H, Kikuchi S, Sugiura Y 2001 Comparison of sensory and sympathetic innervation of the dura mater and posterior longitudinal ligament in the cervical spine after removal of the stellate ganglion. Journal of Comparative Neurology 434(1): 86–100

Yamada S, Zinke D, Sanders D 1981 Pathophysiology of 'tethered cord syndrome'. Journal of Neurosurgery 54: 494–503

Zöch G, Reihsner R, Beer R, Millesi H 1991 Stress and strain in peripheral nerves. Neuro-Orthopaedics 10: 371–382

Zöch G, Reihsner R, Millesi H 1989 Elastic behavior of the median nerve and ulnar nerve in situ and in vitro. Handchirurgie Mikrochirurgie Plastische Chirurgie Nov 21(6): 305–309

Zochodne D 1993 Epineurial peptides: a role in neuropathic pain? Canadian Journal of Neurological Sciences 20(1): 69–72

Zochodne D, Allison J, Ho W, Ho L, Hargreaves K, Sharkey K 1995 Evidence for CGRP accumulation and activity in experimental neuromas. American Journal of Physiology 268(2/2): 584–590

Zochodne D, Ho L 1991a Influence of perivascular peptides on endoneurial blood flow and microvascular resistance in the sciatic nerve of the rat. Journal of Physiology 444: 615–630

Zochodne D, Ho L 1991b Stimulation-induced peripheral nerve hyperemia: mediation by fibers innervating vasa nervorum? Brain Research 12, 546(1): 113–118

Zochodne D, Ho L 1993 Vasa nervorum constriction from substance P and calcitonin gene-related peptide antagonists: sensitivity to phentolamine and nimodipine. Regulatory Peptides 47(3): 285–290

Zochodne D, Huang Z, Ward K, Low P 1990 Guanethidine-induced adrenergic sympathectomy augments endoneurial perfusion and lowers endoneurial microvascular resistance. Brain Research 519(1–2): 112–117

Zochodne D, Low P 1990 Adrenergic control of nerve blood flow. Experimental Neurology 109(3): 300–307

Zochodne D, Theriault M, Sharkey K, Cheng C, Sutherland G 1997 Peptides and neuromas: calcitonin gene-related peptide, substance P, and mast cells in a mechanosensitive human sural neuroma. Muscle and Nerve 1997 20(7): 875–880

Zorn P, Shacklock M, Trott P, Hall R 1995 The effect of sequencing the movements of the upper limb tension test on the area of symptom production. In: Proceedings of the 9th biennial conference of the Manipulative Physiotherapists' Association of Australia: 166–167

Specific neurodynamics

2

The spine – flexion and extension, sliding and convergence, lateral flexion and lateral glide, effect of gravity, contralateral and bilateral neurodynamic tests, neurobiomechanics

Shoulder – scapular depression, glenohumeral abduction, external and internal rotation

Elbow – extension, flexion, supination, pronation

Wrist – flexion , extension, provocative testing, radial and ulnar deviation

Finger – flexion and extension

Hip joint – straight leg raise test, biomechanics, internal rotation, adduction, extension

Knee – extension, flexion (prone knee bend)

Foot and ankle – dorsiflexion, eversion, plantarflexion/inversion, biomechanics of the posterior tibial, peroneal and sural nerves

INTRODUCTION

> **Definition**
> Specific neurodynamics is defined as local effects of body movement on the nervous system in a way that is specific to each region.

The main reason for including this chapter is to provide an updated summary of the subject so that the reader can use this information to understand the mechanical effects of neurodynamic tests for clinical application.

THE SPINE

Flexion and extension

Mechanical interface – spinal canal
Length
Flexion of the whole spine causes elongation of the spinal neural structures because they, and their canal, are located behind the axis of rotation of the spinal motion segments. This places them on the side that elongates and shortens with flexion and extension movements respectively. The spinal canal itself elongates by as much as nine centimetres during flexion of the whole spine (lumbar region – 5 cm) (Louis 1981). Since the neural structures are attached at their caudal end to the coccyx by the highly elastic filum terminale and the rostral end by the dura to the skull, with flexion, the neural structures are pulled from both ends (Fig. 2.1).

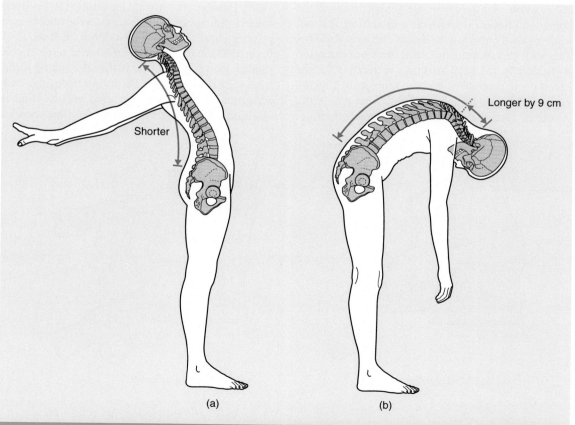

Figure 2.1   Length change in the spinal canal during flexion.

Space around the nervous system

The space around the neural structures in the spine increases with flexion and decreases with extension (Penning & Wilmink 1981). In the cervical spine, the intervertebral foraminae open around the nerve roots by as much as 23% from extension to flexion (Yoo et al 1992). In the lumbar spine, these events also occur at both the central canal and intervertebral foramen (Schonstrom et al 1989). The canal opens by 16% and the area of the intervertebral foraminae increases by as much as 27–30% from full extension to full flexion (Panjabi et al 1983; Inufusa et al 1996). Generally, flexion decreases compressive forces on the spinal neural structures and this is why symptoms of spinal and nerve root stenosis are frequently relieved by flexion (leaning forwards) and provoked by extension (standing and walking) (Fig. 2.2).

Neural tissues

Tension and strain

A key event that occurs in the neural tissues of the spine with flexion is an increase in tension. It is not known exactly how much tension occurs in these tissues with this movement, but strain from extension to flexion in the lumbar dura can reach 30%, the sacral nerve roots 16%, and the spinal cord 10–20% (Adams & Logue 1971; Louis 1981; Yuan et al 1998). As can be seen, the cord and its associated structures

elongate considerably, such that even the blood vessels become uncoiled and elongated. Tension with spinal flexion passes along all the spinal neural tissues, to the point where the filum terminale is elongated as the spinal cord moves in a cephalad direction in the spinal canal (Louis 1981) (Fig. 2.3).

Neck flexion transmits significant tension to the lumbosacral nerve roots (Breig 1978, p. 84), which makes this movement useful clinically in the establishment of a neural aspect to low back pain (Fig. 2.4).

Sliding and convergence

The general mechanisms of sliding and convergence are described in the previous chapter. However, the sliding of neural structures in the spine is complex and not fully understood. Specific sequences of movements produce their own sliding patterns, some of which have been documented. Neck flexion produces cephalad sliding of the neural contents in the lumbar region (Breig & Marions 1963; Breig 1978). However, the straight leg raise (SLR) produces caudad sliding of the nerve roots in the lumbosacral intervertebral foraminae (Goddard & Reid 1965; Breig 1978; Breig & Troup 1979) and cervical cord (Smith 1956). A problem is that the neural structures slide relative to their bony interface differently according to the movement used and location in question. Paradoxically, above the low cervical

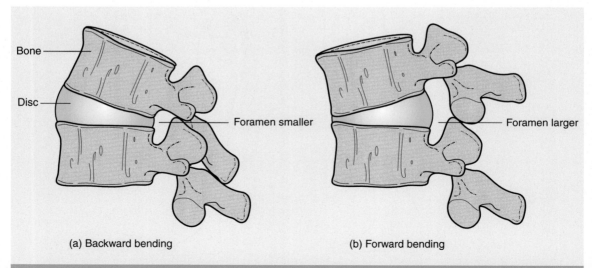

Bone

Disc

Foramen smaller

Foramen larger

(a) Backward bending

(b) Forward bending

Figure 2.2 Effects of spinal movement on the intervertebral foramen. (a) Extension produces closing. Similarly, lateral flexion will produce significant opening and closing effects (discussed later). (b) Flexion produces opening.

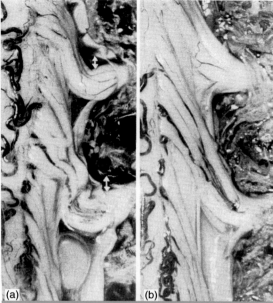

Figure 2.3   Movement, tension and strain in the cervical spinal cord and nerve roots during spinal flexion. Left – (a) Cervical spine in extension showing loose tissue and separation between the neural tissues and the intervertebral foramen (white arrows). Right – (b) Elongation of the neural and vascular tissues, along with sliding and contact of the neural tissues against the structures that form the intervertebral foramen (from Breig 1978, with permission of the author).

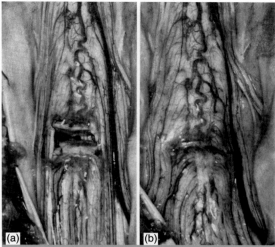

Figure 2.4   Effects of neck flexion on the lumbar cord tissue. Flexion produces a separation of the cut neural tissue (left) whereas the neutral position enables the tissue to approximate (from Breig 1978, with permission of the author).

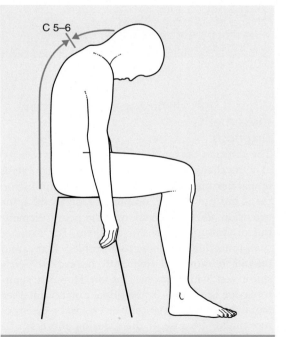

Figure 2.5   Flexion of the cervical spine producing sliding of the neural tissues relative to the spinal canal. Convergence occurs at C5–6 but it does not occur at the low lumbar region because the interface at this site is not moved.

region, flexion of the whole spine and neck flexion alone produce caudad movement of the brain and spinal cord tissue relative to neighbouring bone. Below the low cervical levels, the neural elements move cephalad toward C5 (Adams & Logue 1971; Louis 1981; Yuan et al 1998). The same phenomenon occurs at L4–S1, where the nerves above this level move caudad and those below slide cephalad toward this level (Louis 1981). Movement of the spine around the neural structures, and a complex series of lending and borrowing of neural tissue, produce convergence toward C5–6 and L4–5 the most mobile of spinal segments (Smith 1956; Adams & Logue 1971; Louis 1981).

The above points are particularly important when it comes to understanding neurodynamic sequencing for clinical application (Figs 2.5 and 2.6).

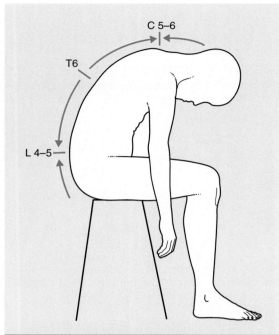

Figure 2.6 Flexion of the whole spine illustrating movement of the neural tissues in the spinal canal relative to the canal. Convergence occurs in the directions indicated.

Clinical uses of flexion and extension movements

Diagnosis

The clinician can apply sagittal movements to arrive at a mechanical diagnosis with spinal problems. Spinal flexion increases tension in the neural structures, but can reduce compression on them. Spinal extension adds compression to the neural elements but produces little tension in them. For instance, symptoms due to a nerve root problem that cannot tolerate tension will frequently be evoked by the slump test, which involves flexion. However, symptoms due to stenosis in the spinal canal or intervertebral foramen will typically be evoked by extension movements because of their closing effects on the neural structures. Hence, a mechanical diagnosis of a tension problem with flexion, or a closing interface problem with extension, can be arrived at with the use of sagittal movements, depending on which manoeuvre evokes or eases symptoms.

Treatment

Mechanical diagnosis leads the therapist toward a specific mechanical treatment. If a tension problem exists, a focus can be on improving the ability of the neural structures to respond to tension. Alternatively, the emphasis may be on preventing tension in the nerves so that they have a chance to settle. If a problem is predominantly one of interface closing, then a treatment technique to improve this mechanism could be performed. Conversely, another choice of treatment for this problem might be to open the interface so that provocation of the neural structures is reduced. These points highlight the need for the clinician to link mechanical diagnosis to the causal mechanisms that produce specific clinical patterns.

Lateral flexion and lateral glide

Mechanical interface

The key event with lateral flexion in relation to the mechanical interface is that the intervertebral foraminae close down around the nerve roots on the ipsilateral side and open up on the contralateral (Fujiwara et al 2001). Increased pressure on the nerve roots will therefore occur on the ipsilateral side and decreased pressure on the contralateral side will result.

Neural effects

Lateral flexion produces increased tension in the neural structures on the convex side of the spine and reduces tension in those on the concave side (Breig 1978; Louis 1981; Selvaratnam et al 1988). In this situation, increased tension in the nervous system occurs through two mechanisms. The first is that lateral flexion itself produces elongation of the interface and neural tissues on the convex side. The second mechanism is by causing an increase in the distance between the spine and periphery by the sideways translation of the vertebrae (lateral glide). This produces mechanical stresses that pass along the peripheral nervous system (Fig. 2.7).

Lateral glide of the spine produces increased tension in the contiguous contralateral nerves and nerve roots. Our observations on dynamic imaging of the brachial plexus and more distal peripheral nerves are that lateral gliding in a contralateral direction can be more effective in producing neural movement at a distal location than contralateral lateral flexion.

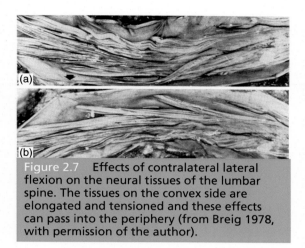

Figure 2.7   Effects of contralateral lateral flexion on the neural tissues of the lumbar spine. The tissues on the convex side are elongated and tensioned and these effects can pass into the periphery (from Breig 1978, with permission of the author).

The effects of contralateral lateral flexion and glide of the spine pass far into the periphery. In the upper limb, the median nerve moves proximally at the wrist as much as several millimetres (McLellan & Swash 1976; Shacklock & Wilkinson 2000 (unpublished sonographic recordings, School of Medical Radiation, University of South Australia)). Similar effects occur in the lower limb, where the sciatic nerve is moved proximally in the pelvis during contralateral flexion of the lumbar spine (Breig 1978).

Clinical use of lateral flexion and lateral glide

Lateral flexion and glide are particularly useful in three capacities; structural differentiation of distal symptoms, sensitization of neurodynamic tests and determination of whether a lateral flexion or lateral translation component exists in the clinical problem.

Structural differentiation

In the upper limb, contralateral lateral flexion is generally more effective in differentiation of a neural component to distal symptoms than ipsilateral lateral flexion, probably because the evoked tension changes pass further along the nerve tract. The question of whether the lateral flexion movements produce isolated movement of the nerves in the upper limb is not completely answered. However, two studies show that this can at times be achieved (McLellan & Swash 1976; Shacklock & Wilkinson 2000 (unpublished

sonographic recordings, School of Medical Radiation, University of South Australia)).

In the lower quarter, contralateral lateral flexion of the lumbar spine can also be used to differentiate a neural component to symptoms, particularly during the straight leg raise (Lew & Puentedura 1985) and slump tests.

Sensitization

In the sensitization of neurodynamic tests, contralateral lateral flexion is frequently essential, again because of its ability to increase tension in the nerves so far along the tract. Lateral flexion has been shown to increase the symptom response to neurodynamic tests in both the upper (Kenneally et al 1988; Selvaratnam et al 1994; Coveney et al 1997) and lower limb (Lew & Puentedura 1985).

Mechanical diagnosis can be greatly enhanced with the use of lateral flexion. Elicitation of pain with ipsilateral lateral flexion can indicate a closing problem in the mechanical interface. Production of pain with contralateral lateral flexion can imply the presence of a tension aspect in which the neural structures on the contralateral side are being stimulated. Hence, lateral flexion can be used to distinguish between different types of neuropathodynamics and can lead the therapist to specific treatment of the relevant component (discussed in more detail in Chapter 4).

Rotation

Mechanical interface

The primary event in the interface with spinal rotation is that the intervertebral foraminae on the ipsilateral side close down whereas, on the contralateral side, they open up (Fujiwara et al 2001). Hence, in assessing closing mechanisms, a small degree of ipsilateral rotation can be combined with flexion or extension movements to ascertain whether a rotational element exists in an interface component of nerve root problems.

Neural effects

The circumference of the spinal cord in the neck reduces with rotation (Breig 1960), as if it were being rung out like a wet towel. It is not clear whether this has any significance for neurodynamic testing but it is possible that, in some patients, rotation can be applied to neurodynamic testing if it meets the patient's needs. An example of this would be the patient in whom a neurogenic symptom is provoked with neck rotation and arm movements. The appropriate upper limb neurodynamic test can be performed with neck rotation as a component of the test. In the lumbar spine, it is common for rotation in combination with the SLR to be an effective treatment technique for low back and posterior thigh pain, given the correct choice of patient.

Effect of gravity

Neurobiomechanics

Breig (1978) showed that the neural contents of the spinal canal droop downwards with gravity. At first, this effect appears to be a trivial epiphenomenon. However, it is actually an important aspect of spinal neurodynamics. In an intelligent and incisive study, Miller (1986) tested the effects of gravity on the response to the SLR in normal subjects. Subjects were positioned on their side and the test on the downward limb was compared with that of the upper side. Even when lateral flexion was neutralized, the test for the downward limb was consistently tighter than the upper one. The reader will notice this in many people in whom straight leg raising of the downward side will usually be tighter, no matter which side the subject lies on. This is conclusive support for gravity being a variable in lumbar neurodynamic testing. The mechanism here is that the neural contents are convex on the downward side and concave on the upper side, producing more tension in the lower SLR (Fig. 2.8).

Clinical application

Gravity can be very useful in clinical neurodynamics. If the desire is to reduce the power of a technique to prevent provocation, the upper side can be tested or mobilized. If the desire is to sensitize the SLR test, then the lower limb on the downward side can be moved. As a useful addition to sensitization, it is also effective and convenient to perform lumbar contralateral lateral flexion with the other elements of the test.

Contralateral neurodynamic tests

Effect on symptom responses

Contralateral movements of the nervous system can produce some fascinating occurrences, not the least

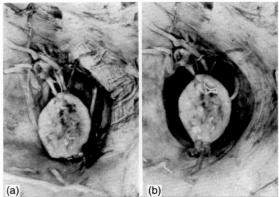

(a)   (b)

Figure 2.8   Effects of gravity on the spinal cord. The neural tissues droop downward with gravity (a. left) and they can be brought back to the centre of the canal with cervical flexion (b. right). These events give therapists new avenues for assessment and treatment of disorders with a neurodynamic component (from Breig 1978, with permission of the author).

of which is the reduction of symptoms during a test. Performance of the median neurodynamic test 1 normally produces symptoms in the ventral elbow and forearm regions (Kenneally et al 1988). When the test is held stationary and the same test is performed on the contralateral upper limb, the symptoms in the held limb often subside (Elvey 1979; Rubenach et al 1985). This is normal and the equivalent events are readily observed to occur with the slump and SLR tests.

Neurobiomechanics

The following is a proposed mechanism for the contralateral neurodynamic test to reduce the response in the held side. It resides in the relationships between the angles of the nerve roots and spinal cord movement.

The cervical and lumbar nerve roots diverge from the spinal cord at an angle. This angle contains two component vectors, horizontal and vertical. The vertical vector is particularly relevant because it is what produces the spinal cord movements necessary to reduce tension in the contralateral nerve root. As the contralateral neurodynamic test is performed, forces enter the spinal cord through the contralateral nerve

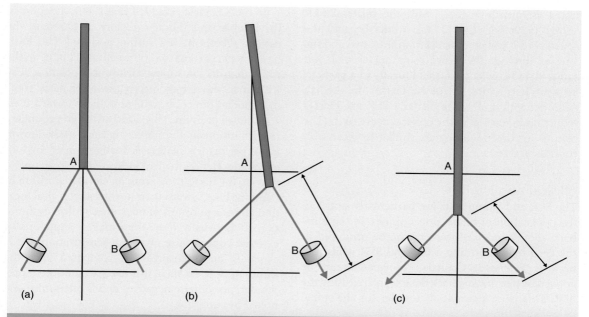

Figure 2.9 (a) Effects on neural tension with application of contralateral neurodynamic testing. (a) Neutral position – A represents the intersection of the nerve root and spinal cord and B indicates the intervertebral foramen. The distance between the two relates to tension in the nerve root. (b) A neurodynamic test is performed as if it were on the patient's left side (viewed from the front), indicated by the arrow at the distal end of the nerve root. The test produces distal movement and tension in the nerve root and migration of the nerve root and spinal cord caudally and ipsilaterally. The new length of the nerve root is indicated by the thin double-ended arrow located adjacent and parallel to the nerve root. (c) A contralateral neurodynamic test (e.g. MNT1 or knee extension in the slump test) is performed. The held nerve root is shortened by virtue of the vertical vector component. The spinal cord has descended in the canal (versus (a) and (b)). The held nerve root is now approximately 10% shorter and possesses less tension than in figure (b).

roots. The vertical component force passing along the contralateral nerve root causes the spinal cord to descend in the canal. The downward movement of the cord is most likely small but is sufficient to transmit a reduction of tension through the vertical component of the ipsilateral held nerve root. The mechanical models that I have made, and geometrical analysis, bear this theory out and it is supported by similar observations in cadavers by Louis (1981) (Fig. 2.9).

Clinical application of contralateral movements

Contralateral movements can be used in mechanical diagnosis and treatment. The event of a contralateral technique producing a change in symptoms in a limb that is held in a neurodynamic position will,

at times, constitute evidence of a neurodynamic mechanism to the symptoms. Treatment with contralateral techniques can be justified in some circumstances, especially if the technique produces an improvement and can be integrated into the rest of patient management.

Bilateral neurodynamic techniques

Neurobiomechanics and symptom responses

Parallels exist between contralateral and bilateral neurodynamic tests. The main point to highlight in this area is that bilateral techniques are particularly useful in producing cephalad and caudad movement of the spinal cord. An example of such effects is that the response to the unilateral median neurodynamic test 1 frequently reduces with the bilateral SLR (Elvey 1979; Bell 1987). This occurs because the spinal cord is pulled downward in the canal and the stresses through the nerve roots are evened out, rather than being concentrated focally in a particular neural structure. In the context of the median neurodynamic test 1, the bilateral SLR produces a reduction in tension in the cervical nerve roots. The reasons for this occurring are similar to those with contralateral tests.

Clinical application

The SLR and slump tests are particularly suited to the application of bilateral techniques. In the lumbar region, caudad movement can be produced in the cord by performing a bilateral SLR whilst the neck is extended. Cephalad movement can be applied by performing neck flexion and releasing the SLR. This is an example of a slider for the spinal neural structures.

A challenge to non-organic contribution to low back pain

A serious issue in relation to the sliding of neural structures in the lumbar spine is the fact that the movement and position of the lumbosacral nerve roots are different between the knee-extension-in-sitting (KEIS) test, the slump test and the straight leg raise (SLR). This is because, if the sequence of movements or the starting position is different, then the test is different. The corollary is that, since symptoms can be specific to the sequence and position used, the evoked symptoms may also be different.

The slump test is primarily a test of tension because the cephalocaudad effects of spinal flexion (including neck flexion) and SLR are in opposition. In the lumbar region, this produces little displacement of the neural structures from their anatomical position but more tension is generated than if forces are applied to the nerve roots from only one end. In the SLR, little pretensioning from a cephalad direction occurs, which allows the nerve roots to displace in a caudad direction further than in the slump test. Hence, if a patient's SLR is more abnormal than the KEIS or slump tests, it means that the problem may be one of loss of, or increased sensitivity to, caudal sliding rather than one of tension.

In the KEIS test (Waddell et al 1980), the spine in the lumbar and thoracic regions is flexed as the patient relaxes in the sitting position. The lumbosacral nerve roots may be positioned higher in the canal than in the supine anatomical position. The KEIS manoeuvre may merely move the nerve roots in a caudad direction, returning them toward their anatomical position. This occurs without producing much tension in the nerves, because neck flexion is not performed, neither is dorsiflexion of the foot and ankle. Hence, the KEIS test is likely to be one of moving the nerve roots from an elevated position in the spine back toward their normal anatomical location and is a poor test of neuromechanical dysfunction. It is usually only abnormal in situations of extreme compromise or severe sensitization and is generally an insensitive test compared with the slump or SLR. As such, it is likely to produce a preponderance of false negatives and is often misinterpreted by clinicians.

Discrepancy between the KEIS test, slump and SLR tests is quite natural and normal (Didben 1996) and is a serious challenge to the notion that such discrepancies are always an indication of non-organic physical signs in low back pain. Many clinicians have encountered patients who can only touch their toes or perform a SLR successfully when their spine is flexed. As soon as they straighten their spine, the SLR becomes restricted.

Clearly, the mechanical effects of the KEIS test, SLR and slump tests are different and can not always be compared on mutual terms. Interpretation of any discrepancy between these tests as a sign of non-organic contribution to low back pain must be executed judiciously, with skill, and in relation to known central, psychosocial and peripheral pain mechanisms (see Waddell 1998; Shacklock 1999a, 1999b, 2000).

For a review of biomechanics of the central nervous system, see Shacklock et al (1994).

UPPER QUARTER

Cervical spine

Cervical lateral flexion

Neurobiomechanics

By way of increasing the distance between the shoulder and neck, contralateral lateral flexion of the neck exerts proximal tensile forces on the brachial plexus (Elvey 1995; Selvaratnam et al 1988; Kleinrensink et al 2000), which is accompanied by movement of the neural structures in the direction of the lateral flexion. The forces of this movement are transmitted as far distally as the radial and ulnar nerves at the elbow (Kleinrensink et al 2000) and median nerve at the wrist (McLellan & Swash 1976, Shacklock & Wilkinson 2000 (unpublished sonographic recordings, School of Medical Radiation, University of South Australia)).

Effect on symptoms

Contralateral lateral flexion of the neck consistently increases symptoms evoked by the median (Kenneally et al 1988; Selvaratnam et al 1994, 1997) and radial (Yaxley & Jull 1991) neurodynamic tests. This movement is a prime one in structural differentiation and sensitization of neurodynamic tests of the upper limb, particularly when the evoked symptoms are located distally.

Ipsilateral lateral flexion frequently reduces the symptoms evoked by all the upper limb neurodynamic tests. However, it is not as useful in structural differentiation as contralateral lateral flexion because tension in the peripheral nerves is sometimes not sufficient to be released further when ipsilateral lateral flexion is applied (Shacklock & Wilkinson 2000 (unpublished sonographic recordings, School of Medical Radiation, University of South Australia)). This is particularly the case when the specific upper limb neurodynamic tests can not be taken to their end range. Hence, false negatives are more common with this movement than contralateral lateral flexion. However, ipsilateral lateral flexion is useful in the case of a sensitive neural problem in which structural differentiation is required. At the point of first onset of symptoms, rather than contralateral lateral flexion being performed, which would further provoke symptoms, ipsilateral lateral flexion can be used to reduce the symptoms. Hence, the main value of ipsilateral lateral flexion is its ability to change symptoms without provoking the problem and is particularly useful in differentiating sensitive neural disorders. Alternatively, release of contralateral lateral flexion is a useful modification of differentiation in sequencing at low level problems (described in more detail in Chapter 6).

Shoulder

Scapular depression
Neurobiomechanics

Scapular depression increases tension in the peripheral nerves of the upper limb by producing an increase in the distance between the neck and arm. The cervical nerve roots move distally with this movement (Frykholm 1951; Smith 1956; Reid 1960; Adams & Logue 1971). Taking neural sliding and convergence into account, the dynamics of scapular depression are complex and probably vary a great deal between individuals and between different locations on the interfacing structures. Proximal sliding of the brachial plexus relative to the glenohumeral joint is likely to occur. From our sonographic recordings on the movements of the median nerve in the forearm and wrist *in vivo*, scapular depression moves the nerve proximally. Depression is not as effective in achieving such excursion as contralateral lateral flexion, but a significant increase in excursion can be achieved when the two movements are combined (Shacklock & Wilkinson 2000 (unpublished sonographic recordings, School of Medical Radiation, University of South Australia)), however this varies between individuals.

Effect on symptoms

Scapular depression consistently produces an increase in symptoms with upper limb neurodynamic tests. As such, the movement can sometimes be used to effectively differentiate a neural component to many upper limb problems.

Glenohumeral abduction

The mechanical interface between the coracoid process and a point midway along the shaft of the humerus increases in length by approximately 2.4 cm with glenohumeral abduction (Elvey 1995). In terms of tension and strain in the neural tissues, abduction causes increased tension in the brachial plexus and the more distal peripheral nerves of the upper limb (Adams & Logue 1971; Wright et al 1996; Selvaratnam et al 1988; Kleinrensink et al 2000). From 0° to 90°, strain in the median nerve at the elbow increases by 4.2%. However, abduction from 90° to 110° produces an even greater increase in strain (9.1%) (Wright et al 1996). In terms of movement, the C5 nerve root slides 4 mm in a distal direction in its intervertebral foramen (Elvey 1979). The median nerve at the level of the shoulder joint moves as much as 1.0 cm (Elvey 1995). We have observed that the median nerve, at a site several centimetres proximal to the elbow, moves proximally by several millimetres.

Clinically, it can be readily observed that the symptoms in response to upper limb neurodynamic testing increase with abduction, illustrating a close relationship between the movement, resultant tension in the nerves and the production of symptoms (Elvey 1979). Glenohumeral abduction produces distal sliding of the nerves located proximal to the shoulder and proximal sliding of the nerves that are located distal to the shoulder, such that they converge toward the shoulder. The median nerve at the wrist slides 8–9 mm proximally with abduction (Wright et al 1996).

External rotation
The effects of glenohumeral external rotation on the nerves are equivocal. Using strain gauges, Ginn (1988) found that the movement did not always produce an increase in tension in the nerve, whereas Selvaratnam et al (1988) showed an increase. Clinically, responses to external rotation during the median neurodynamic test 1 are also variable among individuals.

Horizontal extension
I am not aware of any studies that establish the exact effect of specific glenohumeral horizontal extension on nerve tension. Elvey (1979) mentioned that this movement was related to increased tension in the nervous system. Clinically, the movement increases symptoms with neurodynamic testing, possibly because the nerves pass anterior to the shoulder joint. However, some clinicians do not perform horizontal extension in routine testing (Butler 1991, 2000). This is because, even though it may increase neural tension, it can be a source of inconsistency and is not essential in producing sufficient strain to evoke symptoms in normal subjects. Nevertheless, it may be used to sensitize upper limb neurodynamic tests.

Internal rotation
Internal rotation of the glenohumeral joint increases tension in the radial nerve (Kleinrensink et al 2000) because the nerve passes posterior to the shoulder joint and spirals posterolaterally around the shaft of the humerus. Clinically, it is common for internal rotation to increase the response to the radial neurodynamic test.

Elbow
Extension
Elbow extension increases the length of the bed of the median nerve by 20% (Millesi 1986) which results in an increase in length of the median nerve by 4–5% (Zöch et al 1991). Above the elbow, the median nerve moves distally and, below the elbow, it moves proximally (Wright et al 1996). This is yet another example of the general neurodynamic principle of convergence toward the moved joint.

Flexion
Elbow flexion decreases tension in the median nerve which becomes quite wrinkled at the end range (Wright et al 1996). Conversely, tension in the ulnar nerve at the elbow is increased (Toby & Hanesworth 1998), sometimes by as much as 23% (Grewel et al 2000). The magnitude of strain in the ulnar nerve with elbow flexion varies considerably, depending on the sequence of movements used. More strain can be applied to the ulnar nerve when elbow flexion is the first movement of the ulnar neurodynamic test (Tsai 1995).

In addition to tension being produced in the ulnar nerve by elbow flexion, intraneural pressure rises considerably (Pechan & Julis 1975; Green & Rayan 1999). The retinaculum over the ulnar nerve is stretched by 45% (Schuind et al 1995) and this is associated with a 41% reduction in the space in the cubital tunnel and a 30–50% reduction in cross-sectional area of the nerve. The pressure in the nerve with elbow flexion can rise to 45% higher than the pressure inside the tunnel with flexion (Gelberman et al 1998). The pressure around the ulnar nerve in patients with cubital tunnel syndrome can exceed 200 mmHg (Werner et al 1985a). This is well above systolic blood pressure, which indicates the likelihood of neural ischaemia with cubital tunnel syndrome, especially considering that the pressure threshold for nerve viability is only 30–50 mmHg (Gelberman et al 1983). The elbow flexion manoeuvre, when combined with manual pressure over the nerve at the elbow, is a more sensitive test for cubital tunnel syndrome than the flexion test alone and Tinel's sign (Novak et al 1994).

Supination and pronation
Strain and excursion of the median nerve at the wrist and elbow with pronation and supination are

small, probably because these movements do not produce large changes in the length of the mechanical interface. Also, there appears to be a great deal of variance between individuals (Wright et al 1996). Wright et al (1996) showed that pronation caused an increase in strain in the median nerve at the elbow by 0.6%, whilst, at the wrist, strain decreased by the same amount. The nerve at the elbow at this location also moved proximally by 0.34 mm whereas, at the wrist, it moved distally by 3.9 mm. The total excursion between pronation and supination in the nerve at the wrist amounts to 4.4 mm and, at the elbow, it totals 1.0 mm. These values were measured in cadavera and in a controlled laboratory setting.

Even though it has been shown that only small effects are produced by pronation and supination, a key issue is *when* they are performed. If these movements are part of a whole neurodynamic test at its end range, small changes in the nerves produced by these movements could make a significant difference to the responses. This is because, when the nerves are under tension, only small additional movements can be sufficient to produce significant effects in the system.

A key asset in pronation and supination is the opportunity to apply stresses to the nerves through the mechanical interface. Stretching of the supinator muscle in the form of passive pronation can be used to exert up to 46 mmHg of pressure on the posterior interosseous nerve at the supinator tunnel. Maximal contraction of the supinator muscle exerts up to 190 mmHg (Werner et al 1980). This is support for the idea that active movements can be combined with neurodynamic tests to assess and treat the interfacing structures in conjunction with the nervous system and to localize the application of forces to the nervous system. Interface interactions such as these are a key feature of advanced neurodynamic sequencing discussed later in this book.

Wrist

Flexion and extension
Neurobiomechanics
Flexion of the wrist decreases tension in the median nerve and extension increases tension. The total change in strain in the median nerve at the elbow between the two movements is 14.8%. At the wrist,

the total change in strain of the nerve reaches 9.6%. Excursion of the nerve is proximal with wrist flexion and is distal with extension. The total longitudinal sliding of the nerve at the elbow between flexion and extension is 5.6 mm and, at the wrist, it can reach 19.6 mm (Wright et al 1996). Transverse motion of the median nerve at the wrist occurs and has been measured between 1.5 mm and 3.0 mm (Nakamichi & Tachibana 1992; Greening et al 1999).

Provocative testing
Wrist flexion is used universally as a provocative movement for detection of carpal tunnel syndrome (Phalen 1951, 1970). This is because the manoeuvre applies pressure to the nerve and is likely to produce nerve ischaemia in patients with the syndrome. A nerve that is already ischaemic or under pressure may therefore produce symptoms when additional pressure is applied to it. In normal subjects, pressure as high as 40–50 mmHg can be produced in the carpal tunnel with wrist flexion. Significant variation in the pressure changes with wrist movements occurs in both normal subjects and patients with carpal tunnel syndrome. Sometimes extension of the wrist can produce higher tunnel pressures than flexion (Gelberman et al 1981; Luchetti et al 1998) which means that it too can be used as a physical test.

Radial and ulnar deviation
Radial and ulnar deviation evoke changes in a similar order of magnitude to pronation and supination of the forearm. Once again, the effects being small in magnitude will be caused by the fact that they do not produce much change in the length of the mechanical interface. The total change in strain in the median nerve at the elbow between radial and ulnar deviation is 3.3%. At the wrist, the total change in strain of the nerve reaches 3.8%. Strain in the nerve at the elbow increases with radial deviation and decreases at the wrist. At the wrist, the effects on strain are the opposite, radial deviation producing a decrease in strain and ulnar deviation increasing strain. The total amptitude of longitudinal sliding of the nerve at the elbow between radial and ulnar deviation is only 0.12 mm and, at the wrist, it can reach 0.49 mm (Wright et al 1996). As with pronation and supination, small changes in radial and ulnar deviation may not produce much in the way of mechanical events when they are performed in

isolation. However, when the movements are performed in combination with other components of testing, they can become much more valuable.

Finger flexion and extension
Neurobiomechanics
The patterns of median nerve strain and movement with finger movements are similar to those produced by wrist movements. Flexion of the fingers decreases tension in the median nerve and extension increases tension. The total change in strain in the median nerve at the elbow between the two movements is 10.3%. At the wrist, the total change in strain of the nerve reaches 19.0%. Excursion of the nerve is proximal with wrist flexion and is distal with extension. The total longitudinal sliding of the nerve at the elbow between flexion and extension of the fingers is 3.4 mm and, at the wrist, it can reach 9.7 mm (Wright et al 1996). Extension of the fingers produces between 4.0 mm and 9.5 mm of distal movement in the median nerve at the wrist (Laban et al 1989; Zöch et al 1991).

In terms of transverse displacement in normal subjects, the median nerve at the wrist usually moves in a radial direction (approximately 1.55 mm) with finger extension (Erel et al 2003).

Provocative testing
The performance of passive extension of the index finger for diagnosis of chronic carpal tunnel syndrome has been termed the 'Tethered median nerve stress test' (Laban et al 1986) and may be used in the examination of patients with symptoms suggestive of the problem. However, it is frequently rather provocative and should be used with caution. This might be due to the fact that finger extension produces significant strain in the median nerve.

THE LOWER LIMB

Hip

Flexion – straight leg raise (SLR) test
The SLR has been researched extensively and it has long been confirmed that the manoeuvre produces a great deal of movement and tension in the lumbosacral nerve roots and sciatic nerve (Charnley 1951; Goddard & Reid 1965; Breig 1978).

Mechanical interface
In terms of the interface, hip flexion produces increased tension in the hamstring muscles, an effect that then produces posterior rotation of the pelvis as early as 10° of hip flexion (Bohannon et al 1985). This in turn produces flexion of the lumbar spine (Breig 1978) and moves all the local musculoskeletal and neural structures in the lumbopelvic region. Hence, the SLR per se does not distinguish between neural and musculoskeletal structures. Always therefore, structural differentiation is a necessary addition in performance of the test.

Neural tissues
It was often thought by clinicians that the SLR pulls and moves the sciatic nerve distally through the whole length of the lower limb. It is true that tension is applied to the nerve with the use of hip flexion. However, this action is in fact caused by the interface elongating around the sciatic nerve at the hip and, instead of producing widespread distal movement of the sciatic nerve in the limb, convergence of the nerve toward the hip joint occurs (Smith 1956). Because elongation is initiated at the hip joint, the neural structures above and below the hip slide distally and proximally toward the hip respectively. Once again, convergence participates in the movement of nerves. Since the tibial nerve slides proximally up the leg, this effect will evoke movement in a similar direction in the plantar nerves (Fig. 2.10).

Distal movement of the lumbosacral nerve roots in their foraminae can amount to 9–10 mm, whilst the lumbosacral trunk in the pelvis also moves in this

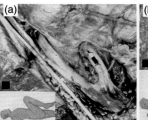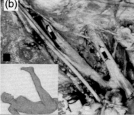

Figure 2.10   Effect of hip flexion on the spinal nerves and lumbosacral trunk. Distal movement of these neural structures occurs and sometimes this can amount to almost 1 cm (from Breig 1978, with permission of the author).

direction (Goddard & Reid 1965). The magnitudes of tension and strain that occur during the SLR have not been established. However, the nerve bed between the hip and ankle elongates by as much as 124 mm (Beith et al 1995) which, in a person of average height, can be calculated to be between 10% and 17%. Hip flexion accounts for 44% of the change in nerve bed length with the SLR (Beith 1995).

Medial rotation

Medial rotation of the hip increases tension in the lumbosacral plexus and its related nerve roots and also in the sciatic nerve (Breig & Troup 1979). This is because the neural structures pass posterior to the joint. Medial rotation is a valuable sensitizing movement for the SLR and slump tests, with its ability to increase the response to the test in patients and normal subjects.

Adduction

Adduction of the hip increases the response to the SLR (Sutton 1979). However, to my knowledge, direct measurement of tension in the neural tissues during adduction has not been performed. Hip adduction may be used to sensitize the SLR in certain circumstances.

Extension

In normal subjects, hip extension increases the response to the prone knee bend (Davidson 1987). However, it is likely that this is via movement of the iliopsoas muscle, through which the lumbar plexus passes. Even though hip extension increases the symptom response, it is possible that, in some subjects, the response is no more neural in nature than the standard prone knee bend because the increase in symptoms with hip extension is not always influenced by neural differentiation movements eg. neck flexion (Davidson 1987).

Knee

Extension

Knee extension increases the length of the sciatic nerve bed by up to 60 mm, and accounts for 49% of nerve bed elongation (Beith et al 1995). The sciatic and tibial nerves converge toward the knee, sliding distally and proximally respectively (Smith 1965).

This will cause the plantar nerves to slide proximally. Knee extension is useful clinically because the joint offers a large range of motion through which changes in symptoms can be easily observed. Hence, this movement can be used to mobilize nerves that are located a large distance from the knee, such as the posterior tibial nerve (Shacklock 1995) or the lumbosacral nerve roots, without producing excessive mechanical stresses in these structures.

Flexion – prone knee bend

The prone knee bend is used clinically to apply tension to the mid-lumbar nerve roots and femoral nerve (O'Connell 1943) by virtue of the quadriceps muscle pulling on the terminations of the femoral nerve. However, the standard prone knee bend is not a definitive neural test. This is because, through the connection of the rectus femoris muscle to the pelvis, anterior rotation of the pelvis occurs and therefore potentially implicates any of the lumbopelvic structures as a source of pain in the back or pelvis. Therefore further differentiating manoeuvres are used to take the prone knee bend into the realm of neural differentiation. These are described in Chapter 7.

Foot and ankle

Dorsiflexion

Dorsiflexion of the ankle has been shown to increase tension in the tibial nerve (Beith et al 1995) and, at the height of the SLR, has at surgery been observed to produce movement in the lumbosacral nerve roots (Macnab 1988, personal communication). Clinically, dorsiflexion is frequently a valuable differentiation and sensitizing manoeuvre for the SLR because of its ability to produce movement in the sciatic nerve tract as far proximally as the lumbosacral nerve roots.

Eversion

The posterior tibial nerve is tensioned by eversion of the ankle (Daniels et al 1998) because the nerve courses along the medial aspect of the ankle, albeit behind the medial malleolus. Pressure on the nerve during eversion rises to 32 mmHg, between seven and 16 times that which occurs in the neutral position (Trepman et al 1999). It is clear that mechanical function of the lower limb is important in managing neural problems in this region.

Dorsiflexion/inversion – sural nerve

Dorsiflexion/inversion of the ankle and foot tensions the sural nerve because of its posterolateral course around the ankle joint. This nerve may become damaged in cases of sprained ankle in which the injuring movement involves these specific movements.

Plantarflexion/inversion – peroneal nerve

Because of the passage of the superficial peroneal nerve over the anterolateral aspect of the ankle, the nerve is tensioned and moves distally in the leg with plantarflexion/inversion of the foot and ankle (Kopell & Thompson 1976; Shacklock 1989 (unpublished data)). In cadavers, I have observed that the movement can amount to several millimetres with more movement occurring at the level of the superficial peroneal nerve immediately proximal to the ankle and less movement occurring at the level of the head of the fibula. The nerve tends to move with, although not as much as, the adjacent tendons.

Some ankle sprains produce damage in this nerve (Nobel 1966; Streib 1983; Kleinrensink et al 1994). This may account for peroneal neurodynamic tests (slump and SLR versions) becoming abnormal (Mauhart 1989; Pahor & Toppenberg 1996) in some patients with sprained ankle.

Plantarflexion/inversion of the ankle is valuable in the sensitization (Slater 1988; Mauhart 1989) and differentiation of peroneal involvement in lower limb pain. Plantarflexion/inversion is also relevant to the piriformis syndrome because the manoeuvre may produce specific forces in the peroneal part of the sciatic nerve up to the pelvis in those who have a high division of the sciatic nerve into its peroneal and tibial components (Shacklock 1989).

References

Adams C, Logue V 1971 Studies in cervical spondylotic myelopathy: 1 Movement of the cervical roots, dura and cord, and their relation to the course of the extrathecal roots. Brain 94: 557–568

Bell A 1987 The upper limb tension test and straight leg raising. In: Proceedings of the 5th Biennial Conference of the Manipulative Therapists' Association of Australia, Melbourne: 106–114

Beith I, Robins E, Richards P 1995 An assessment of the adaptive mechanisms within and surrounding the peripheral nervous system, during changes in nerve bed length resulting from underlying joint movement. In: Shacklock M (ed), Moving in on Pain, Butterworth-Heinemann: 194–203

Bohannon R, Gajdosik R, LeVeau B 1985 Contribution of pelvic and lower limb motion to increases in the angle of passive straight leg raise. Physical Therapy 65(4): 474–476

Breig 1960 Biomechanics of the central nervous system. Almqvist and Wiksell, Stockholm

Breig A 1978 Adverse mechanical tension in the central nervous system. Almqvist and Wiksell, Stockholm

Breig A, Marions O 1963 Biomechanics of the lumbosacral nerve roots. Acta Radiologica. Diagnosis 1: 1141–1160

Breig A, Troup J 1979 Biomechanical considerations in the straight leg raising test. Cadaveric and clinical studies of medial hip rotation. Spine 4(3): 242–250

Butler D 1991 Mobilisation of the Nervous System. Churchill Livingstone, Edinburgh

Butler D 2000 The sensitive nervous system. NOI Group Publications, Adelaide

Charnley J 1951 Orthopaedic signs in the diagnosis of disc protrusion. Lancet 1: 186–192

Coveney B, Trott P, Grimmer K, Bell A, Hall R, Shacklock M 1997 The upper limb tension test in a group of subjects with a clinical presentation of carpal tunnel syndrome. In: Proceedings of the 10th Biennial Conference of the Manipulative Physiotherapists' Association of Australia, Melbourne: 31–33

Daniels T, Lau J, Hearn T 1998 The effects of foot position and load on tibial nerve tension. Foot and Ankle International 19(2): 73–78

Davidson S 1987 Prone knee bend: an investigation into the effect of cervical flexion and extension. In: Proceedings of the 5th Biennial Conference of the Manipulative Therapists'Association of Australia. Melbourne: 235–246

Dibden K 1996 A comparison of the straight leg raising manoeuvres in supine and sitting in an asymptomatic population. Graduate Diploma thesis, University of South Australia

Elvey R 1979 Brachial plexus tension tests and the pathoanatomical origin of arm pain. In: Idczak R (ed) Aspects of manipulative therapy. Lincoln Institute of Health Sciences, Melbourne: 105–110

Elvey R 1995 Peripheral neuropathic disorders and neuromusculoskeletal pain. In: Shacklock M (ed) Moving in on Pain. Butterworth-Heinemann: 115–122

Erel E, Dilley A, Greening J, Morris V, Cohen B, Lynn B 2003 Longitudinal sliding of the median nerve in patients with carpal tunnel syndrome. Journal of Hand Surgery 28B(5): 439–443

Frykholm R 1951 The mechanism of cervical radicular lesions resulting from friction or forceful traction. Acta Chirurgia Scandinavica 102: 93–98

Fujiwara A, An H, Lim T, Haughton V 2001 Morphologic changes in the lumbar intervertebral foramen due to flexion-extension, lateral bending, and axial rotation an in vitro anatomic and biomechanical study. Spine 15/26(8): 876–882

Gelberman R, Hergenroeder P, Hargens A, Lundborg G, Akeson W 1981 The carpal tunnel syndrome. A study of carpal canal pressures. Journal of Bone and Joint Surgery 63A(3): 380–383

Gelberman R, Szabo R, Williamson R, Hargens A, Yaru N, Minteer-Convery M 1983 Tissue pressure threshold for peripheral nerve viability. Clinical Orthopaedics and Related Research 187: 285–291

Gelberman R, Yamaguchi K, Hollstien S, Winn S, Heidenreich F, Bindra R, Hsieh P, Silva M 1998 Changes in interstitial pressure and cross-sectional area of the cubital tunnel and of the ulnar nerve with flexion of the elbow. An experimental study in human cadavera. Journal of Bone Joint Surgery 80A(4): 492–501

Ginn K 1988 An investigation of tension development in the upper limb soft tissues during the upper limb tension test. In: Proceedings of the International Federation of the Orthopaedic Manual Therapists, Cambridge: 25–26

Goddard M, Reid J 1965 Movements induced by straight leg raising in the lumbo-sacral roots, nerves and plexus, and in the intrapelvic section of the sciatic nerve. Journal of Neurology, Neurosurgery and Psychiatry 28: 12: 12–18

Green J, Rayan G 1999 The cubital tunnel: anatomic, histologic, and biomechanical study. Journal of Shoulder and Elbow Surgery 8(5): 466–470

Greening J, Smart S, Leary R, Hart-Craggs M, O'Higgins B, Lynn B 1999 Reduced movement of the median nerve in carpal tunnel during wrist flexion in patients with non-specific arm pain. Lancet 354: 217–218

Grewal R, Varitimidis S, Vardakas D, Fu F, Sotereanos D 2000 Ulnar nerve elongation and excursion in the cubital tunnel after decompression and anterior transposition. Journal of Hand Surgery 25B(5): 457–460

Inufusa A, An H, Lim T, Hasegawa T, Haughton V, Nowicki B 1996 Anatomic changes of the spinal canal and intervertebral foramen associated with flexion-extension movement. Spine 1, 21(21): 2412–2420

Kenneally M, Rubenach H, Elvey R 1988 The upper limb tension test: the SLR test of the arm. In: Grant R (ed) Physical Therapy of the Cervical and Thoracic Spine, Clinics in Physical Therapy 17. Churchill Livingstone, New York: 167–194

Kleinrensink GJ, Stoeckart R, Meulstee J, Kaulesar Sukul DM, Vleeming A, Snijders CJ, van Noort A 1994 Lowered motor conduction velocity of the peroneal nerve after inversion trauma. Medicine and Science in Sports and Exercise 26(7): 877–883

Kleinrensink GJ, Stoeckart R, Mulder PG, Hoek G, Broek T, Vleeming A, Snijders C 2000 Upper limb tension tests as tools in the diagnosis of nerve and plexus lesions.

Anatomical and biomechanical aspects. Clinical Biomechanics 15(1): 9–14

Kopell H, Thompson W 1976 Peripheral Entrapment Neuropathies. Robert Krieger Publishing Company, Malabar, Florida

Laban M, Friedman N, Zemenick G 1986 'Tethered' median nerve stress test in chronic carpal tunnel syndrome. Archives of Physical Medicine and Rehabilitation 67: 803–804

Laban M, MacKenzie J, Zemenick G 1989 Anatomic observations in carpal tunnel syndrome as they relate to the tethered median nerve stress test. Archives of Physical Medicine and Rehabilitation 70: 44–46

Lew P, Puentedura E 1985 The straight leg raise test and spinal posture. In: Proceedings of the 4th Biennial Conference of the Manipulative Physiotherapists' Association of Australia, Brisbane: 183–205

Louis R 1981 Vertebroradicular and vertebromedullar dynamics. Anatomia Clinica 3: 1–11

Luchetti R, Schoenhuber R, Nathan P 1998 Correlation of segmental carpal tunnel pressures with changes in hand and wrist positions in patients with carpal tunnel syndrome and controls. Journal of Hand Surgery 23B(5): 598–602

McLellan D, Swash M 1976 Longitudinal sliding of the median nerve during movements of the upper limb. Journal of Neurology, Neurosurgery and Psychiatry 39: 556–570

Mauhart D 1989 The effect of chronic ankle inversion sprain on the plantarflexion/inversion straight leg raise. Graduate Diploma thesis, University of South Australia

Miller A 1986 The straight leg raise test. Graduate Diploma Thesis, University of South Australia

Millesi H 1986 The nerve gap: theory and clinical practice. Hand Clinics 4: 651–663

Nakamichi K, Tachibana S 1992 Transverse sliding of the median nerve beneath the flexor retinaculum. Journal of Hand Surgery 17B: 213–216

Nobel W 1966 Peroneal palsy due to hematoma in the common peroneal nerve sheath after distal torsional fractures and inversion ankle sprains. Journal of Bone and Joint Surgery 48A(8): 1484–1495

Novak C, Lee G, Mackinnon S, Lay L Provocative testing for cubital tunnel syndrome 1994 Journal of Hand Surgery 19A(5): 817–820

O'Connell J 1943 Sciatica and the mechanism of the production of the clnical syndrome in protrusion of the lumbar intervertebral discs. British Journal of Surgery 30: 315–327

Pahor S, Toppenberg R 1996 An investigation of neural tissue involvement in ankle inversion sprains. Manual Therapy 1(4): 192–197

Panjabi M, Takata K, Goel V 1983 Kinematics of the lumbar intervertebral foramen. Spine 8(4): 348–357

Pechan J, Julis I 1975 The pressure measurement in the ulnar nerve. A contribution to the pathophysiology of cubital tunnel syndrome. Journal of Biomechanics 8: 75–79

Penning L, Wilmink J 1981 Biomechanics of the lumbosacral dural sac. A study of flexion-extension myelography. Spine 6(4): 398–408

Phalen G 1951 Spontaneous compression of the median nerve at the wrist. Journal of the American Medical Association 145(15): 1128–1133

Phalen G 1970 Reflections on 21 years' experience with the carpal-tunnel syndrome. Journal of the American Medical Association 212(8): 1365–1367

Reid J 1960 Ascending nerve roots. Journal of Neurosurgery. 23: 148–155

Rubenach H 1985 The upper limb tension test – the effect of the position and movement of the contralateral arm. In: Proceedings of the 4th Biennial Conference of the Manipulative Therapists' Association of Australia: 274–283

Schonstrom N, Lindahl S, Willen J, Hansson T 1989 Dynamic changes in the dimensions of the lumbar spinal canal: an experimental study in vitro. Journal of Orthopaedic Research 7(1): 115–121

Schuind F, Goldschmidt D, Bastin C, Burny F 1995 A biomechanical study of the ulnar nerve at the elbow. Journal of Hand Surgery 20B(5): 623–627

Selvaratnam P, Cook S, Matyas T 1997 Transmission of mechanical stimulation to the median nerve at the wrist during the upper limb tension test. In: Proceedings of the 10th Biennial Conference of the Manipulative Physiotherapists' Association of Australia: 182–188

Selvaratnam P, Glasgow E, Matyas T 1988 Strain effects on the nerve roots of brachial plexus. Journal of Anatomy 161: 260–264

Selvaratnam P, Matyas T, Glasgow E 1994 Noninvasive discrimination of brachial plexus involvement in upper limb pain. Spine 19: 26–33

Shacklock 1989 The plantarflexion inversion straight leg raise. Master of Applied Science Thesis. University of South Australia, Adelaide

Shacklock M 1995 Clinical application of neurodynamics. In: Shacklock M (ed) Moving in on Pain. Butterworth-Heinemann, Sydney: 123–131

Shacklock M 1999a Central pain mechanisms; a new horizon in manual therapy. Australian Journal of Physiotherapy 45: 83–92

Shacklock M 1999b The clinical application of central pain mechanisms in manual therapy. Australian Journal of Physiotherapy 45: 215–221

Shacklock M 2000 Balanced on a tight rope between low back pain and evidence-based practice. New Zealand Journal of Physiotherapy 28(3): 22–27

Shacklock M, Butler D, Slater H 1994 The dynamic central nervous system: structure and clinical neurobiomechanics. In: Boyling G, Palastanga N (eds), Modern Manual Therapy of the Vertebral Column, Churchill Livingstone, Edinburgh: 21–38

Slater H 1988 The effect of foot and ankle position on the 'normal' response to the SLR test, in young, asymptomatic subjects. Master of Applied Science thesis, University of South Australia

Smith C 1956 Changes in length and position of the segments of the spinal cord with changes in posture in the monkey. Radiology 66: 259–265

Streib E 1983 Traction injury of peroneal nerve caused by minor athletic trauma: electromyographic studies. Archives of Neurology 40(1): 62–63

Sutton J 1979 The straight leg raising test. Graduate Diploma in Advanced Manipulative Therapy Thesis, University of South Australia

Toby E, Hanesworth D 1998 Ulnar nerve strains at the elbow. Journal of Hand Surgery 23A(6): 992–997

Trepman E, Kadel N, Chisholm K, Razzano L 1999 Effect of foot and ankle position on tarsal tunnel compartment pressure. Foot and Ankle International 20(11): 721–726

Tsai Y-Y 1995 Tension change in the ulnar nerve by different order of upper limb tension test. Master of Science Thesis, Northwestern University, Chicago

Waddell G 1998 The back pain revolution. Churchill Livingstone, Edinburgh

Waddell G, McCulloch J, Kummel E, Venner R 1980 Nonorganic physical signs in low back pain. Spine 5(2): 117–124

Werner C, Haeffner F, Rosén I 1980 Direct recording of local pressure in the radial tunnel during passive stretch and active contraction of the supinator muscle. Archives of Orthopaedic and Traumatic Surgery 96: 299–301

Werner C, Ohlin P, Elmqvist D 1985a Pressures recorded in ulnar neuropathy. Acta Orthopaedica Scandinavica 56(5): 404–406

Werner C, Rosén I, Thorngren K 1985b Clinical and neurophysiologic characteristics of the pronator syndrome. Clinical Orthopaedics and Related Research 197: 231–237

Wright T, Glowczewskie F, Wheeler D, Miller G, Cowin D 1996 Excursion and strain of the median nerve. Journal of Bone and Joint Surgery 78A(12): 1897–1903

Yaxley G, Jull G 1991 Adverse tension in the neural system: a preliminary study of tennis elbow. Australian Journal of Physiotherapy 39: 15–22

Yoo J, Zou D, Edwards W, Bayley J, Yuan H 1992 Effect of cervical spine motion on the neuroforaminal dimensions of human cervical spine. Spine 17(10): 1131–1136

Yuan Q, Dougherty L, Margulies S 1998 In vivo human cervical spinal cord deformation and displacement in flexion. Spine 23(15): 1677–1683

Zöch G, Reihsner R, Beer R, Millesi H 1991 Stress and strain in peripheral nerves. Neuro-Orthopaedics 10: 371–382

General neuropathodynamics

3

Classifications of neurodynamic disorders

Expanding the boundaries

Defining relationships between neuropathodynamics and clinical problems

Mechanical interface dysfunctions – definitions, closing and opening dysfunctions (reduced and excessive), pathoanatomical, pathophysiological

Neural dysfunctions – sliding, tension, hypermobility/instability, pathoanatomical, pathophysiological

Innervated tissue dysfunctions – motor control (hyperactivity protective, localized hyperactivity, hypoactivity, inflammation (decreased and increased)

Case histories

General points

General and specific neuropathodynamics

As was the case with neurodynamics, neuropathodynamics has been divided into general and specific domains. General neuropathodynamics refers to abnormalities in function of the nervous system that are fundamental and can occur at many sites in the body. Specific neuropathodynamics relates to dysfunctions that occur in specific parts of the body and is influenced by local anatomy and biomechanics. This aspect is presented in the chapters on particular syndromes that take place clinically.

The need for new classifications of neural disorders

Peripheral neuropathies have in the past been classified according to their related pathoanatomical and pathophysiological changes and clinical correlates. The two most notable classifications were proposed by Seddon and Sunderland. The familiar terms neurapraxia, axonotmesis and neurotmesis were presented to illustrate three types of neuropathy (Seddon 1943). In addition, Sunderland (1951) proposed five different subtypes that involved damage to specific parts of the nerve and was an advance on Seddon's classification because it took injury to the axons and neural connective tissues into more detail (reviewed in Sunderland 1991). These classifications are appropriate in patients whose lesion is severe enough to produce gross anatomical and neurological changes. Despite this, patients whose problem fits these categories form only a small number seen by therapists. Many of the remaining neural disorders are of a different *kind* from those classified by current methods. In these cases, usually no obvious pathology or neurological loss exists, but the problem is still caused by mechanical or physiological

> ### Definition
> **Neurogenic pain** – pain that is initiated or caused by a primary lesion, dysfunction, or *transitory perturbation* in the peripheral or central nervous system (Merskey & Bogduk 1994).

dysfunction (neuropathodynamics) that is usually intermittent, dynamic and related to perturbations in *movement and sensitivity* rather than being caused by pathology. The International Association for the Study of Pain has published an expansive classification of painful disorders, including those that arise from the nervous system (Merskey & Bogduk 1994).

Historically, the above definition was influenced by previous research into pain neurophysiology. However, since mechanics of the nervous system influences nervous system physiology, now is the time to include mechanical aspects within this definition.

Expanding the boundaries

The above definition allows for intermittent dysfunction in the nervous system to be a cause of pain without the presence of pathology or loss of nerve conduction. As mentioned, it is now necessary to take this definition into the mechanical domain because of the relationships this parameter has with physiology of the nervous system. Once the prospect of mechanical dysfunction being a potential cause of pain is embraced, more classifications for neural problems are revealed in which the specific elements of mechanical dysfunction can be placed into distinct components, or diagnostic categories. Such a classification must produce diagnostic categories that take into account several key factors.

1. The fact that mechanical dysfunction in the nervous system can cause pain.
2. Neural dysfunctions are intertwined with dysfunction in the tissues around the nervous system (mechanical interface) and the tissues innervated by the nervous system (innervated tissues). For that reason, diagnostic categories must cater for the interactions between the three types of structures; mechanical interface, neural and innervated tissue.
3. The relevant anatomical and neurophysiological aspects must be included in clinical analysis for reasons of safety and for the completion of an approach that integrates neurodynamics with the musculoskeletal system.

The following is a classification, or set of diagnostic categories, of disorders that affect the nervous system. It achieves the goal of linking pathodynamics in the nervous system with treatment. A key feature is that it integrates nervous system function with that of the musculoskeletal system.

The existence of different types of mechanical dysfunction

As mentioned, neuropathodynamic mechanisms can be divided into those that affect the nervous system through three main components; mechanical interface, neural structures and innervated tissues.

In some patients, specific mechanical dysfunctions can present in a manner that distinctly reflects the pathomechanics. For instance, a problem with closing of the mechanical interface around the nervous system will present differently from an opening problem. The problem of impaired neural sliding will manifest itself differently from the one of altered tension behaviour in a nerve.

Different mechanisms interact

In almost every case, interactions will occur between the different elements of pathodynamics. Interface components will interact with the neural components that may then interact with innervated tissue components. To complete the cycle, innervated tissue components may then influence other aspects of pathodynamics. In most patients, a contribution by more than one component mechanism occurs and these are classifiable. The following is a classification of neurodynamic problems that forms the cornerstone of mechanical diagnosis and treatment in this book.

Defining relationships between neuropathodynamics and clinical problems

In defining dysfunction categories that form the basis for diagnosis, words such as normal, abnormal, desirable (optimal) and undesirable (suboptimal) will be used. They relate to the notion of whether the function of a part of the body is adequate, such that symptoms do not occur. In the lucky few, body function is so good (optimal) that even high stresses and strains pose no problem, such as elite athletes and asymptomatic workers in repetitive environments. Everyday normal body function is somewhat different. It is rarely perfect or optimal but has desirable and undesirable features that influence the likelihood of problems developing. Normality generally produces nothing in the way of symptoms until the part

is subjected to sufficient mechanical stress. In those whose body occupies the lower range of normal or possesses an anomaly or subtle pathological process, symptoms may not occur but are more likely to do so in the presence of provocation. This can be classified as undesirable or, in the words of Jenny McConnell, 'suboptimal'. Improving function to a more desirable level (i.e. optimizing function) may be an essential aspect of treating the problem. Effectively we try to place the nervous system in as good an environment as possible to facilitate optimal function. This is as long as the signs, symptoms and patient behaviour form an appropriate match.

The inclusion of the above terms makes diagnosis more complex, but the benefit of such a method is that it encourages the clinician to consider the *relevance* and *role* of pathodynamics in relation to the whole patient problem. This is a deliberate departure from the old concepts of normal and abnormal as being black and white categories that either fulfill or fail our patients. For instance, a problem could exhibit a subtle imperfection of nerve or interface dynamics that might be considered to be within normal limits, but at the lower end of the scale. When related to an athlete, in whom a high level of function is required, this might be particularly relevant and need treatment. Conversely, in the patient who experiences severe and disabling pain dominated by central and behavioural aspects, a small imperfection in function might not be so relevant. The following is an illustration of a suboptimal problem that is not relevant to the patient's current problem.

Clinical case

In November 2001, I had occasion to examine an elite boxer. He was experiencing pain in both his ventromedial forearms during and after training. The most significant trigger was boxing against the heavy punching bag. After training, he noticed that his forearms would be quite swollen and felt pumped full of blood. Tenderness was present along the anteromedial muscles of both forearms. The right median neurodynamic test 1 was distinctly abnormal in being slightly tight and producing a stinging pain in the anterior shoulder region. It was positive to structural differentiation but produced nothing like the pain he had been experiencing. At this point, it became apparent that a previous injury was related to his abnormal test but was *not* related to the current problem. The injury was a labral tear in the right glenohumeral joint (diagnosed with radiological imaging) that had in the past produced this same anterior shoulder pain but was not at this time symptomatic. With palpation, the anterior shoulder region was tender. Pathomechanics, inflammation and scarring around the shoulder could have produced secondary subclinical neuropathodynamics (Levin & Dellon 1992). This is an example of a suboptimal or abnormal problem that was not related to the current forearm pain. Procedures to investigate the basis for the forearm pain may then consist of intramuscular pressure tests and bone scans and others to ascertain if a local problem existed.

On that account, the terms normal, abnormal, optimal and suboptimal are used in the classification of dysfunction related to the nervous system. The final benefit of this aspect is that these terms mark an intentional divergence from classifying neurodynamic tests in terms of 'positive' and 'negative' which so commonly occurs and is entirely inaccurate. Rather than there being a black and white separation between normal and abnormal (alias negative and positive), there is a spectrum of alterations in the nervous system that should be included in the analysis. This is discussed in more detail in Chapter 5.

Optimal/desirable – when the neuromusculoskeletal system behaves exceedingly well and does not produce symptoms in situations of high stress.

Suboptimal – when the neuromusculoskeletal system behaves imperfectly, to the point where the likelihood of symptoms increases but symptoms do not necessarily result until an adequate trigger (or provocation) occurs. Depending on the state of the tissues, it can be relevant, irrelevant, symptomatic or asymptomatic.

Normal – when the function of the neuromusculoskeletal system is within normal values. However,

whether the tissues are subjected to normal or abnormal mechanical stresses will influence the likelihood of symptoms developing.

Abnormal – when the function of the neuromusculoskeletal system is distinctly outside the normal range. This can be caused by pathology or abnormality in mechanics or physiology. However, since neuropathies may not always produce symptoms (Neary et al 1975), the abnormal category can be symptomatic, asymptomatic, relevant or irrelevant.

Relevant – when pathodynamics are causally linked to the clinical problem.

Irrelevant – when pathodynamics are not causally linked to the clinical problem.

The above categories of problem are not mutually exclusive and will interact in many cases.

MECHANICAL INTERFACE DYSFUNCTIONS

Definition
Mechanical interface dysfunctions occur when the forces exerted on the nervous system by the interfacing movement complex are abnormal or undesirable.

Pressure exerted on the nervous system could be intermittent or sustained, depending on the behaviour of the disorder. Dysfunction in the mechanical interface can be divided into different types. Naturally, the clinician must be proficient in mechanical testing and treatment of the musculoskeletal system because they are key parts of dealing with interface problems.

1. Closing dysfunctions

Definition
The closing dysfunction is defined as an alteration in the closing mechanism of the movement complex (joints, muscles or other tissues) around the nervous system, producing abnormal or undesirable forces on the adjacent neural structures.

As with all dysfunctions, suspicion about the existence of a closing dysfunction is raised during the verbal interview and is based on the history, behaviour of symptoms, radiological investigations and manual examination. The closing dysfunction in the mechanical interface is one of the most common forms of pathodynamics.

A. Reduced closing

Definition
The reduced closing dysfunction occurs when the movement complex lacks appropriate movement in the closing direction (Fig. 3.1).

Since closing is a normal aspect of movement complex and nervous system function, it is possible that the nervous system needs to be subjected to regular appropriate elevations in pressure for normal nutrition to occur and to prevent the development of stiffness and hypersensitivity to closing. Hence, if the diagnosis is reduced closing, improvement of the closing mechanism may be a necessary part of treatment, particularly if the problem is mechanical in origin. However, due to the risks attached to increasing pressure on the nervous system, the clinician must be absolutely sure that treatment with a closing technique is likely to be safe, effective and actually necessary. The reduced closing dysfunction is often caused by a protective response due to the presence of pathology. Disc bulges, swollen posterior intervertebral joints, osteophytes tumours and abscesses are pathologies that can cause reduced closing and must always be borne in mind when considering this dysfunction. Frequently in this dysfunction it is actually better to open around the neural structures to reduce pressure on them in the early stages. For more detail on treatment, see Chapter 8 onwards.

B. Excessive closing

Definition
When the interfacing movement complex demonstrates more movement than normal, or is undesirable, in the closing direction (Fig. 3.2).

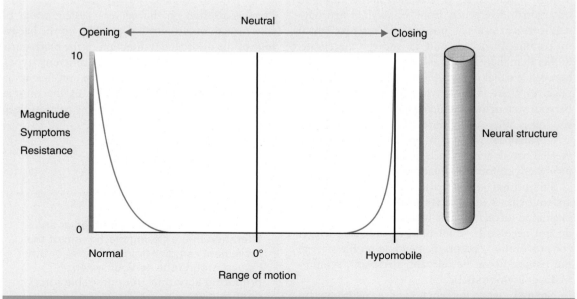

Figure 3.1   Movement diagram of the reduced closing dysfunction.

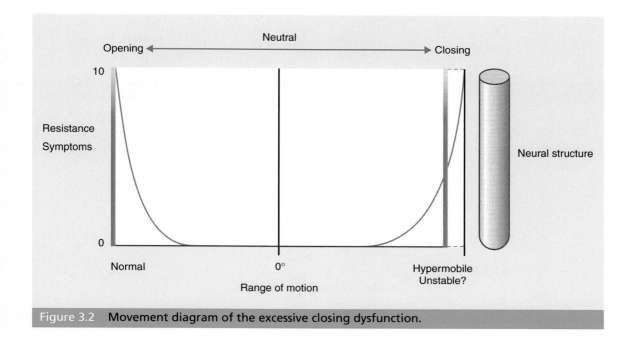

Figure 3.2   Movement diagram of the excessive closing dysfunction.

When excessive closing occurs in a joint, it must in some way be related to hypermobility or instability. This is frequently a result of tissue disruption, altered motor control, inappropriate use or variation in anatomy of the movement complex. If the closing dysfunction resides in a structure other than a joint, for instance, a muscle, then it may need treatment through soft tissue releases or motor control techniques. In any case, the excessive closing dysfunction relates closely to instability and motor control, which must be addressed in order to reduce the closing effects on the nervous system.

2. Opening dysfunctions

Definition
The opening interface dysfunction is defined as an abnormality in the opening mechanism of the movement complex that is located adjacent to the nervous system. As with the closing dysfunction, it also houses two subtypes, reduced opening and excessive opening.

A. Reduced opening

Definition
When the movement complex around the nervous system does not open sufficiently, or in a desirable manner (Fig. 3.3).

In the spine, the opening mechanism around a nerve root may be abnormally reduced due to stiffness in the local motion segment. In this case, the nerve root may never be completely relieved of pressure and may become sensitized and painful due to subtle perturbations in its blood flow. This is different from the closing problem because it is one of *reduced opening* rather than excessive closing. An example of insufficient opening is the C5–6 segment that can laterally flex and rotate normally toward the ipsilateral side but the intervertebral foramen does not open fully with lateral flexion and rotation in the contralateral direction.

In the extremities, the same kind of mechanism can operate. An example of this would be carpal tunnel syndrome in which the tunnel pressures may not be very high, but they could be sufficient to

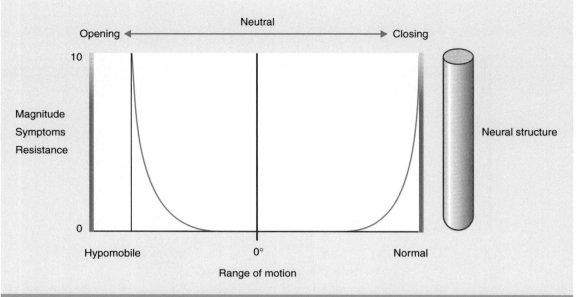

Figure 3.3   Movement diagram of the reduced opening dysfunction.

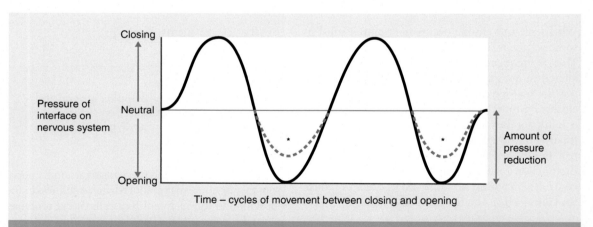

Figure 3.4   Effects of the reduced opening dysfunction on pressure changes around neural structures. The bold line indicates the pressure changes with cyclic movement in the opening and closing directions. The broken line adjacent the asterisks represents the impairment in reduction of pressure with opening and closing movements.

produce mild obstruction of venous return and cause a mild neuropathy that, if sustained, may progress to a more severe problem. Reduced range of horizontal flexion after wrist trauma illustrates this kind of dysfunction (Fig. 3.4).

Key point
The key pathological mechanism in the reduced opening dysfunction is that of impairment of *reduction* in pressure rather

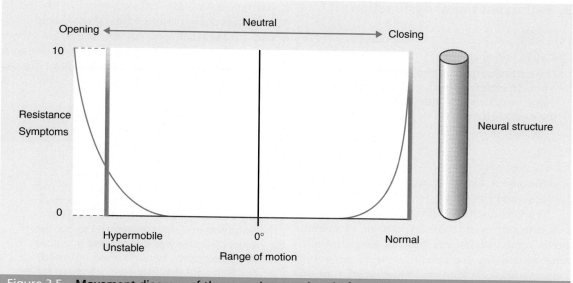

Figure 3.5   Movement diagram of the excessive opening dysfunction.

than elevated peak pressure. This may produce a lack of recovery of the neural structure to normal pressures.

B. Excessive opening

Definition

The excessive opening dysfunction occurs when the opening of the interfacing movement complex around the nervous system is greater than normal, or is undesirable, thereby exerting undesirable forces on the neural ElemEmts (Fig. 3.5).

In the problem of excessive opening, it is possible that the nervous system is stretched excessively by traction on the tissues that pass between the interface and neural tissues. This type of dysfunction relates specifically to the spine where contralateral lateral flexion plays a key role. Forceful lateral flexion of the neck during injury, or repeated lateral flexion during an occupational or athletic movement are such examples. In this dysfunction, the movement of the spinal structures imparts excessive tension on the contralateral nerve roots and plexus. This kind of problem is not uncommon in injuries that involve forceful sideways movement, particularly trauma in contact sport and high velocity vehicle accidents. The excessive opening dysfunction is closely related to instability.

Comments on Instability

Instability is at present a topical subject and has distinct effects on the nervous system. Instability of the ankle has been shown to impart increased mechanical stresses onto the posterior tibial nerve at the tarsal tunnel (Daniels et al 1998). In the spine, such a dysfunction may subject the nerve roots to excessive compression, strain or shear. The cause of neural stresses with instability is likely to be via the neutral zone of the motion segment expanding or altering its position on the opening and closing spectrum and poor control of movement. If this produces a problem in neural tissues, it is probably through mechanical irritation. In terms of treatment, it would be essential to improve the mechanical function of the interface as the main component of treatment. This illustrates the notion that it is not necessary to mobilize all neural problems. Protection of the nervous system should at times be a focus and will necessitate improving motor control.

3. Pathoanatomical dysfunction

Definition

The pathoanatomical dysfunction occurs when an interfacing structure of abnormal shape or size exerts undesirable pressure on the neural elements.

Characteristics

Pathologies in the mechanical interface that can compress and irritate the nervous system consist of, in the spine, disc protrusions, swollen joints, stenosis, osteophytes and tumours, to name a few. In the limbs, some pathologies consist of ganglia, swollen tendons and synovial sheaths, stenosed nerve tunnels, anomalous tendons and muscles, bony protuberances and growths and foreign bodies (reviewed in Shacklock 1996).

In the pathoanatomical dysfunction, movement in the closing direction provokes pain or is lacking. This dysfunction is frequently produced by space occupying lesions in which pain is provoked by closing movements as they exert excessive pressure on the neural structure. Consequently, the body sometimes adopts a position of reduced closing (or even frank opening) in order to protect the local neural and musculoskeletal structures.

Precautionary issues

It is important to acknowledge the pathoanatomical type of disorder because it influences prognostic factors that link to the limitations of physical treatment and safety issues. In patients whose basis for their problem is pathoanatomical, the response to mechanical therapy is usually poorer than the problem that is caused by an intermittent dysfunction that does not include a pathology. This is because of the continuous, progressive and sometimes serious nature of the pathology and the general inability of physical therapies to directly alter pathology. Patients in whom this type of problem is suspected to exist should be promptly referred for medical investigation and management. In such cases, direct neurodynamic techniques that increase forces on the nervous system are often contraindicated. However, given the right conditions and carefully applied, techniques that open the interface, and reduce pressure on the nervous system and reduce tension in the neural structures can be performed and given as home exercises for the relief of symptoms, as long as safety is the primary concern. Exercises for the protection of the nervous system through motor control can also be administered.

Clinical example

Patient presentation

A middle aged man who experienced pain and spasms in his left lumbar and buttock regions, accompanied by neurological symptoms and signs, presented to our sports injury clinic. He was due to have a lumbar microdiscectomy because a sequestrated disc fragment was lodged in his spinal canal near the intervertebral foramen and was compressing his left S1 nerve root, as shown by magnetic resonance imaging. He appeared to have weak plantarflexion and his calf muscles were slightly wasted. The reason he sought treatment was because, even though surgery was planned in the next six weeks, he wanted to at least obtain some relief of his symptoms so that he could walk and sleep with less pain.

Pulling occurred in his left lower back and left leg with lumbar flexion and these symptoms increased with the addition of neck flexion. Lumbar extension was restricted to one quarter of the normal range and evoked back pain. The L4–S1 segments showed severe loss of extension and ipsilateral lateral flexion and these movements reproduced his back and buttock pain. Right lateral flexion revealed little in the way of symptoms, however there was mild localized restriction in the low lumbar segments. This is an example of the pathoanatomical dysfunction linking to the reduced closing dysfunction. Neurological examination revealed weak calf muscles, an absent ankle jerk reflex and loss of vibration sense in his foot. The left straight leg raise test was restricted to approximately 30° and this reproduced his low back and leg pain, whereas the right straight leg raise was normal. Dorsiflexion at the top of the left straight leg raise was positive for the back pain.

Clinical reasoning

This problem represents a pathoanatomical disorder in the mechanical interface that was probably causing pressure ischaemia of the S1 nerve root and loss of conduction, along with mechanosensitivity of the nerve root and pain in its distribution. As mentioned, this resulted in a reduced closing dysfunction. Based on the pathoanatomy, closing manoeuvres would be contraindicated because of the potential to aggravate symptoms and cause further neurological changes. However, opening techniques could be of some benefit, particularly if they were successful in producing temporary reductions in pressure on the nerve root. Opening techniques are certainly not contraindicated and may at least offer the patient a means of giving himself temporary relief so that he could function reasonably well prior to having his surgery.

Treatment and results

Treatment consisted of a trial of static openers (see Chapter 11) in which the patient was shown how to open the left lumbar intervertebral foraminae himself. He was given a position that consisted of lying on the right (contralateral) side with his hips and knees at right angles and his lower legs hanging over the side of the bed. This produced right lateral flexion (opening the ipsilateral intervertebral foraminae) and, since he was lying down with his intervertebral discs in a non-weight bearing position, he could maintain this position for sustained periods. A bolster was placed under his waist so that this further opened the left lumbar intervertebral foraminae. After several successful trials of sustaining this position for one minute, he then adopted this position for several minutes any time he needed to relieve his symptoms or whenever it was convenient. No movements that produced pressure or excessive tension in the neural structures were performed in treatment. At the first consultation, the patient obtained instant relief of his pain and even his neurological signs improved slightly. After several treatments of holding this position whilst the lumbar spine was gently mobilized into right lateral flexion, he had felt such an improvement in pain and spasms that he no longer needed treatment. He rated the improvement between 60% and 80%. His vibration sense improved dramatically to be almost normal but the motor signs remained impaired. He subsequently managed normally in his daily activities until he had his surgery.

Clinical case

The following case illustrates the potential for pathoanatomical and pathophysiological dysfunctions in the interface to affect the neural tissues. A 68 year old woman presented with severe pain and pins and needles in the medial aspect of her right upper arm and these symptoms spread to the thumb, thenar eminence and index finger. She had several days earlier received an investigation of her kidney function in which a catheter had been inserted into her brachial artery, after which considerable bleeding occurred. The development of neural symptoms was based on the pathoanatomy (haematoma) and pathophysiology (bleeding and inflammation) around the median nerve. Clearly, the treatment through a tension technique could be inappropriate and sliders to maintain neural movement through a bleeding nerve bed may be necessary (Fig. 3.6).

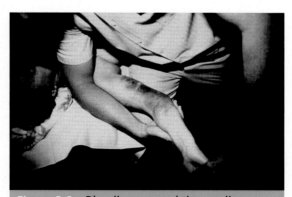

Figure 3.6   Bleeding around the median nerve. Similar cases in which muscle injury (e.g. hamstring strain) could produce similar consequences and will need appropriate treatment (with permission, Mr Paul Ryan, Musculoskeletal Physiotherapist).

4. Pathophysiological dysfunction

Definition

The pathophysiological dysfunction occurs when pathophysiological changes in the mechanical interface produce pathodynamics in the adjacent neural structures.

The reason for including the pathophysiological dysfunction generally is that it connects with pain mechanisms, the understanding of which is essential in the sound application of clinical neurodynamics.

The pathophysiological problem in the mechanical interface is presented as a specific category of problem because, like the pathoanatomical interface disorder, it can also produce adverse consequences in the nervous system. For instance, inflammation in musculoskeletal structures will produce swelling and may exert pressure on the nervous system.

Another mechanism by which pathophysiological changes in the interface can affect neural elements is that caused by protrusion of nucleus pulposus. Within minutes, chemicals located in the epidural region can seep into the nerve roots through small veins that connect the epidural space with the intraneural capillaries in the nerve roots (Byrod et al 1995). When nucleus pulposus is positioned next to the nerve root, without increasing pressure on the root, the physiology of the nerve root can become profoundly disturbed. This is by way of impaired conduction and development of intraneural oedema and Schwann cell swelling (Olmarker et al 1994; Olmarker et al 1996; Byrod et al 1998). This is effectively an inflammatory response triggered by the mere presence of a specific foreign substance and occurs in the *absence* of increased pressure on the neural structure (Olmarker & Rydevik 1998).

Key point

Mere exposure of the nerve root to nucleus pulposus material sensitizes the nerve root.

Clinical comment

The above mechanisms explain the occurrence of patients with neurogenic pain in spite of their radiological report stating '… the observed disc bulge is of doubtful clinical significance because no significant pressure is exerted on the nerve root'.

NEURAL DYSFUNCTIONS

1. Neural sliding dysfunction

Definition

The neural sliding dysfunction occurs when a neural structure demonstrates reduced excursion compared with normal, or is hypersensitive to sliding movements.

Key point

Reduced sliding of nerves produces increased tension and strain in the neural tissues and has been shown to be related to the production of symptoms.

Evidence

In the case of spinal cord and dural tissue being tethered to the spinal canal, the contiguous neural tissue elongates internally more than normal as a means of compensating for the loss of movement (Adams & Logue 1971). Spinal cord tethering is a model for the effects of neuromechanical dysfunction in which impaired sliding of the cord in its canal differentiates patients with and without neurological symptoms. Interestingly, those with malformed connective tissue around the cord and who still have normal cord movement do not report neurological symptoms whereas those whose spinal cord can not move adequately report neurological symptoms (Levy 1999). Hence reduction in movement of the cord correlates more closely with the presence of neurological symptoms than the mere presence of scarring around the cord i.e. pathology.

Even though not yet fully proven (Erel et al 2003), the extremities also sometimes demonstrate the above principles. In cases of carpal tunnel syndrome, longitudinal excursion of the median nerve at the wrist is significantly reduced (Valls-Sollé et al 1995). In relation to the transverse movement of the nerve, normally it is measured at values between 1.5 mm and 3.0 mm (Nakamichi & Tachibana 1992; Erel et al 2003). However, in patients with carpal tunnel syndrome, the transverse sliding can be reduced by between 43% (Erel et al 2003) and 75% (Nakamichi & Tachibana 1995) of its normal amount. Furthermore, this lack of nerve movement has, at surgery, been linked to tethering of the nerve to its interface by connective tissue (Nakamichi & Tachibana 1995). Transverse movement of the median nerve is also reduced in patients with non-specific upper limb pain related to occupational overuse (Greening et al 1999). Paraneural scarring that reduces neural movement occurs in many peripheral nerve problems (Kalb et al 1999) and is linked to friction irritation (Sakurai & Miyasaka 1986; Sunderland 1991; Skalley et al 1994; Petersen et al 1996; Gorgulu et al 1998). Nerve root adhesions are also associated with reduced movement of the nerve roots in cases of chronic radicular pain (Frykholm 1951a, b; Murphy 1977).

On some occasions, it is possible to ascertain whether clinical evidence in support of the neural sliding dysfunction exists.

Clinical case

A case of tarsal tunnel syndrome that I encountered in a female athlete illustrates the above. She experienced burning pain in the region of the plantar fascia. When neurodynamic testing in the following order: dorsiflexion/ eversion, straight leg raise was performed, her pain was reproduced. Flexion of the toes at this point produced an *increase* in her pain. This is a proximal sliding dysfunction either in the form of reduced sliding as the nerve passed through the tarsal tunnel or it was hypersensitive to this movement. Palpation

of the nerve at the distal edge of the tunnel also reproduced her pain which matched the nerve rubbing up against the tunnel's edge when it slid proximally.

Adherence of paraneural scar tissues in the case of neural tethering will also increase tension in the tissues that form the adhesion, making them another potential source of symptoms. Furthermore, a key issue is that restriction of nerve excursion through scarring between the epineurium and its adjacent tissues can occur without axonal damage (Weller 1974). This highlights the value of mechanical tests that produce *sliding* as opposed to tension in the nervous system.

2. Neural tension dysfunction

Definition

Tension dysfunction in the neural tissues occurs when the tension dynamics of the nervous system are abnormal or undesirable, giving rise to abnormal tension in the neural structures, or when they are abnormally sensitive to such events.

Since its inception, the tension dysfunction has gone through quite a pendular effect with early proponents changing their opinion on whether it exists or not, or even whether it is relevant in the clinical context. The big challenges have been the rise of popularity in central pain mechanisms and their potential to produce false positive effects in neurodynamic testing and the confusion about what is a normal and abnormal neurodynamic test. My position is that neural tension dysfunction exists in some people. The problem was that it was in the past diagnosed too frequently and inappropriately.

Tension dysfunction in nerves is related to a number of variables. As mentioned, reduced neural sliding will produce increased tension in the nerves. Also present is the possibility that internal scarring of a nerve may reduce the ability of a nerve to elongate. The following is an example of neural tension dysfunction (Fig. 3.7).

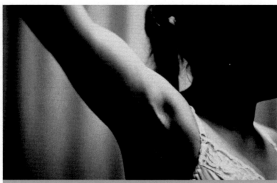

Figure 3.7   Tension dysfunction in the median nerve.

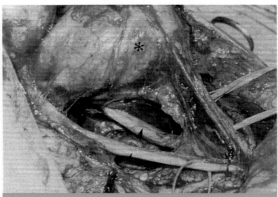

Figure 3.8   A tumour around the brachial plexus as a pathoanatomical cause of neuropathy (Mackinnon & Dellon, 1988 Surgery of the Peripheral Nerve. Thieme, ch.19, p. 544. Reprinted with permission).

Clinical features

The physical findings related to the neural tension dysfunction are simply that the patient's symptoms are provoked by movements that place the relevant neural structure on tension. Clearly, movements that elongate the nerve will therefore be relevant and sometimes it is appropriate and necessary to perform tensioner techniques in the treatment of these problems. Appropriate selection of techniques is discussed in Chapter 6 and the respective chapters on specific clinical syndromes.

3. Neural hypermobility – instability

Definition
Neural instability occurs when the excursion of the neural elements is greater than normal or is desirable.

Clinical note
Nerves can displace in and out of their normal position. The typical example of nerve instability is the clicking ulnar nerve with flexion/extension movements of the elbow. With repetition, ulnar neuritis can result and, if conservative management fails, the nerve can be surgically translocated to the anterior aspect of the elbow. I have also seen cases of clicking median nerve at the elbow.

4. Pathoanatomical dysfunction

Definition
The pathoanatomic neural dysfunction occurs when disturbance of nervous system function is caused by pathology in the nervous system.

Such pathologies can consist of those in the classifications of Seddon and Sunderland, as mentioned previously. In these cases, clear changes in neurological function will be evident. In addition, pathologies within the nervous system itself, such as meningiomas, Schwannomata, arachnoiditis producing meningeal scarring, spinal dysraphism and anomalies (even two nerve roots can pass through one foramen, leaving the adjacent foramen vacant) can occur. This would render the nerve root complex disadvantaged or in a suboptimal state. Since therapists do not perform diagnostic imaging techniques for these problems and symptoms and physical examination are not diagnostic for pathologies, there is potential for the therapist to overlook the possibility of a serious pathoanatomical cause of symptoms (Fig. 3.8).

5. Pathophysiological dysfunction

Definition

The neuropathophysiological dysfunction occurs when an aspect of the physiology of the nervous system is abnormal.

Intraneural blood flow – elevated pressure and the tourniquet effect

The effect of pressure on the flow of blood through the nervous system is quite graded. At tissue pressures as low as 30–50 mmHg (Gelberman et al 1983), pressure on the neural structure rises and the flow of blood through the veins that remove fluid from the nerve is reduced (discussed in Sunderland 1976). Venous fluid stagnates, causing the pressure in the nerve to rise further and oedema to form around the axons. Since fluid can not leave the nerve and arterial blood can still enter, swelling develops further and the provision of oxygenated blood to the nerve becomes impossible. This is similar to gently applying a tourniquet around the arm. Because arterial pressure is higher than venous pressure, blood can enter the limb but it can not leave. The veins in the limb bulge and, if the tourniquet is held for long enough, blood flow through the limb will reduce and the limb will turn blue and become hypoxic (Fig. 3.9).

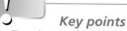

Key points

Two important variables in pressure are magnitude and time. The higher the pressure or the longer its duration, the longer the nerve takes to recover.

Causes of elevated pressure on neural structures consist of constricted tunnels, spinal canal and intervertebral foraminae; swelling of structures adjacent to the nerves e.g. tendons and excessive contraction of muscles that approximate the peripheral nerves (Werner et al 1980, 1985a, 1985b). Pressures exerted on nerves in patients with peripheral neuropathies can range from 30 mmHg to 240 mmHg (Gelberman et al 1981; Werner et al 1985a). The latter pressure is well above normal venous pressure and sometimes higher than arterial pressure.

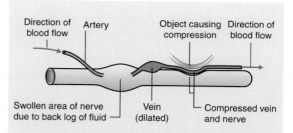

Figure 3.9 Tourniquet effect in which the blood flow out of the nerve is reduced due to pressure on the vein. Internally, a pressure back log builds up and the nerve becomes swollen and oedematous.

Mechanical irritation

As discussed in Chapter 1, the connective tissues of the nervous system are innervated by C nociceptors. In addition to having afferent functions, they also act in an efferent direction and influence inflammation in the tissues that they innervate. One of the tissues innervated by these nociceptors happens to be the connective tissues of the neural structure itself, in which the nociceptive axons pass. The nociceptive axons that pass in the nerve provide branches that terminate in the epineurium or dura and are sensitive to mechanical events. When the nerve's nociceptors are stimulated by potentially harmful forces, such as excessive friction or repeated compression, they initiate an inflammatory response in the nerve by releasing calcitonin gene-related peptide and substance P which are intensely vasoactive and give rise to local inflammation. This illustrates the notion that, like musculoskeletal structures that contain connective tissue and are innervated by C nociceptors, so too can nerves become inflamed through mechanical irritation (Zochodne & Ho 1991).

The inflammatory response being produced by activation of the nociceptors in the peripheral nerve presents a couple of points that are important for the clinician. The more intense the stimulation, the greater is the endoneurial blood flow. Endoneurial flow can increase by as much as 43% above resting levels during stimulation of the nerve's nociceptors. Also, the blood flow increases with the duration of stimulation. One minute of stimulation produces a 10% increase in endoneurial blood flow and stimulation for 15 minutes results in a 50% increase (Zochodne & Ho 1991).

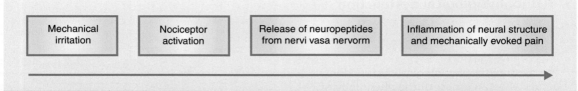

Figure 3.10   The process by which mechanical irritation causes inflammation and pain from neural structures. This is effectively neurogenic inflammation in nerve tissue.

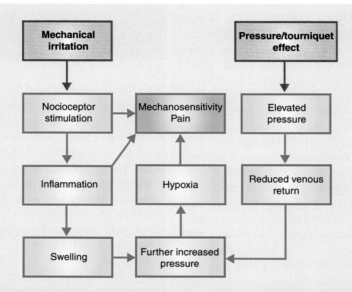

Figure 3.11   Interactions between the pressure (tourniquet) effect in neural tissues and mechanical irritation. Inflammation may paradoxically lead to ischaemia and hypoxic changes in neural tissue through the production of swelling and excess pressure.

Mechanical irritation produces inflammation of nerves (Sunderland 1991) and has many parallels with the compression type of neuropathy. The inflammation that ensues is associated with endoneurial oedema. The formation of oedema in the neural structure is common to both inflammatory and compressive neuropathies because, just as the compressive problem produces intraneural oedema by obstruction of venous return, so does mechanical irritation through the production of inflammation. In the words of the late Emeritus Professor Sir Sydney Sunderland, 'fibroblasts love oedema'. Endoneurial oedema then provides an ideal environment for fibroblasts to proliferate and produce scarring, which can then produce loss of neural excursion and pain with movement. Friction and pressure with repetitive

daily movements initiate inflammation in the connective tissues of the nerve, as would be the case with connective tissue in any other type of structure. Inflammatory scarring due to mechanical irritation occurs in both peripheral nerve (Laban et al 1989) and nerve roots (Frykholm 1951a, 1951b; Murphy 1977) (Figs 3.10 and 3.11).

Mechanosensitivity
Overview
Mechanosensitivity is the chief mechanism by which the nervous system becomes a source of pain with movements and postures. This is because it allows the production of afferent impulses from the neural structure for processing in the central nervous system.

Definition

Mechanosensitivity is the ease with which the neural tissues become active when mechanical force is applied to them. The more mechanosensitive the nerve is, the less force is needed to elicit activity and the more intense is the response. Two types of responses occur, impulse based ones and chemical ones.

Normal versus abnormal mechanosensitivity

Two divergent positions on the subject of mechanosensitivity have been adopted in the literature. The first is that nerves are never mechanosensitive and therefore could not be a source of pain. This is clearly incorrect and deserves no further attention. The second is that normal nerves are not mechanosensitive and damaged or inflamed ones are. Neither does this statement fully bear out the research and, instead, subtleties in the phenomenon should be borne in mind. High intensity force evokes much activity in undamaged axons and this is more significant in injured nerves (Gray & Richie 1954; Lindquist et al 1973; Howe et al 1976, 1977; Burchiel 1984). It is a matter of taking into account several variables simultaneously in each case. These variables consist of the magnitude of the mechanical trigger and the state of the neural tissue. In the studies that directly investigate mechanosensitivity in which strong stretch or compression are applied to neural tissue, the axons respond intensely with many impulses in quick succession (Howe et al 1977). This applies to sensory, motor, autonomic and spinal cord axons (Lindquist et al 1973; Nordin et al 1984). Nerve cells are in fact mechanical transducers and *normally* become active in response to high intensity mechanical stimuli (Rosenblueth et al 1953; Julian & Goldman 1962). One can test this by performing a neurodynamic test strongly, or tapping a nerve vigorously, both of which can produce pins and needles in normal subjects. In the abnormal situation, in which the neural tissues are sensitized by injury or inflammation, impulses can be more readily activated with the application of only gentle mechanical forces that are likely to occur during normal daily movement (Howe et al 1977; Calvin et al 1982).

One exception to the above is the dorsal root ganglion because it normally produces impulses spontaneously and in response to mechanical events such as the straight leg raise. However, it too becomes more mechanosensitive in response to injury (Howe et al 1977; Wall & Devor 1983). In pathological states, increased mechanosensitivity occurs in peripheral nerves (Nordin et al 1984), nerve roots (Howe et al 1977), the dorsal root ganglion (Wall & Devor 1983) and the spinal cord (Smith & McDonald 1980). In the inflamed state, nerves can even become active as pressure is removed from them (Howe et al 1977). This could be interpreted as dynamic hyperalgesia or allodynia and may manifest itself in the patient on whom applying and releasing tension from sensitized neural structures produces pain. Also, in nerve injured animals, cross-talk between nerve cells in the dorsal root ganglion increases considerably, possibly giving rise to abnormal and confused afferent input to the central nervous system which may be part of the dysaesthesiae seen in patients with neural disorders (Devor & Wall 1990). Mechanosensitivity may well be influenced by axonal transport (Devor & Govrin-Lippmann 1983), possibly through altered delivery of abnormal amounts of receptors to specific locations along the axon.

Chemical mechanosensitivity

Another element of mechanosensitivity that is usually not taken into account is that of chemical and cytoskeletal sensitivity. Probably in response to mechanical compression and tension, cytoskeletal elements such as neurofilaments accumulate at the nodes of Ranvier where the Schwann cells that make up the myelin sheath leave the axon exposed to mechanical forces. This is thought to be an adaptive mechanism to accommodate to, and protect the nerve cell from, mechanical stresses (Price et al 1993). For this to occur, mechanosensitivity must be a built-in natural mechanism that responds to all manner of normal forces, even though these effects may not be perceptible. This type of slow response to mechanical stimulation is likely to extend to the connective tissue of the nervous system in the form of increased connective tissue attachments between the neural elements and their interfacing tissues with age (Goddard & Reid 1965). The final element of mechanosensitivity ought to include the phenomenon of thixotropy. This is when the axoplasm in the nerve becomes thinner and flows more easily with movement (Baker et al 1977) and relates to viscoelastic function of nerve cells. It is possible that nerves that do not move become less pliable and may need appropriate movement, including compression and tension for maintenance of good health.

Hence, an element of mechanosensitivity is the slow adaptive response to natural movement and is worth bearing in mind in patients in need of long term rehabilitation.

Clinical correlates of mechanosensitivity

The clinical correlates of heightened mechanosensitivity are the production of symptoms, such as pain and paraesthesiae, with mechanical stresses in the nerves induced by normal body movements. Mechanosensitivity as a direct response to mechanical loading of the neural structures has been correlated with the production of symptoms at the exact time at which mechanical force was applied. This has been achieved in two ways. The first was by direct mechanical stimulation of the neural tissues in patients whose nerve roots were observed at surgery to be inflamed and scarred due to disc protrusion. Gently moving a thin nylon thread that was placed around the nerve root reproduced patients' sciatic pains (Smythe & Wright 1958). The second was, whilst under mechanical tension, measurement of electrical activity in the axons of the neural structure from which the symptoms arose, was achieved using needle microelectrodes placed in the nerve. The impulse traffic in the neural structure increased at the same time as mechanical stress was applied and the patients' reported symptoms. These events occurred with the ulnar nerve, cervical and lumbar nerve roots and spinal cord (Nordin et al 1984).

On that account, mechanosensitivity in relation to the production of symptoms and clinical analysis should now be considered with the following points in mind.

> **Key points**
> 1. Normal nerves subjected to normal forces are less likely to produce symptoms.
> 2. Normal nerves under abnormal mechanical forces are more likely to produce symptoms.

> 3. Sensitized nerves subjected to normal forces may produce symptoms.
> 4. Sensitized nerves that are subjected to abnormal forces are likely to produce symptoms.
> 5. Consequently, an aspect of assessing for the presence of a symptomatic neural structure in patients is to understand whether the mechanical stresses to which the patient's nervous system is subjected are normal or ideal (optimal) or not and ascertain if any sensitization is likely to have occurred. Consistent with the concept of neurodynamics, the clinician must now view mechanosensitivity as part of a continuum of interactions between the state of the neural structure and the related mechanical events.

Metabolic disorders

Although only briefly mentioned, metabolic and endocrine diseases are an important aspect of the neural disorder. Many diseases influence nutrition and mechanical function of peripheral nerves. Diabetes is a particularly common one in which the peripheral nerve in a diabetic person is more susceptible than normal to compression (Dellon et al 1988). Others to be aware of are alchohol toxicity, HIV/aids (Fuller et al 1991), thyroid disease and many more.

INNERVATED TISSUE DYSFUNCTIONS

Starting summary

1. The abnormal nervous system can cause dysfunction in the innervated tissues via its outward actions.
2. Changes in the innervated tissues produced by the abnormal nervous system include hyperactivity and hypoactivity of muscles, trigger point-like tenderness and alterations in inflammation in the musculoskeletal structures.
3. Since nervous system dysfunction can express itself in the body, the innervated tissues can be used as a looking glass for understanding nervous system dysfunction and may require direct treatment in the presence of neuropathodynamics.

1. Motor control dysfunctions

Importance of motor control

Motor control dysfunction is very important in relation to the nervous system because, if the musculoskeletal system does not move optimally, forces exerted on the nervous system by the mechanical interface will become disadvantageous. Much is known about neurodynamics and it is possible to link this dimension to aspects of motor control in the improvement of forces on the nervous system.

Relationships of motor control to neurodynamics

Muscles form a key interface to the nervous system, but they are also an innervated tissue. Hence, when considering its interactions with the nervous system, the muscular system can be classified in two ways.

If a muscle malfunctions, the forces exerted on the adjacent neural structures may become abnormal. The thoracic outlet where the scalene and pectoralis minor muscles relate to the brachial plexus is a good example of this. Here, the muscles are an *interface* to the nervous system. However, it would be different in the case of an S1 nerve root problem causing alterations in function in the calf muscle. In this case, the muscle is an *innervated tissue* and it will be necessary to adapt treatment accordingly. Hence the following statement applies.

> **Key point**
>
> In classifying a motor control problem that relates to neurodynamics, it is essential to establish whether the muscles in question are an interface or innervated tissue and how their function relates to the nervous system.

The next step is to classify the kind of motor control dysfunction. The categories of dysfunction are as follows. Clearly, the dysfunctions are not mutually exclusive and considerable overlap between dysfunctions will exist. Some will be simple and others more complex, involving many spatially remote muscle groups.

A. Protective muscle hyperactivity dysfunction

> **Definition**
>
> The protective muscle hyperactivity dysfunction occurs when abnormally increased muscle contraction occurs in a pattern that protects a neural structure.

Overview

Contraction of certain muscles, for instance upper trapezius, during the median neurodynamic test 1, is quite normal (Balster & Jull 1997; Coppeiters et al 1999, 2003; van der Heide et al 2001). However, hyperactivity of muscles in the presence of neuropathic problems has been demonstrated (Hall et al 1995, 1998; Coppeiters et al 2003) and in my opinion is very common. This activity probably occurs as a series of central reflexes in order to protect the related neural structure from potentially harmful physical forces. To illustrate, hyperactive contraction of the trapezius muscle during the median neurodynamic test 1 would prevent excessive depression of the scapula and over-straining the brachial plexus and cervical nerve roots. Hence, this motor action is a protective one.

In the presence of neural problems, the muscles that protect a neural structure can contract earlier and more strongly than normally. For instance, the S1 nerve root problem could trigger a protective response in the hamstrings or calf muscles because stretching these muscles also stretches the nerve root. However, a tight quadriceps muscle would not constitute a protective dysfunction because, due to its lack of mechanical association with the S1 nerve root, it does not provide a guarding effect.

> **Key point**
>
> The essential feature of the protective motor control dysfunction is that the hyperactive muscles contract in a pattern that protects a specific neural structure.

Clinical example – treatment after carpal tunnel release

History

A middle-aged woman attended our sports injury clinic for treatment following a recent surgical release of her carpal tunnel for carpal tunnel syndrome. As far as she was concerned, her main problem was constant burning pain in her first three digits and wrist and loss of movement of her hand. Prior to the surgery, she had experienced only pins and needles that worsened with use of her hand and at night when she slept. The symptoms were continuous and severe much of the time and were provoked by use of her hand. Among other findings, the leading physical finding was spasm of her wrist and finger flexor muscles with extension movements of the hand and fingers. The muscular changes varied. At times of greatest severity, they took the form of a sudden rigidity that prevented any extension of the wrist or fingers past the point of onset of pain. When the symptoms were milder, more movement could be performed.

Analysis and treatment

This particular problem was a hyperactivity protective dysfunction. The dysfunction was most likely related to motor control changes in relation to pain and was dealt with as such. Treatment consisted of motor control education with the use of electromyographic (EMG) biofeedback in which the sensor pad was placed on the flexors in the forearm. To this point, the patient thought that the loss of movement was purely due to the tissues being too tight and stretching them would cause further damage. She never realized that hyperactive muscles contributed to the problem. Furthermore, she avoided movement because it hurt and she was frightened by it, showing signs of fear-avoidance and kinesiophobia. Interestingly, she paid great attention to her hand by looking at it very closely as she moved it. Muscle contraction occurred when she anticipated that pain was about to occur, producing a bracing action immediately prior to movement. Effectively, the patient was protecting her median nerve excessively and this kinesiophobia was expressed in terms of changes in motor control and reduced neural mobility and related to hypersensitivity of the nerve.

So that the patient would focus on motor control as the primary event and avoid paying undue attention to the pain, the EMG monitor was placed in such a position that she was unable to see her hand whilst it moved. She was then asked to keep the reading on the machine as low as possible (without being aware of the therapeutic techniques, namely passive wrist and finger extension movements). Fortunately, the patient was particularly successful at this task and after several repetitions, a vastly improved range of motion was achieved without evoking pain. When the wrist and fingers were toward end range of extension, and the reading on the EMG machine was at a low value, the patient was then instructed to look at her hand because, to this point, she had not been watching. She was surprised to see that it had moved almost fully without hurting. Treatment then proceeded along the lines of explaining that movement is not necessarily painful and it depended on how she could control it. She was also told that, nerve movement was a powerful way of stimulating healing in the nerve because nerves contain connective tissue that needs moulding with movement and this moulding influences the outcome. She could then control her motor response and thus mobilize the nerve more effectively than before. Less pressure would be subsequently exerted on the median nerve because the tendons (mechanical interface) were more relaxed. Also, the nerve could most likely move transversely more easily, thus taking a shorter longitudinal course during movement and encountering less tension. It was then possible to apply other neurodynamic exercises as part of her rehabilitation. After six weeks of regular treatment she returned to her normal job as a room cleaner at a local international hotel.

B. Muscle imbalance dysfunction

Types of muscle imbalance that have been described by clinicians and researchers are numerous, to the point where the problem seems to be ubiquitous in the physical therapies. This is not a criticism, but it does illustrate the difficulty in classifying motor control dysfunctions and this is compounded further when they are integrated with the nervous system. The central nervous system undoubtedly plays a key role in the generation of such dysfunctions and this is where the clinician must classify the motor problem and establish its relationship to neurodynamics. For instance, a tight pectoralis minor muscle with a hypoactive lower trapezius that causes the scapula to exert excessive force on the brachial plexus at the thoracic outlet is a good example of an interface problem caused by muscle dysfunction. Treatment of scapular movement dysfunction for this problem is naturally important. Depending on assessment findings, it may also be useful to make sure that the brachial plexus can slide and cope with tension in the presence of improving muscle function.

It is beyond the scope of this book to discuss altered motor control in detail and the reader is referred to other well known sources such as Sahrmann, Janda, McConnell, Hodges and Comerford for more information.

C. Localized muscle hyperactivity dysfunction (Alias–Trigger Point)

> **Definition**
> The localized hyperactivity dysfunction occurs when activity in a muscle is increased compared with normal due to increased efferent actions of the nervous system.

Mechanisms

Injured mechanosensitive peripheral nerves produce efferent impulses that pass to the muscles supplied by the damaged nerve. The passing distally of impulses in motor fibres with mechanical stimulation of the nerve distinguishes the nerve as being pathological because this event does not occur in normal nerves. The production of muscle contraction in response to tapping a sensitized nerve at the site of injury is the motor equivalent of Tinel's sign and can be used in assessment of neural disorders (Kingery et al 1995).

During daily movements, mechanical stimulation of sensitized neural structures may activate impulses that pass to the innervated muscles to produce muscle hyperactivity. This can be quite localized to a part of a muscle and may produce trigger point-like changes that are quite palpable. Sometimes a thorough examination of the muscles that relate to a particular neural structure should be performed as part of establishing what kind of neural dysfunction is present. This would involve specific muscle testing and palpation for local thickness, tenderness and trigger points.

A typical example of the above neuropathodynamics is that of the S1 radiculopathy. After several treatments, the back pain and thigh symptoms improve and the patient reports being left with a localized patch of pain in the posterolateral aspect of their calf. On palpation, this is often exquisitely tender and hardened due to local muscle tissue contraction. In the past, this might have been interpreted as peripheralization of pain but in fact it is not. This may be an efferent mechanism that needs treatment designed to relieve the muscle dysfunction through local techniques. Such techniques could consist of massage, trigger point therapy, acupuncture and muscle stretches, to name a few, but also specific neurodynamic techniques.

D. Muscle hypoactivity dysfunction

> **Definition**
> The muscle hypoactivity dysfunction occurs when the activity in muscle is reduced compared with normal due to decreased efferent actions of the nervous system. This is not paralysis. Instead, it is probably due to altered central drive of muscle function. This pattern can produce reduced protection of the neural structures. For instance, the upper trapezius muscle that is hypoactive in the presence of a thoracic outlet syndrome may cause reduced protection of the brachial plexus and cervical nerve roots by permitting excessive scapular depression during daily activities.

E. Paralysis

In cases of neuropathy characterized by severe loss of conduction, muscle weakness and wasting is common. The relevant muscles will therefore be hypoactive and this should be detectable with muscle testing, neurological examination and observation of muscle bulk.

2. Inflammation dysfunction

It is well known that efferent actions are produced by the autonomic and motor elements of the nervous system. Although more recently, the sensory part of the peripheral nervous system in the production of such effects has been taken more seriously.

Neurogenic inflammation
Release of inflammatory substances

As discussed earlier in Chapter 1, calcitonin gene-related peptide (CGRP) and substance P are produced by C nociceptive nerve fibres at their cell bodies in the dorsal root ganglion, after which these substances are transported along their axons in the peripheral nerve to their distal terminals. C fibres release these substances tonically from their terminals as they control vasodilation and inflammation (Sann et al 1988) and, on stimulation, larger amounts are released into the tissues (Kenins 1981; White & Helme 1985). Inflammation in the innervated tissues results from increased release of these substances which can result in fierce vasodilation, leakage of plasma from blood vessels into the tissues, degranulation of mast cells and increased motility of white cells in the area (Lembeck & Holzer 1979; Dimitriadou et al 1991; O'Halloran & Bloom 1991). The appearance of red blood cells in the joint from stimulation of the relevant nerve (Ferrell & Russell 1986) is an illustration of the power of this phenomenon. Long term potentiation of fibroblasts and priming of white cells can also result from stimulation of C fibres (Kimball & Fisher 1988; Perianin et al 1989). All this provides a mechanism for neural disorders to produce inflammation in musculoskeletal tissues (even synovial joints, Levine et al 1984) and to make these tissues mechanically hypersensitive in response to a current or prior neural disorder. The musculoskeletal tissues could also become more likely to develop inflammation due to a mild insult when a neural disorder has predated the insult (Fig. 3.12).

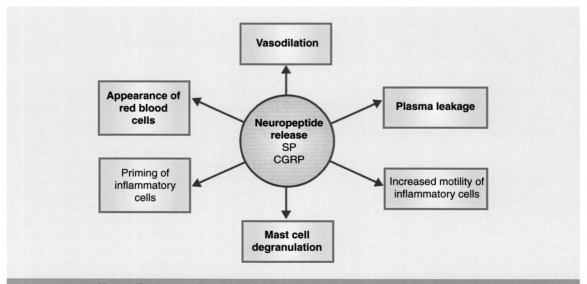

Figure 3.12 Effects of release of neuropeptides by antidromic stimulation of peripheral nerves and nerve roots, resulting in inflammation in the innervated tissues.

Stimulation of inflammation from neural structures

Mechanical or electrical stimulation of a damaged neural structure can be the trigger for inflammation (Bayliss 1901; Langley 1923). In the presence of neuropathy, dorsal nerve root stimulation produces dermatomal inflammation (Pintér & Szolcsàni 1988) and activation of the peripheral nerve produces inflammation in the field of the nerve (Chahl & Ladd 1976). Antidromic impulses arise from the dorsal root ganglion and peripheral nerve in cases of neuropathy (Wall & Devor 1983) and could be involved in the production of symptoms in the extremities in such circumstances (Xavier et al 1990). At times, the mechanosensitive neural structure will produce inflammation in the innervated tissues by depolarizing and releasing CGRP and substance P when movement in the neural structure occurs.

Clinical research

> **Key points**
> 1. Patients with entrapment neuropathies have been shown to exhibit impairment in function of C fibres that regulate inflammation (Cline et al 1989; Goadsby & Burke 1994; Lax & Zochodne 1995).
> 2. The cause of the inflammatory dysfunction in the innervated tissues has been localized to C fibres (Cline et al 1989; Goadsby & Burke 1994; Lax & Zochodne 1995).
> 3. The vascular and inflammatory changes in the innervated tissues can reflect directly the state of the neuropathy (Lax & Zochodne 1995).

Implications and subcategories

Neurogenic inflammation has two particularly important clinical implications. It means that attention must at times be directed at inflammatory mechanisms in the innervated tissue as an aspect of treating the neural problem. Also treatment of a nerve or nerve root problem may form an integral part of treating an inflammatory problem in a musculoskeletal structure.

A. Increased inflammation

> **Definition**
> The increased inflammation dysfunction occurs when the inflammatory mechanisms in the innervated tissues are increased due to increased efferent activity in the nervous system.

> **Clinical case – heel pain**
> A case that illustrates the effect of neural dysfunction on inflammation of innervated tissues is that of heel pain. A middle-aged man sought treatment of pain in the under surface of his heel. It had developed gradually over the last three months and was continuing to worsen, being provoked by the heel strike component of walking. He had inserted padding in the sole of his shoe to reduce the impact of walking but this produced no change in his symptoms. Interestingly, non-steroidal anti-inflammatory drugs did not help his pain. He had in the past experienced low back pain that spread into the ipsilateral buttock but he was not currently experiencing any difficulties with this, other than occasional aches with activities that involved sustained flexion. He was also not currently experiencing any symptoms suggestive of a neural problem, such as pins and needles, loss of sensation or weakness.
>
> The man's heel pain could be reproduced by pressing his heel on the ground and palpation of a small tender spot under his heel. Further examination revealed several clues to neural involvement. The straight leg raise and slump tests with dorsiflexion were significantly tight compared to the contralateral tests and, in the slump test, knee extension and dorsiflexion ranges of motion and manually detected resistance to movement improved with releasing neck flexion. Interestingly, passive stretch of the calf muscles in isolation was normal, but the muscles tightened excessively when the straight leg raise and slump tests were

added to testing. This clearly represented an abnormal nervous system in which there were a number of concerns – protective hyperactivity dysfunction and possibly neurogenic inflammation. In considering the role of the innervated tissues, palpation of the patient's gastrocnemius muscle was performed and this revealed some findings that turned out to be crucial. The lateral head of the muscle was hard and tender compared with the contralateral one and application of firm manual pressure evoked local pain that spread down the leg and in fact reproduced his heel pain. This was a trigger point problem created by a quiescent, but sustained, neural disorder.

Treatment initially consisted of trigger point therapy and deep massage to his calf region (working out the hardened and tender spots), ultrasound and interferential therapy. At the beginning, it was explained that the problem most likely arose from the lumbar neural problem and that it would probably need treatment in order to produce a satisfactory outcome. However, it was justifiable to treat the calf problem at first, as long as an improvement occurred. After seven treatments, he described his symptoms as having reduced by 80% and the calf muscle was much softer and less tender. Walking produced only slight discomfort in the patient's heel and, on gait analysis, he bore weight more normally than before. The tenderness and hardness of the muscle had reduced and it was becoming more difficult to reproduce the heel pain with manual pressure. Nevertheless, progress in the previous two treatments had stopped. Treatment was then directed simultaneously at the neural and muscular components by performing hold/relax stretch techniques to the calf muscles in the position of straight leg raise. Over the next four treatments, the straight leg raise and slump tests with dorsiflexion improved considerably and the calf muscle was much softer and only slightly tender. The heel pain could no longer be reproduced without excessive pressure being applied to the trigger point and the patient could walk normally without pain and did not need the padding in his shoe. He was discharged with the advice that he had an

inherent back problem that might need maintenance therapy with his own home exercises (the stretching and neurodynamic techniques performed in the clinic). He was free to return for more treatment if he could not control the problem himself.

The above was a case of distal innervated tissue dysfunction and pain produced by the efferent actions of the nervous system. Such involvement of nociceptive fibres is supported by the fact that anaesthetizing a distal area in a limb can abolish pain that follows radiculopathy in humans (Xavier et al 1990). This inflammation dysfunction can occur in disorders such as specific plantar fasciitis and heel pain and can respond well to clinical neurodynamics (Shacklock 1995).

B. Reduced inflammation

Definition
The reduced inflammation dysfunction occurs when the inflammatory mechanisms in the innervated tissues are decreased due to decreased efferent activity in the nervous system.

The dysfunction of reduced inflammation is in exact contrast to the previous one. In the profoundly damaged nerve, characterized by denervation and hypoactivity, the inflammatory response is impaired, showing a distinct lack of rubor and a poorer healing response than normal (Lewis 1927). In fact, neurological deficits have been correlated in patients with a reduced inflammatory response (Courtright & Kuzell 1965) (Fig. 3.13).

Based on the above, in addition to the usual manual testing of the musculoskeletal innervated tissues, physical examination may also include analysis of the inflammatory response. Observation of the colour, temperature, sweating and nutrition are part of this. However, in extending evaluation to the *dynamics* of blood flow in relation to neuropathy, other clinical tests can be performed. Stimulation of innervated tissues, such as mechanical stimulation (Lynn & Cotsell 1992) in the form of scratching the skin 5–10 times

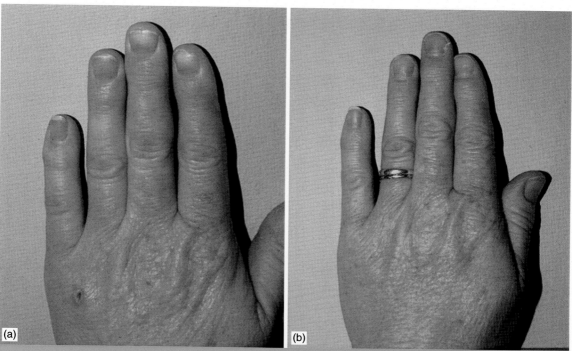

Figure 3.13   Reduced healing and nutrition of the tissues in the hand related to carpal tunnel syndrome. (a) There is pallor in the nail beds of the second and third digits, suggesting reduced perfusion in these regions. The nails of the index and middle fingers are chipped. An ulcer is located in the ulnar aspect of the hand. (b) Good healing after treatment. The colour in the hand and nail beds has improved, the nails have healed and the ulcer has disappeared.

with something mildly noxious such as the back of a fingernail, can be a part of advanced innervated tissue examination. Normally, vasodilation occurs within seconds and is usually symmetrical. However, in cases of altered inflammation due to neuropathy, the reaction time, degree, or extent of redness can be asymmetrical and these changes can be localized to the innervation zone of the peripheral nerve or nerve root. Vasodilatory responses can exhibit variations as the scratching movement is passed across adjacent normal and abnormal dermatomes or peripheral nerve fields.

Role of the sympathetic nervous system

In addition to the C fibres mediating inflammation in the innervated tissues, so do sympathetic axons in peripheral nerves. This is by way of releasing prostaglandins and substances such as noradrenaline from the sympathetic terminals (Levine et al 1986; Coderre et al 1989). Inflammation in the innervated tissues is balanced by sympathetic and C fibre systems. Alterations in function of the sympathetic axons can occur with excessive pressure on peripheral nerves (Lindquist et al 1973) and may affect inflammation.

References

Adams C, Logue V 1971 Studies in cervical spondylotic myelopathy: 1 Movement of the cervical roots, dura and cord, and their relation to the course of the extrathecal roots. Brain 94: 557–568

Baker P, Ladds M, Rubinson K 1977 Measurement of the flow properties of isolated axoplasm in a defined chemical environment. Journal of Physiology 269: 10–11P

Balster S, Jull G 1997 Upper trapezius muscle activity during the brachial plexus tension test in asymptomatic subjects. Manual Therapy 2(3): 144–149

Bayliss W 1901 On the origin from the spinal cord of the vaso-dilator fibres of the hind-limb, and on the nature of these fibres. Journal of Physiology 26(3):173–209

Burchiel K 1984 Effects of electrical and mechanical stimulation on two foci of spontaneous activity which develop in primary afferent neurons after peripheral axotomy. Pain 18: 249–265

Byrod G, Olmarker K, Konno S, Larsson K, Takahashi K, Rydevik B 1995 A rapid transport route between the epidural space and the intraneural capillaries of the nerve roots. Spine 20(2): 138–143

Byrod G, Rydevik B, Nordborg C, Olmarker K 1998 Early effects of nucleus pulposus application on spinal nerve root morphology and function. European Spine Journal 7(6): 445–449

Calvin W, Devor M, Howe J 1982 Can neuralgias arise from minor demyelination? Spontaneous firing, mechanosensitivity, and after discharge from conducting axons. Experimental Neurology 75: 755–763

Chahl L, Ladd R 1976 Local oedema and general excitation of cutaneous sensory receptors produced by electrical stimulation of the saphenous nerve in the rat. Pain 2: 25–34

Cline M, Ochoa J, Torebjork H 1989 Chronic hyperalgesia and skin warming caused by sensitized C nociceptors. Brain 112(3): 621–647

Coderre T, Basbaum A, Levine J 1989 Neural control of vascular permeability: interactions between primary afferents, mast cells, and sympathetic efferents. Neurophysiology 62(1): 48–58

Coppetiers M, Stappaerts K, Staes F 1999 A qualitative assessment of shoulder girdle elevation during the upper limb tension test 1. Manual Therapy 4: 33–38

Coppieters M, Stappaerts K, Wouters L, Janssens K 2003 Aberrant protective force generation during neural provocation testing and the effect of treatment in patients with neurogenic cervicobrachial pain. Journal of Manipulative and Physiological Therapeutics 26(2): 99–106

Courtright L, Kuzell W 1965 Sparing effect of neurological deficit and trauma on the course of adjuvant arthritis in the rat. Annals of Rheumatic Diseases 24: 360–367

Daniels T, Lau J, Hearn T 1998 The effects of foot position and load on tibial nerve tension. Foot and Ankle International 19(2): 73–78

Dellon A, Mackinnon S, Seiler W 1988 Susceptibility of the diabetic nerve to chronic compression. Annals of Plastic Surgery 20(2): 117–119

Devor M, Govrin-Lippmann R 1983 Axoplasmic transport block reduces ectopic impulse generation in injured peripheral nerves. Pain 16: 73–85

Devor M, Wall P 1990 Cross-excitation in dorsal root ganglia of nerve injured and intact rats. Journal of Neurophysiology 64(6): 1733–1746

Dimitriadou V, Buzzi M, Moskowitz M, Theoharides T 1991 Trigeminal sensory fiber stimulation induces morphological changes reflecting secretion in rat dura mater mast cells. Neuroscience 44(1): 97–112

Erel E, Dilley A, Greening J, Morris V, Cohen B, Lynn B 2003 Longitudinal sliding of the median nerve in patients with carpal tunnel syndrome. Journal of Hand Surgery 28B(5): 439–443

Ferrell W, Russell N 1986 Extravasation in the knee induced by antidromic stimulation of articular C fibre afferents of the anaesthetized cat. Journal of Physiology 379: 407–416

Frykholm R 1951a Cervical nerve root compression resulting from disc degeneration and root-sleeve fibrosis. Acta Chirurgia Scandinavica, Suppl. 160

Frykholm R 1951b The mechanism of cervical radicular lesions resulting from friction or forceful traction. Acta Chirurgia Scandinavica 102: 93–98

Fuller G, Jacobs J, Guiloff R 1991 Subclinical peripheral nerve involvement in aids: an electrophysiological and pathological study. Neurology, Neurosurgery and Psychiatry 54: 318–324

Gelberman R, Hergenroeder P, Hargens A, Lundborg G, Akeson W 1981 The carpal tunnel syndrome. A study of carpal tunnel pressures. Journal of Bone and Joint Surgery 63A: 380–383

Gelberman R, Szabo R, Williamson R, Hargens A, Yaru N, Minteer-Convery M 1983 Tissue pressure threshold for peripheral nerve viability. Clinical Orthopaedics and Related Research 187: 285–291

Goadsby P, Burke D 1994 Deficits in the function of small and large afferent fibers in confirmed cases of carpal tunnel syndrome. Muscle and Nerve 17: 614–622

Goddard M, Reid J 1965 Movements induced by straight leg raising in the lumbo-sacral roots, nerves and plexus, and in the intrapelvic section of the sciatic nerve. Journal of Neurology, Neurosurgery and Psychiatry 28(12): 12–18

Gorgulu A, Imer M, Simsek O, Sencer A, Kutlu K, Cobanoglu S 1998 The effect of aprotinin on extraneural scarring in peripheral nerve surgery: an experimental study. Acta Neurochirgica (Wien) 140(12): 1303–1307

Gray J, Ritchie J 1954 Effects of stretch on single myelinated nerve fibres. Journal of Physiology 124: 84–99

Greening J, Smart S, Leary R, Hart-Craggs M, O'Higgins B, Lynn B 1999 Reduced movement of the median nerve in carpal tunnel during wrist flexion in patients with non-specific arm pain. The Lancet 354: 217–218

Hall T, Zusman M, Elvey R 1995 Manually detected impediments during the straight leg raise test. In: Jull G (ed) Clinical Solutions. Ninth Biennial Conference of the Manipulative Physiotherapists Association of Australia, Gold Coast, Queensland: 48–53

Hall T, Zusman M, Elvey R 1998 Adverse mechanical tension in the nervous system? Analysis of the straight leg raise. Manual Therapy 3(3): 140–146

Howe J, Calvin W, Loeser J 1976 Impulses reflected from dorsal root ganglia and from focal nerve injuries. Brain Research 116: 139–144

Howe J, Loeser J, Calvin W 1977 Mechanosensitivity of dorsal root ganglia and chronically injured axons: a physiological basis for the radicular pain of nerve root compression. Pain 3: 25–41

Julian F, Goldman D 1962 The effects of mechanical stimulation on some electrical properties of axons. Journal of General Physiology 46(1): 297–313

Kalb K, Gruber P, Landsleitner B 1999 Compression syndrome of the radial nerve in the area of the supinator groove. Experiences with 110 patients. Handchirurgie Mikrochirurgie Plastische Chirurgie 31(5): 303–310

Kenins P 1981 Identification of the unmyelinated sensory nerves which evoke plasma extravasation in response to antidromic stimulation. Neuroscience Letters 25: 137–141

Kimball E, Fisher C 1988 Potentiation of IL-1-induced balb/3T3 fibroblast proliferation by neuropeptides. Journal of Immunology, 141: 4203–4208

Kingery W, Park K, Wu P, Date E 1995 Electromyographic motor Tinel's sign in ulnar mononeuropathies at the elbow. American Journal of Physical Medicine and Rehabilitation 74(6): 419–426

Laban M, MacKenzie J, Zemenick G 1989 Anatomic observations in carpal tunnel syndrome as they relate to the tethered median nerve stress test. Archives of Physical Medicine and Rehabilitation 70: 44–46

Langley J 1923 Antidromic action. Journal of Physiology 57: 428–446

Lax H, Zochodne D 1995 'Causalgic' median mononeuropathies: segmental rubror and edema. Muscle and Nerve 18: 245–247

Lembeck F, Holzer P 1979 Substance P as neurogenic mediator of antidromic vasodilation and neurogenic plasma extravasation. Naunyn-Schmiedeberg's Archives of Pharmacology 310: 175–183

Levin L, Dellon A 1992 Pathology of the shoulder as it relates to the differential diagnosis of thoracic outlet compression. Journal of Reconstructive Microsurgery 8(4): 313–317

Levine J, Clark M, Devor M, Helms C, Moskowitz M, Basbaum A 1984 Intraneuronal substance P contributes to the severity of experimental arthritis. Science 226: 547–549

Levine J, Dardick S, Roizen M, Helms C, Basbaum A 1986 Contribution of sensory afferents and sympathetic efferents to joint injury in experimental arthritis. Journal of Neuroscience 6(12): 3423–3429

Levy L 1999 MR imaging of cerebrospinal fluid flow and spinal cord motion in neurologic disorders of the spine. Magnetic Resonance Imaging Clinics of North America 7(3): 573–587

Lewis T 1927 The Blood Vessels of the Human Skin and Their Responses. Shaw and Sons, London.

Lindquist B, Nilsson B, Skoglund C 1973 Observations on the mechanical sensitivity of sympathetic and other types of small-diameter nerve fibres. Brain Research 49: 432–435

Lynn B, Cotsell B 1992 Blood flow increases in the skin of the anaesthetized rat that follow antidromic sensory nerve stimulation and strong mechanical stimulation. Neuroscience Letters 137: 249–252

Mackinnon S, Dellon A 1988 Surgery of the Peripheral Nerve. Thieme, New York

Merskey H, Bogduk N 1994 Classification of Chronic Pain: Definitions of Chronic Pain Syndromes and Definitions of Pain Terms, 2nd edition. IASP Press, Seattle: 212

Murphy R 1977 Nerve roots and spinal nerves in degenerative disk disease. Clinical Orthopaedics and Related Research 129: 46–60

Nakamichi K, Tachibana S 1992 Transverse sliding of the median nerve beneath the flexor retinaculum. Journal of Hand Surgery 17B: 213–216

Nakamichi K, Tachibana S 1995 Restricted motion of the median nerve in carpal tunnel syndrome. Journal of Hand Surgery 20B: 460–464

Neary D, Ochoa J, Gilliatt R 1975 Sub-clinical entrapment neuropathy in man. Journal of the Neurological Sciences 24: 283–298

Nordin M, Nystrom B, Wallin U, Hagbarth K 1984 Ectopic sensory discharges and paresthesiae in patients with disorders of peripheral nerves, dorsal roots and dorsal columns. Pain 20: 231–245

O'Halloran D, Bloom S 1991 Calcitonin gene related peptide: a major neuropeptide and the most powerful vasodilator of all. British Medical Journal 302: 739–740

Olmarker K, Nordborg C, Larsson K, Rydevik B 1996 Ultrastructural changes in spinal nerve roots induced by autologous nucleus pulposus. Spine 21(4): 411–414

Olmarker K, Rydevik B 1998 New information concerning pain caused by herniated disk and sciatica. Exposure to disk tissue sensitizes the nerve roots. Lakartidningen 95(49): 5618–5622

Olmarker K, Rydevik B, Nordborg C 1994 Autologous nucleus pulposus induces neurophysiologic and histologic changes in porcine cauda equina nerve roots. Spine 19(20): 2369–2370

Perianin A, Snyderman R, Malfroy B 1989 Substance P primes human neutrophil activation: a mechanism for neurological regulation of inflammation. Biochemical and Biophysical Research Communications 161(2): 520–524

Petersen J, Russell L, Andrus K, MacKinnon M, Silver J, Kliot M 1996 Reduction of extraneural scarring by ADCON-T/N after surgical intervention. Neurosurgery 38(5): 976–983

Pintér E, Szolcsànyi J 1988 Inflammatory and antiinflammatory effects of antidromic stimulation of dorsal roots in the rat. Agents and Actions, 25(3/4): 240–242

Price R, Lasek R, Katz M 1993 Neurofilaments assume a less random architecture at nodes and in other regions of axonal compression. Brain research 607:125–133

Rosenblueth A, Buylla A, Ramos G 1953 The responses of axons to mechanical stimuli. Acta Physiologica Latinoamericana 3(2): 204–215

Sakurai M, Miyasaka Y 1986 Neural fibrosis and the effect of neurolysis. Journal of Bone and Joint Surgery 68B(3): 483–488

Sann H, Pintér E, Szolcsányi J, Pierau F-K 1988 Peptidergic afferents might contribute to the regulation of skin blood flow. Agents and Actions 23(1/2): 14–15

Seddon H 1943 Three types of nerve injury. Brain 66(4): 237–288

Shacklock M 1995 Clinical application of neurodynamics. In: Shacklock M (ed) Moving in on Pain. Butterworth-Heinemann, Sydney: 123–131

Shacklock M 1996 Positive upper limb tension test is a case of surgically proven neuropathy: analysis and validity. Manual Therapy 1: 154–161

Skalley T, Schon L, Hinton R, Myerson M 1994 Clinical results following revision tibial nerve release. Foot and Ankle International 15(7): 360–367

Smith K, McDonald W 1980 Spontaneous and mechanically evoked activity due to central demyelinating lesion. Nature 286: 154–155

Smythe M, Wright V 1958 Sciatica and the intervertebral disc. Journal of Bone and Joint Surgery 40A(6): 1401–1418

Sunderland S 1951A classification of peripheral nerve injuries producing loss of function. Brain 74: 491

Sunderland S 1976 The nerve lesion in the carpal tunnel syndrome. Journal of Neurology, Neurosurgery and Psychiatry 39: 615–626

Sunderland S 1991 Nerve Injuries and Their Repair: A Critical Appraisal. Churchill Livingstone, Edinburgh

Valls-Sollé J, Alvarez R, Nuñez M 1995 Limited longitudinal sliding of the median nerve in patients with carpal tunnel syndrome. Muscle and Nerve 18: 761–767

van der Heide B, Allison G, Zusman M 2001 Pain and muscular responses to a neural tissue provocation test in the upper limb. Journal of Manual Therapy 6(3): 154–162

Wall P, Devor M 1983 Sensory afferent impulses originate from dorsal root ganglia as well as from the periphery in normal and nerve injured rats. Pain 17: 321–339

Weller R 1974 Localised hypertrophic neuropathy and hypertrophic polyneuropathy. Lancet 2: 592–593

Werner C, Haeffner F, Rosén 1980 Direct recording of local pressure in the radial tunnel during passive stretch and active contraction of the supinator muscle. Archives of Orthopaedic and Traumatic Surgery 96: 299–301

Werner C, Ohlin P, Elmqvist D 1985a Pressures recorded in ulnar neuropathy. Acta Orthopaedica Scandinavica 56(5): 404–406

Werner C, Rosén I, Thorngren K 1985b Clinical and neurophysiologic characteristics of the pronator syndrome. Clinical Orthopaedics and Related Research 197: 231–237

White D, Helme R 1985 Release of substance P from peripheral nerve terminals following electrical stimulation of the sciatic nerve. Brain Research 336: 27–31

Xavier A, Farrell C, McDanal J, Kissin I 1990 Does antidromic activation of nociceptors play a role in sciatic radicular pain? Pain 43(2): 259–262

Zochodne D, Ho L 1991 Stimulation-induced peripheral nerve hyperemia: mediation by fibers innervating vasa nervorum? Brain Research 546(1): 113–118

Diagnosis of specific dysfunctions

4

Matching clinical features with specific dysfunctions – diagnosis

Mechanical interface – closing and opening dysfunctions, pathoanatomical and pathophysiological

Neural dysfunctions – sliding, tension, hypermobility (instability), pathoanatomical and pathophysiological

Subjective features – symptoms and their behaviour, history, clinical examples, radiological investigation

Innervated tissue dysfunctions – motor control (protective, muscle imbalance, localized hyperactivity, hypoactivity), inflammation dysfunction (increased and decreased)

Physical findings – active movements, manual testing, palpation, neurodynamic testing and neurological examination

Interface versus neural problem?

Case histories

GENERAL POINTS

Matching clinical features with specific dysfunctions

Diagnosis of neuropathodynamics naturally involves a verbal interview and physical examination that are personalized for the patient. During the appraisal, which continues throughout the duration of management, the patient is escorted through a series of procedures ranging from diagnostic questioning to physical testing for detection of specific dysfunctions. This chapter completes the topic of general pathodynamics. In doing so, the diagnostic categories mentioned in the previous chapter are repeated, although this time they are matched with their respective clinical features, with the addition of some patient illustrations.

MECHANICAL INTERFACE DYSFUNCTIONS

General features

Symptoms
Quality
In the mild closing dysfunction, the most common quality of symptom is aching and pains. This is probably because the problem mainly resides in the musculoskeletal tissues around the nervous system and, to a lesser extent, the connective tissues of the nervous system, and is therefore predominantly nocigenic. Neurological and dysaesthetic symptoms are less common than aches and pains because frank damage and malfunction of the axons are not usually present. With increasing severity, neurological symptoms such as pins and needles, tingling and burning pains become more of a problem and probably represent an intensification of the abnormalities in the interface as they exert their effects on the neural structures. In the most severe cases of interface dysfunction, neurological symptoms in the form of numbness and weakness of muscles also appear.

Distribution
The symptoms of an interface problem occur in the distribution of the involved interface and neural structures. For instance, in the case of reduced closing,

a disc bulge may cause discogenic referred pain in addition to producing pain from the related neural structure. A posterior intervertebral joint problem that produces irritation of the neighbouring nerve root complex may also produce a pain pattern that relates to both the joint and the nerve root.

Behaviour
Generally, the symptoms of a mechanical interface disorder fluctuate with postures and movements that increase pressure or tension in the interfacing structures. In minor cases, in which the problem is subtle and difficult to detect, the problem might only manifest itself as an inability to move into or out of, repeat, or hold, a posture for sustained periods in a direction that closes down or opens around the neural structure in question. It is also possible that movements in a closing or opening direction can be performed easily by the patient, but it is just that pain is provoked or distal referral of symptoms occurs with such a manoeuvre.

Symptoms and signs of inflammation in the interface are frequently present in the interface dysfunction. The associated symptoms can exhibit a circadian pattern with increased pain at night and morning stiffness and the problem frequently responds to anti-inflammatory medication. Also, the inflamed structures will show the usual signs of inflammation, such as swelling, localized tenderness and loss of function.

Interestingly, interface disorders can produce painful arcs when the nervous system is moved. For instance, knee extension in the slump position can produce low back pain through an arc of, say 120°–150°. This can indicate that a neural structure has come into contact with the interface for a short period of time during the manoeuvre. The structures in this case could be a disc bulge or pedicle. However, it is important to realise that painful arcs during a neural movement are not pathognomic of an interface problem because this pattern of symptom behaviour could also be triggered by a sensitive area in a neural structure sliding past an interfacing structure.

History
Frequently, the patient reports a history of injury or hosts a pathology, disease process or malfunction in the mechanical interface. These can be in the form of spondylolisthesis, traumatic arthritis or repetitive use in movements and postures that apply pressure

or tension to the nervous system. Frequently, a provoking movement, usually in a closing direction, has been performed habitually or in an unaccustomed fashion prior to the onset of symptoms. The symptoms may also have developed after a recent minor injury that produces a localization of forces on the interface and neural elements.

Clinical example

A typical history of an interface dysfunction is a patient who jumped from a small boat as it was approaching the shore. The water was shallower than he expected, so the patient did not brace his neck before a jarring impact occurred as he landed unexpectedly on the ground. His neck was forcibly compressed vertically into a lordotic position, resulting in a closing mechanism around the nerve roots. He developed a C5–6 nerve root problem that was predicated on the presence of degenerative changes at this level. Clearly, three coexisting factors were responsible for the problem.

1. The injuring mechanism was a closing one.
2. Prior degenerative changes existed in the musculoskeletal structures around the nerve root.
3. The patient's bracing mechanism was not in action at the time of the impact.

Radiological investigation

Sometimes radiological evidence of pathology in the interface exists. When an association occurs between constant or severe neurological symptoms and a closing dysfunction, the possibility of a pathoanatomical cause rises considerably, and should always be taken seriously.

In the spine, radiological investigations can show early degenerative changes that may be associated with a sustained presence of instability. In hypermobile people, sometimes a hyperlordosis is apparent which would cause the intervertebral foraminae and spinal canal to close excessively. In the extremities, radiological investigation only occasionally reveals relevant abnormalities. Ultrasound scanning of the tissues around the nerves can be performed but,

even though capable of detecting soft tissue abnormalities that relate to neuropathy, ultrasound can be a relatively insensitive procedure in comparison with neurodynamic testing. This is because pathology can be found at surgery when the ultrasound scan is negative and neurodynamic tests are abnormal (Shacklock 1996).

Physical findings

Active movements and protective deformity

The patient may show an inability to move in directions related to opening or closing. Such dysfunctions can be generalized, extending over many joints, or they may be quite localized to a spinal level or one peripheral joint or muscle. In some of the more severe cases, a protective deformity can be observed. The distortion is in the direction of reduced closing or opening, depending on the pathodynamics. In the right patient, it can be important to correct the deformity manually so that its role in the problem can be established. It is also useful in some instances to perform the corrective technique in a position in which the deformity is most accentuated. Changes in pain associated with such corrective procedures indicate the significance of the deformity.

Manual testing

Several possibilities in relation to manual testing of the mechanical interface can occur with an interface dysfunction. In terms of abnormalities related to passive movement and palpation, the chief findings are altered pain production (mechanical allodynia and hyperalgesia), thickening of soft tissues including muscles, stiffness or even hypermobility and instability. Frequently, increased resistance to passive movement in a closing or opening direction is apparent. The pattern of findings with manual examination will depend on whether the dysfunction is one of reduced or increased opening or closing, which is covered later in this section.

In interface dysfunctions generally, there exists a continuum of responses that ranges from a sensitive or more irritable problem to a relatively insensitive and non-irritable one (see Maitland 1986). The symptoms of a highly sensitive problem are easily reproduced with interface manoeuvres. In this case, it is necessary to limit the performance of physical tests for safety reasons. In problems of moderate sensitivity, the patient's symptoms are not as easily reproduced and physical testing is less limited than in the first instance. In the least sensitive problem characterized by only subtle changes, slight abnormalities in function and sensitivity in the interface and nervous system may be the only physical findings. This may necessitate a more extensive manual examination and can involve combining movements of both neural and musculoskeletal systems. Neurodynamic sequencing becomes a key aspect in diagnosis of this type of problem.

Palpation

Palpation is an essential aspect of differentiating between interface and neural components. In the interface dysfunction, palpation of the interface frequently reveals more in the way of abnormalities than palpation of the local nerves, even though both components can be symptomatic. The interfacing structures, if in the limbs, are frequently more thickened, swollen or tender than the neighbouring nerves. In the spine, the offending structure and spinal level can often be detected with palpation and passive movements.

Neurodynamic testing

In cases of mild to moderate severity, abnormalities in the neurodynamic tests tend to be less significant than abnormalities in the interface. However, in cases of a severe interface problem, neurodynamic tests may be profoundly abnormal, in which case a pathoanatomical basis for the problem should always be suspected. In cases of obscure or subtle changes in neurodynamic tests, alterations in sequencing can be used to detect the elusive pathodynamics.

Neurological examination

Frequently, the mild and moderate interface dysfunctions produce nothing in the way of neurological changes because the forces on the nervous system are only intermittent and the neurological examination is usually performed in a position in which the interface is not pressing on the nervous system. Neurological changes are usually only detected in the severe interface dysfunction, in which case, the clinician should consider the possibility of a pathoanatomical cause and exercise caution.

1. Closing dysfunctions

A. Reduced closing

Symptoms and their behaviour

The key behavioural aspect of the reduced closing dysfunction is that the symptoms increase with closing movements.

History

Frequently a history of an injury to the interface exists. The consequent inflammation and biomechanical changes then exert effects on the neural elements. Alternatively, a habitual activity that involves closing may provoke neural symptoms and will need rectifying. Movements that involve a repeated closing action, such as squeezing during gripping as part of being on a factory production line or weeding the garden are common examples. The pronator or supinator muscles as they compress their respective nerves would be implicated in this scenario. By the time the therapist encounters the problem, the closing is reduced by pain avoidance.

Radiological investigation

An anomalous musculoskeletal system may be present, such as a narrow trefoil spinal canal or a shallow trochlea for the ulnar nerve. Even though pathology in the interface can exist, patients with neurogenic pain do not always undergo radiological investigation. The incidence of symptomatic interface pathologies may be higher than supposed.

Physical findings

Posture

In acute and severe disorders caused by a reduced closing dysfunction, a protective deformity is frequently apparent. The deformity is always in the opening direction so as to reduce pressure on the adjacent neural structure. Accordingly, a spinal manifestation of the reduced closing dysfunction is a contralateral list. If the list is relevant to the current problem, manual correction will increase the patient's symptoms.

Active movements

In the reduced closing dysfunction, active movements reveal reduced range of motion in the closing direction. In the spine, these movements naturally consist of extension, ipsilateral lateral flexion and, to a lesser extent, ipsilateral rotation. In the limbs, closing is influenced by the location of the nerve relative to the joint axis and behaviour of the neighbouring joint, muscles and tendons. Two closing movements for carpal tunnel syndrome would be wrist flexion or active finger flexion. A closing movement for the posterior interosseous nerve would be active supination, which applies pressure to the nerve by contraction of the supinator muscle. Pronation would also constitute a closing movement for the nerve, but it would achieve this through stretching supinator. For a review of biomechanics, see Chapter 2.

Manual testing
In the mild dysfunction, it is possible that the only conclusive abnormality to exist in the interface is reduced active or passive segmental movement in the closing direction. Even in the disorder of moderate severity, passive tests do not usually reproduce the patient's entire constellation of symptoms. However, it is sometimes possible to elicit them when an interface test is combined with a neurodynamic test, for instance in a lumbar problem, passive ipsilateral lateral flexion at the same time as performing a straight leg raise. In cases in which the dysfunction is more apparent, the restriction of closing movements is easily detectable and can reproduce the patient's symptoms, or at least evoke symptoms that bear some relationship to the problem.

Clinical example – reduced closing dysfunction

Clinical features
A middle-aged patient with a cervical joint dysfunction serves as a good example of a reduced interface closing dysfunction. Pain and pins and needles developed in the right side of the patient's neck, ipsilateral forearm and hand the evening after he had spent the afternoon painting a ceiling. In spite of him having never performed this activity before, he endured some neck discomfort for several hours during the activity. Interestingly, on the evening of the onset of his symptoms, the patient could read in bed without provocation (neck flexion is an *opening* movement).

Approximately 18 months earlier, the patient sustained a neck injury at social football by way of a heavy fall on his right shoulder, illustrating a closing mechanism for the right side.

On physical examination, the patient's distal symptoms could be reproduced with cervical extension, ipsilateral lateral flexion and rotation, in the sitting position. The median neurodynamic test 1 was only slightly more uncomfortable and mildly tighter than that of the asymptomatic side. Restriction of passive right lateral flexion of C5–6 was present, but the movement did not reproduce the distal symptoms because the technique was performed in supine, that is, without weight bearing. The neurological status was normal. Palpation of the neck revealed thickening and tenderness over the right C4–5–6 posterior intervertebral joints and laminae, producing a small degree of local muscle spasm, particularly over C5–6.

Analysis
The patient was right-handed and it appeared that looking upwards and toward the right side during the painting triggered the problem. This constituted a repeated closing action on the C6 nerve root and, in the presence of a quiescent closing dysfunction from the injury at football, probably triggered inflammation, oedema and increased mechanosensitivity in the nerve root. There may also be a disc bulge or thickened posterior intervertebral joint. However, no radiological tests had been performed to this point.

Key points
1. The symptoms were
   a. well localized
   b. provoked with a closing action
   c. related to a previous closing problem
   d. appeared to be caused by a reduced closing dysfunction.
2. The abnormal physical signs were balanced toward the interface, with only mild neural signs being evident.

B. Excessive closing

Symptoms and their behaviour

Symptoms of the excessive closing disorder are provoked by closing movements. However, the difference between this dysfunction and the reduced closing disorder is that the amount of closing is excessive. Hence, elements of hypermobility, instability or habitual closing exist. A common form of this problem is the hyperlordotic lumbar spine in which backache increases with standing, walking and running activities. The patient's abdominal and gluteal muscles do not adequately keep the lumbar spine in a neutral position. This can exert undesirable forces on the neural elements at the spinal canal and intervertebral foraminae. Another example is when the maintenance of a flexed elbow for too long a time during sleep provokes the symptoms of cubital tunnel syndrome. Even though the ulnar nerve may be normal and is subjected to normal force (elbow flexion is a normal movement), the nerve is compressed for an undesirable duration. This is a problem of excessive closing along temporal lines and can be easily treated.

In cases of musculoskeletal instability, the nerves may be subjected to excessive force and will need protecting. An example of this is perilunate instability in which, in the presence of a positive Watson's test, the median nerve may be subjected to excessive force induced by bony movement.

History

In the excessive closing dysfunction, a history of habitual use of the body or postural imperfection is common. This relates to how the person uses and moves their body during daily activities. It could be that the body is actually normal structurally but is being moved inappropriately, such that neural irritation occurs. Sometimes a history of trauma and features of instability are present also.

Key point

The provoking movement is in a closing direction and is excessive in magnitude, frequency or duration.

Physical findings

Active movements and posture

Analysis of posture and functional movements can reveal that the neutral zone used by the patient is biased toward the closing position. This results in more sustained or repeated closing movements compared with normal. Again, the hyperlordotic lumbar spine will show an increased lumbar lordosis in the standing position and active posterior and anterior pelvic rotation will be unequal (Fig. 4.1).

In general, even though a relative discrepancy between opening and closing movements can exist, when these movements are examined in isolation, they can appear quite normal. If these movements are normal, habitual use in the closing direction and hypersensitivity of the local structures due to mechanical irritation should be suspected. If active movement reveals greater than normal closing movement, instability may be a possible cause, particularly if the increased movement is well localized and related to previous trauma or a disease process such as arthritis or arthrosis.

Manual testing

Manual testing of movement segments in the excessive closing dysfunction often reveals no physical abnormality or can show excessive segmental movement.

Palpation

Palpation of the segments related to this dysfunction often reveals localized tenderness and slight protective muscle contraction. The palpated structures can also appear to be quite normal in the event that they are not particularly irritated.

Neurodynamic testing

Neurodynamic tests in the excessive closing dysfunction are frequently normal or only slightly abnormal. This is probably because the problem is usually one of transient mechanical irritation rather than frank compression or pathology and the neural structures are not under any great strain at the time of testing. Sometimes it is necessary to modify the neurodynamic sequence and incorporate interface and neural testing simultaneously to detect covert pathodynamics in the nervous system.

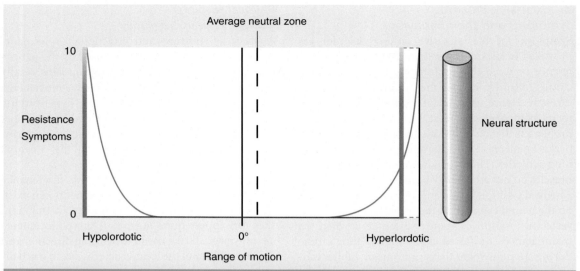

Figure 4.1 Movement/postural diagram of the effects of the hyperlordotic lumbar spine. The pelvis is situated in anterior rotation which produces increased closing around the lumbar nerve roots. The average neutral zone migrates in the direction of the nerve roots.

2. Opening dysfunctions

A. Reduced opening

Subjective findings

Symptoms and their behaviour

The symptoms of a reduced opening dysfunction are usually aches and pains that are local and may occur with or without referred pain. Opening movements provoke the patient's symptoms and are usually restricted.

History

Frequently, a history of trauma exists in which the patient has been forced into an opening position. The body then compensates during the healing process to produce inflammation and muscular bracing, such that opening movements are reduced to avoid further provocation. As far as other causes are concerned, an activity that produces habitual opening movements can also be a stimulus for this dysfunction by producing mechanical irritation.

As an example in the spine, the neck could be forced into contralateral lateral flexion during an event such as a vehicle accident in which the side of the patient's car collides with a cliff or tree whilst sliding off the road. Here, the head would continue moving sideways whilst the body decelerates, producing forced lateral flexion.

Physical findings

Protective deformity and posture

In cases involving the spine, the reduced opening dysfunction can produce a protective deformity of ipsilateral listing. This is the opposite to a reduced closing dysfunction, which, as mentioned, can produce a deformity in the contralateral direction. Like other deformities, those of the reduced opening dysfunction can extend over many levels or it may be localized to a specific segment. The deformity is specifically designed to reduce tension in the interfacing and neural tissues. The reduced opening problem can also be one of traction on the neural structures and links to whether they are hypersensitive due to injury or mechanical irritation. Hence, one could say that a tension component can exist with these disorders which makes use of the term 'tension dysfunction' appealing. This would depend on which component, interface or neural, dominates the clinical picture. In the most severe cases, ipsilateral listing is often accompanied by other compensatory movements such as elevation of the scapula in the case of cervicobrachialgia or hitching and external rotation of the hip during the straight leg raise in lumbar disorders.

Manual testing

Manual testing of the mechanical interface with passive physiological and accessory movements reveals reduced opening. Sometimes these movements reproduce the patient's symptoms. However, since the patient is often in a non-weight bearing position during testing, the only physical sign here may be loss of movement.

Palpation

Palpation in the reduced opening dysfunction often reveals changes in the interfacing structures. These changes come in the form of tenderness, muscle tightness and local thickening. The key point is that, for the problem to be one of reduced interface opening, the changes on palpation must be in the tissues whose function is to limit opening movements. For instance, in the lumbar spine, reduced opening of L4–S1 segments may be accompanied by tenderness and tightness of the ipsilateral erector spinae muscles because they limit contralateral lateral flexion in a manner that protects the neural elements.

Neurodynamic tests

Neurodynamic tests are more likely to be abnormal in the reduced closing problem than many other types of interface dysfunction. This is because, opening often increases tension in the neural tissues and, if they are sensitized, may be provoked by opening movements and postures. Hence, the reduced opening dysfunction often houses a neural component.

Case example – diagnosis of reduced opening dysfunction

History and symptoms

A man in his late thirties was playing soccer when, at speed, he fell on his right shoulder. A graze was sustained in the skin over the acromioclavicular joint and there was also a bruise on the ipsilateral parietal region of his head. Immediately on impact, he experienced severe burning pain that extended from the right side of his neck, past his shoulder down the C6 dermatome to his thumb. At the same time, he noticed paralysis in his arm, particularly with loss of active shoulder abduction and external rotation, elbow flexion and extension, supination and wrist and finger extension. This is commonly called a 'stinger'.

On physical examination, neurological changes matched a mixed brachial plexus lesion with a focus in the C6 spinal nerve. It was probably produced by extreme contralateral lateral flexion whilst the shoulder was forcefully depressed during the accident. The existence of the neurological loss was confirmed with nerve conduction studies, even though no abnormality in the brachial plexus could be detected with magnetic resonance imaging (MRI). However, X-rays showed only disc space narrowing at C5–6 and C6–7. Interestingly, neurodynamic tests were normal.

After two years, the patient's main problems were an incomplete recovery of muscle power accompanied by weakness of wrist extension with heavy use of his right arm and constant loss of sensation, as originally. There was also a variable feeling of dysaesthetic numbness in the tip of his right thumb and pain in his thumb when he touched warm objects (probably thermal allodynia due to central sensitization). At this time, the patient's main symptoms were pain and stiffness in the right side of his neck, provoked by sustained flexion or right rotation. When these symptoms were severe, a right sided (ipsilateral) list would develop which, when corrected manually, reproduced his right neck and shoulder pain. For the first six months or so after the accident, the neck pain and stiffness were very mild and had disappeared for a time. Whereas now, the neck symptoms were more apparent, such that it seemed that an additional neck problem was developing insidiously. In fact, this is what prompted the patient to seek further medical advice and opt for an MRI scan of his neck.

The MRI scan of the neck revealed left sided (contralaterally located) ossified disc bulges at C5–6–7 that caused an indentation in the spinal cord and displaced it toward the symptomatic side. There was also foraminal stenosis at C5–6–7 on the left and this resulted in pressure being exerted on the left C5–6–7 nerve roots. Interestingly, the patient never experienced any symptoms on the left side! The main physical findings with manual testing and palpation at this stage were stiffness to contralateral lateral flexion, pain and stiffness from C4–7 on the right side and tightness and tenderness in the right upper trapezius and scalene muscles. The neurological changes apparent at this stage were of the same kind and were in the same distribution as at the beginning, but they were now less severe. The patient could function normally in daily activities except for heavy lifting and prolonged writing which evoked weakness in the muscles used. He was a physiotherapist. There was a subtle discomfort in the whole upper quarter with the median neurodynamic test 1 and this symptom decreased with release of wrist extension. During episodes of increased pain, the development of an ipsilateral list was associated with a mild deterioration in the neurodynamic test. At these times, the median neurodynamic test 1 would reproduce part of the right neck pain, but the test was not grossly tight or restricted in range of motion. The main tightness was in scapular depression and contralateral lateral flexion, both of which changed with wrist movements at the end range of the test (positive to structural differentiation). The response of the ipsilateral list with the median neurodynamic test 1 was absent when the patient was examined at the beginning.

Interpretation
This is a reduced opening dysfunction caused by trauma in an opening direction. Even though a definite neurological problem exists, the mechanical function of the nerves is actually quite good. The bulk of the mechanical findings are located in the interface and they show themselves as local musculoskeletal changes and intermittent ipsilateral listing. It is likely that the forced contralateral lateral flexion that occurred during the accident produced disc bulges on the left side and they were ultimately asymptomatic, until four years after the injury, when he started to experience weakness in his left wrist extensors with heavy or repeated use of his left arm. Clearly, the injury triggered a pathological process in the interface that grew insidiously to produce significant interface changes but

only subtle neurodynamic abnormalities. Behaviourally, the neurodynamic tests were more closely linked to the interface problem in the right side of the neck rather than the neurological one in the brachial plexus.

B. Excessive opening
Subjective findings
Symptoms and their behaviour
In many respects, the symptoms of an excessive opening dysfunction are similar in kind to all the other interface dysfunctions. They consist of aching and pains, often in the region of the structure in question and can produce referred pain. Symptoms are provoked by opening movements, at least partly because the movements produce increased tension in the musculoskeletal and neural tissues. The problem often has aspects of hypermobility, inappropriate use or excessive postures. Dysaesthesiae, pins and needles and numbness can occur with this dysfunction, but they tend to be less common than in the closing dysfunctions. The symptoms are usually intermittent and are dependent on what provoking movements are performed by the patient. It is common for the neural component to be rather subtle with this dysfunction. Detailed physical examination that incorporates different sequencing options is often warranted.

History
The excessive closing dysfunction can generally be divided into two types. The first involves traumatic stretch of the neural and musculoskeletal tissues in an opening direction. This produces inflammation and hypersensitivity. The second type involves habitual or inappropriate use and is sometimes associated with hypermobility or instability in the opening direction. The patient may not report a particular history of injury.

Physical findings
Protective deformity and posture
By definition, no protective deformity in the opening direction occurs with this disorder. Opening movements are instead increased, since this is what causes the problem. The neck is a common region for this to occur whereby contralateral lateral flexion and

rotation are hypermobile and place strain on the brachial plexus. Sometimes, the patient is a thin female with a neck that has the appearance of being long due to low riding shoulders and hypoactive upper trapezius muscles.

Manual testing
Manual testing in the form of passive physiological and accessory movements shows plenty of movement generally and, hypermobility in the opening direction. In the extremities, the excessive opening disorder may occur in conditions such as recurrent sprained ankle and other hypermobility syndromes.

Palpation
Tenderness over specific irritated sites is often present. This is because the hypermobility produces mechanical irritation of the relevant structures. The tenderness in these patients is frequently along the joint line, whether the problem is in the spine or extremities. In any case, the tenderness is usually localized to the specific sites of irritation. Palpation of the nerves can reveal tenderness along their course from the site of irritation.

Neurodynamic tests
Neurodynamic tests in this dysfunction are often normal or only show subtle abnormalities. This is where it can be important to modify the neurodynamic sequencing so as to test the interface and neural system at the same time (level/type 3c testing, see Chapter 6).

3. Pathoanatomical dysfunction

Pathology as a cause of neuropathodynamics warrants specific attention for several reasons.

1. Anatomical abnormalities in the musculoskeletal and nervous systems can produce movement-evoked pain, which is of particular importance to the therapist.
2. Detection and appropriate treatment of patients with pathologies must be instigated as early as possible.

Table 4.1   Summary of clinical features of the mechanical interface dysfunctions

MECHANICAL INTERFACE DYSFUNCTIONS IN GENERAL

Symptoms and their behaviour
- aches and pains more prominent than dysaesthetic symptoms
- occur in the distribution of the related musculoskeletal structure +/− neural structure
- provoked by movements of the interface that are related to the specific dysfunction e.g. opening/closing
- inflammatory or degenerative component is common

History
- disease process, trauma or habitual irritating movement in interface

Physical examination
- interface findings more prominent than neural findings
- neurodynamic tests often only reveal covert abnormal findings (see Chapter 5)

1A. REDUCED CLOSING	1B. EXCESSIVE CLOSING
Closing movements provoke symptoms (active and/or passive) Closing movements often restricted Contralateral list possible Pathology, disease process or derangement more likely	Usually no great restriction of closing movements Hypermobility in closing direction often present No list Often habitual movement or posture in closing direction

2A. REDUCED OPENING	2B. EXCESSIVE OPENING
Opening movements provoke pain Ipsilateral list possible Trauma or dysfunction in opening direction Neurodynamic tests often abnormal	Provoked by opening movements Often hypermobility/postural/repetitive component Neurodynamic tests often normal or only subtle abnormalities are present

3. The presence of pathology can at times indicate a poor prognosis or give rise to the potential for harm with manual treatment. Consequently, it is always important that the clinician come to an understanding of the basis for the neuropathodynamics (Elvey 1998).

A typical illustration of the pathoanatomical diagnostic category is that of ulnar neuritis that produces an abnormal response to the neurodynamic test for the ulnar nerve. Problems in nerves generally can be produced by a large number of pathologies, some of which include anomalous tendons, scar tissue across the nerve and ganglia protruding from the neighbouring joint, or even a Pancoast tumour (Shacklock 1996; Elvey 1998). The spinal equivalent of such a problem would be a disc bulge, swollen or degenerative posterior intervertebral joint, stenosis or a spondylolisthesis that causes instability and neural irritation. Also, the possibility of more sinister pathologies, such as haematomas, meningiomas bony disorders and malignancy must always be kept in mind.

Subjective features

Symptoms

Quality

The symptoms of pathoanatomical origin vary widely and will be influenced by, among other biopsychosocial factors, the structure in which the pathology is situated. The symptoms typically have aching and paining qualities and can be associated with dysaesthesiae, paraesthesiae and loss of sensation. It is crucial that the reader understand that the quality of symptoms will not necessarily offer anything valuable about whether pathology is their cause. The whole clinical picture must be weighed up before key clinical decisions are made.

Distribution

The distribution of symptoms with a pathoanatomical problem does not usually differ from that of any other interface or neural problem because the nocigenic mechanisms involved are common to all groups of dysfunctions. However, one difference is that sometimes pathologies such as malignancy and amyotrophy produce more diffuse neurological changes. Widespread neurological signs should therefore make the clinician suspicious of pathology. An excellent book on pathological causes of neuromusculoskeletal pain is that written by Boissonnault (1994).

Behaviour

The symptoms of a pathoanatomical problem are often provoked by the same events as other interface dysfunctions, depending on which structure is affected and which dysfunction category it occupies. This makes it difficult to discern whether the symptoms are caused by pathology as opposed to benign dysfunction. However, symptoms with a pathological disorder can be recalcitrant, progressive or unremitting, and sometimes bear little relationship to movement and postures, for instance, spinal malignancy.

History

The history with the pathoanatomical dysfunction is often one of insidious and progressive onset of symptoms with no mechanical trigger, or the trigger might have been quite innocuous, such that the problem is merely 'tipped over the edge'. Asking about the patient's general health, medical history and medical tests is crucial in implicating the pathoanatomical disorder. If medical evaluation has not been administered, it is important that the patient be referred to a doctor for evaluation. Furthermore, lack of improvement is a warning that a pathological problem might be the basis for the symptoms.

4. Pathophysiological dysfunction

Symptoms and their behaviour

The pathophysiological interface type of problem relates closely to all the other categories of interface dysfunction because mechanical disorders generally relate to the physiology of the musculoskeletal system. For instance, an injury to, or a dysfunction in, a musculoskeletal structure can produce changes in its physiology by way of inflammation initially and, in the longer term, a degenerative process.

In relation to inflammation, pain is the key symptom. One of the behavioural aspects of the inflammatory disorder is a circadian pattern of pain. Night pain or morning stiffness indicates that inflammation may be present. Also, pain that worsens during or after rest is very common and it is eased with gentle repeated movement. Being chemical in nature, the pain can also be continuous, even though it may vary with movements, postures and time of day.

In relation to degeneration, pain tends to be provoked with movement and sustained postures and does not worsen at night or with rest. Instead, rest eases the pain of degeneration.

History

Frequently, there is a history of prior injury or prolonged mechanical dysfunction. There may also be radiological evidence of a pathological interface with conditions such as, narrowed spaces, bulges or swollen joints. Sometimes a rheumatological problem exists in which inflamed musculoskeletal structures have an impact on the nervous system. Carpal tunnel syndrome is such a condition in which rheumatoid disease produces swollen tendon sheaths that in turn apply pressure on the median nerve at the wrist.

Physical examination

Examination of the interface reveals changes that would be compatible with pathophysiology. Tenderness, loss of movement, thickening, swelling and sometimes reproduction of pain can be features of this problem. The examination findings will match those of the specific interface dysfunctions, as described above.

Neurodynamic tests in the pathophysiological problem can be deceptive. Sometimes the pathophysiological problem can produce genuine changes in neurodynamics and these are expressed in the neurodynamic testing. A problem is that because inflammatory problems can produce central sensitization, false positive results can occur with neurodynamic tests.

Clinical example of false positive neurodynamic tests

A young man attended our sports injury clinic for pain in the right inguinal region. There was no other symptom. It came gradually the afternoon following a game of ice hockey. During the game, he had fallen heavily on his right side and noticed some mild pain after this. His first examination was two days after the incident, at which point, physical testing revealed that the hip was painful to move in every direction, particularly flexion/adduction. Interestingly, the prone knee bend reproduced his pain, as did the dorsiflexion component of the straight leg raise and the neck flexion component of the

slump test. Mechanically this does not make sense in view of the fact that, to palpation, his lumbar spine was completely normal. At the third visit, he appeared pale and light headed and had beads of sweat on his forehead. He was referred to his doctor for a full medical assessment when it was revealed that an abscess was present inside his hip joint (found on CT scans). The abscess was surgically drained and all the patient's symptoms disappeared. This is a case of a major pathophysiological problem causing central sensitization and false positive neurodynamic tests. I have encountered the same thing with a patient who suffered from an abscess in her coccyx. The slump test was markedly positive and this problem needed medical management.

NEURAL DYSFUNCTIONS

1. Neural sliding dysfunction

On some occasions, it is possible to ascertain whether neuropathodynamics exist in relation to excursion of a nerve or whether it is hypersensitive to sliding. This is particularly easy to achieve in the case of the superficial peroneal nerve as it passes subcutaneously over the dorsum of the ankle and slides transversely with foot movements. In cases of sprained ankle, the nerve can show abnormal responses to its neurodynamic test (Mauhart 1989), and I have also observed its movement to be reduced. In the patients that I have observed this to be the case, the cause of reduced nerve excursion was scarring over the ankle joint from a severe inflammatory response. Another cause of impaired sliding that I have observed clinically, is that of the young man who fell through a glass sliding door. In the process of passing through the breaking glass, a large fragment cut into the medial aspect of his arm, completely severing his ulnar nerve. It was surgically repaired and he was referred to physiotherapy. On examination, the scar that connected the skin to the nerve could be seen to be pulled distally and proximally with sliding techniques for the ulnar nerve.

Symptoms and their behaviour

It is likely that the symptoms of the neural sliding dysfunction consist of aches and pains at the site of the problem and possibly along the course of the nerve. This is because the place of tethering is likely to be a point of peak stress in the neural and neighbouring tissues. The symptoms along the line of the neural tract are likely to correlate with a spread of stress and strain along the nerve. The distance along the nerve tract passed by the symptoms would be influenced by the degree of fixation, spread of pathodynamics and the sensitivity of the neural structure.

If the symptoms are isolated to tethering around the neural structure, theoretically, they will be intermittent and mechanically evoked, particularly by movements that produce stress at the tethered site. Of course, sliding techniques for the neural structure may evoke symptoms and so may tension based techniques, depending on the local dynamics. Dysaesthetic and paraesthetic symptoms can also occur with the neural sliding dysfunction.

History
Patients with the neural sliding dysfunction may have a history of an interface dysfunction, as mentioned earlier. There might also be a history that suggests that tethering between the interface and neural system has occurred, such as that involving repetitive movements and a subsequent inflammatory reaction accompanied by acute pain and loss of movement.

Physical findings
Neurodynamic tests
Neurodynamic tests show specific abnormalities that have in the past mystified clinicians. The key event is that, in a neurodynamic position, the addition of a further neurodynamic movement produces a reduction in symptoms. In illustrating this point, several clinical examples are noteworthy:

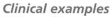

> **Clinical examples**
> 1. The addition of knee extension after the neck flexion component of the slump test produces a reduction in low back pain.
> 2. Neck flexion reduces the symptoms produced by knee extension.
>
> In each of the above cases, the neural elements are returned toward their starting position, and even though tension in them

has increased, they have been taken away from the provoking direction.

3. Piriformis syndrome in which internal rotation of the hip produces a reduction of pain and permits a greater range of straight leg raise. It is possible that the sciatic nerve comes out of contact with a neighbouring structure. The patient in mind went to surgery and a scar across the sciatic nerve was detected and removed.
4. A case of heel pain that was reproduced by the straight leg raise and further *increased* with the toe flexion. The leg raise pulls the posterior tibial nerve proximally and toe flexion permits further proximal sliding, therefore the disorder was possibly one of proximal sliding.
5. A decrease in upper limb symptoms with the addition of contralateral lateral flexion.

Palpation
The involved neural structure is often sensitive along a portion of its length, starting from the point of fixation and spreading proximally and distally from this point. Palpation can also be used to test lateral movement in the nerves and, in those that are accessible, sometimes this lateral movement can be palpably and visibly reduced. Sometimes tissue changes in and around the nerve can be detected and these are in the form of swelling and thickening.

2. Neural tension dysfunction
Symptoms and their behaviour
The neural tension dysfunction can produce a constellation of symptoms that range from aches and pains to pins and needles and dysaesthesiae. Effectively the problem is one of lack of elongation of the neural structure or increased sensitivity to tension during daily movements. Stretching out a limb or reaching are often problematic, whereas sliding movements tend to be less of a problem.

Physical examination
Active and passive movements
Active and passive movements reveal loss of range of motion *when the nerve is under tension*. This point is important because, when the nerve is not under

tension, movement of related joints and muscles normalizes.

Neurodynamic tests

Neurodynamic tests show reduced range of motion compared with the patient's normal and they often reproduce the patient's symptoms or at least produce subtle abnormalities in the form of the covert abnormal response (discussed in Chapter 5). The reason that the neurodynamic tests are more likely to be abnormal in the case of the tension dysfunction than the hypomobility dysfunction is that tension is the primary mechanism of the standard tests. Impairments in tension function of the nervous system can therefore be readily detected.

Palpation

Palpation often reveals tenderness along the line of the neural structure. This is probably because tension also operates along the neural tract and mechanical irritation due to overstress could produce diffuse changes.

3. Hypermobility – nerve instability

Symptoms and their behaviour

As mentioned earlier, nerve hypermobility can occur. It is manifested as a clicking nerve as the limb is taken through an arc of movement. The clicking is usually dull and does not sound like the high pitched articular 'snap'. Instead, it tends to be quite dull and is often only heard by the patient. If symptomatic, the click can be accompanied by local pain or discomfort. In more severe cases, pins and needles can occur momentarily in the distribution of the nerve.

The most common example of the hypermobility/ instability dysfunction is the clicking ulnar nerve, which occurs during elbow flexion/extension. When tension in the nerve is taken up from remote sites, the clicking can accentuate. The nerve can become inflamed (e.g. ulnar neuritis) with repetitive movements. The clicking nerve can also occur in the carpal tunnel when patients occasionally say that a twang occurs in their wrist as they perform a gripping action. This can occur in the course of activities such as weeding the garden. Pins and needles shoot momentarily into the first three digits during this event. Patients sometimes describe it as a 'zap in the fingers'. The same can occur with the sciatic nerve with hamstring contraction. Here, a click occurs and symptoms shoot down the leg.

Physical examination

Neurodynamic tests

Neurodynamic tests can be normal or abnormal. The tests are more likely to be abnormal if the nerve is sensitized. If tests do show abnormalities, they tend to produce only the covert abnormal response rather than an overt one (discussed in Chapter 5). Hence, the deviations from normal are usually rather subtle. If the nerve is not sensitized, neurodynamic tests are usually normal because nothing in particular reduces movement of the nerve.

Palpation

When the nerve is accessible, the jumping of the nerve can sometimes be palpated and even seen under the skin.

Neurological examination

Usually neurological examination is normal. However, if the nerve shows reduced conduction, surgical intervention may be necessary. This is if therapy that is designed to reduce movement of the nerve is unsuccessful.

4. Pathoanatomical dysfunction

Symptoms and their behaviour

The symptoms of a pathoanatomical dysfunction in the nervous system tend toward pain, dysaesthesia, paraesthesia and neurological impairment. This is because the problem usually invades intraneural structures such as axons, blood vessels and nociceptors. Pathoanatomical problems in the nervous system produce persistent symptoms that, in the long term, do not respond well to therapy, even though temporary relief of symptoms can sometimes occur. The symptoms of pathoanatomy can be provoked and eased with movement but they also often develop a constancy and persistence that are not as common in more benign conditions. Persistent paraesthesia, loss of sensation, and motor weakness are key symptoms that should raise concern.

Physical examination

Neurodynamic tests

Even though pathology is present with the neural dysfunction, responses to neurodynamic tests can vary from being quite abnormal to appearing normal.

This is probably related to physiology of the problem and pain mechanisms, which are entirely variable between individuals. I suspect that a neuropathology that results in a reduction in sensitivity in the nerves would produce less in the way of neurodynamic tests abnormalities. The pathology that produces hypersensitivity in the nerves is more likely to produce abnormalities in neurodynamic testing. In any case, the neurodynamic tests should be performed appropriately so that their relationship to the pathology can be understood.

Palpation

Palpation may reveal a sensitive nerve but it is unlikely to detect the pathology unless the nerve is very accessible and the changes in the nerve are rather gross. A large Schwannoma in the radial sensory nerve would fall into this category.

Neurological examination

Neurological examination can reveal abnormalities for the reason that the pathology is often located inside the neural structure and is in a good position to impair conduction.

Clinical example

An example of the pathoanatomical dysfunction is a middle-age woman who attended for treatment of pins and needles in her axilla and down the medial aspect of her arm to her elbow. Neurodynamic tests were mildly abnormal and so was neurological examination in the form of reduced sensation down the medial aspect of her arm. Neurodynamic treatment gave her a 40–50% improvement in her symptoms after each treatment but the problem returned within a day or so after each treatment. After five treatments, there was no lasting improvement so, in view of her past history of ipsilateral breast cancer and mastectomy, she was referred to her doctor. Magnetic resonance imaging showed that a secondary malignancy had invaded her brachial plexus.

5. Pathophysiological dysfunction

Overview

A reason for including pathophysiological mechanisms of the nervous system in clinical reasoning is that they form an important part of what is wrong in the patient. However, a difficulty in interpreting their relevance is that they are not always specific to the mechanical problem. An example of this is the fact that over stretching a peripheral nerve, to the point of slight failure of the epineurium, will produce many changes in physiology that will also occur with other kinds of mechanical insult. Over stretch produces rupture of connective tissue, intraneural oedema and inflammation, mechanosensitivity and scarring (Denny-Brown & Doherty 1945; Sunderland 1981). Just like a patient whose primary mechanism is compression, a patient with this neuropathy may find it painful to move. Moderate compression can also cause intraneural oedema, inflammation and mechanosensitivity and movement evoked pain and paraesthesiae. For therapeutic purposes, it is therefore vitally important that hypothesized changes in physiology be placed in the context of mechanical dysfunctions. Hence, a compressive problem might be diagnosed as a closing dysfunction that produces various changes in physiology in the nervous system. Then the likely changes in physiology would be used by the clinician for the purpose of evaluating the effects of treatment.

Another reason for including pathophysiology is that a primary event in this domain might be responsible for symptoms, but the problem may not have any relationship to abnormality in mechanical function. The diabetic nerve whose neurodynamic tests and palpation findings are normal is a good illustration of this statement. Another example is the patient who undergoes a neural compression injury that is instantaneous and short-lived. Instead of an interface dysfunction persisting, the problem may have only been an isolated incident in which the interface resumes normal function. Yet another alternative is one in which the patient experiences a back injury in the direction of flexion, after which nerve root pain persists. It is possible that the nerve root remains inflamed long after the musculoskeletal component has resolved.

The key elements of pathophysiology to consider in relation to mechanical dysfunctions are presented in Chapter 3. However, a couple of examples of how to include physiology in clinical reasoning are as follows.

Mechanosensitivity

This is a key mechanism in clinical neurodynamics because, it is the means by which the nervous system can be a source of pain with movement. It is also a good yardstick for pathophysiological changes to be monitored in order to judge progress.

Clinical example

A patient presents with pain down his right leg that you have determined is arising from the S1 nerve root. The straight leg raise is limited to 30° and this reproduces the patient's back, buttock and thigh pain. At this same point, muscle holding in the hamstrings commences (a protective component of motor control changes) and isolated dorsiflexion increases the back pain. The analysis in terms of mechanosensitivity is that the nerve root has become sensitized (for whatever reason) and produces afferent impulses with movement. The threshold for mechanosensitivity is located at 30° straight leg raise. After treatment, the straight leg raise then reaches 40° before pain and hamstring bracing commence, therefore the threshold for mechanosensitivity has improved by 10°, or 33%.

Alternatively, the range of straight leg raise at which the mechanosensitivity and muscle holding arise could reduce to 20°. In this case, a worsening in the radiculopathy may have occurred and would indicate that continuing with the same treatment may not be appropriate.

Intraneural pressure and blood flow

Clinical example

The case of carpal tunnel syndrome serves as a good example for analysis of pressure in the median nerve at the wrist.

The patient states that her symptoms worsen acutely at night whilst she is asleep. She is woken by pins and needles several times each night between the hours of

3.00 am and 5.00 am and is compelled to flick her hand repeatedly for approximately a minute to obtain relief. After treatment, the time at which their onset occurs extends to 4.00 am and the need to flick her hand reduces to just a few seconds. This may indicate a significant improvement (reduction) in intraneural pressure at night and might be linked to increased venous return and improved arterial flow through the nerve. It is possible that treatment assisted in reducing the pressure around the nerve by improving the flow of fluid through the carpal tunnel.

INNERVATED TISSUE DYSFUNCTIONS

1. Motor control dysfunctions

A. Protective dysfunction

The key feature of the protective motor control dysfunction is that the altered muscle activity occurs in a pattern that protects a specific neural structure. Hence, diagnosis involves examination of the nervous system, in such a way as to determine which neural structure is at fault, and the musculoskeletal structures that protect neural structure. The findings of increased muscle contraction and resistance to movement in the muscles that offer a protective role would then be compared with those that would not. In effect, both the musculoskeletal and nervous systems are examined to establish if a patho*dynamic* link between the two exists. In the process of investigating such interactions, the clinician also ascertains whether the muscles currently function in a protective fashion by testing them independently of neural tension, then in a position that applies tension to the nerves to see if any change in muscle function between the two positions occurs. In the protective dysfunction, the activity in the protective muscles will be greater in the neurodynamic position. Even though this phenomenon is normal, it will be seen by the clinician that the relevant muscles are excessively active in the abnormal situation with bilateral comparison and knowledge of normal and optimal function. Furthermore, in the event that they are significant, their activity will correlate with production of relevant symptoms.

Key points in physical examination

Stage 1. The muscles are tested in a position in which tension in the nervous system is minimal.

Stage 2. The muscles are then tested in a position that adds tension to the nervous system and any changes in the symptom response and resistance to movement noted. An increase in both symptom response and activity in the muscle suggests that it is exerting a protective effect. Care is taken not to mistake this for a normal response by comparing the events with the same test performed on the opposite side. Examination of the unaffected side first is often preferred because this gives a good indication of normal prior to testing the affected side.

Stage 3. If necessary, muscles that do not offer a protective effect for the neural structure in question are then tested for comparison. However, this is not usually necessary.

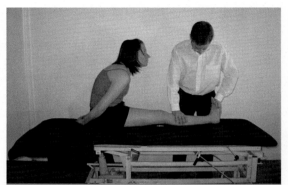

Figure 4.2   Starting position for the neurodynamic and muscle tests combined. Long sitting slump position for a calf muscle problem.

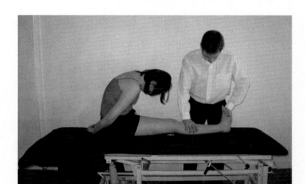

Figure 4.3   Differentiating manoeuvre for assessment of the effect of neck movements on the muscle response.

Clinical example

A patient describes feeling cramping discomfort in the calf region with walking for lengthy periods. There is a past history of sciatica on this side that has been no problem for quite some time. The slump test reveals a covert abnormal response (see Chapter 5) in the form of pulling in the calf at the dorsiflexion phase of the test and this reduces with release of neck flexion. It is not the patient's exact clinical symptom but it is in the right area and the dorsiflexion seems slightly tighter than on the unaffected side. When comparing the same manoeuvre on the unaffected side, the calf muscle does not tighten up as much with neck flexion as on the affected side and there is not as much stretch in this region (Figs 4.2 and 4.3).

B. Muscle imbalance dysfunction

It is not my intention to discuss muscle imbalance comprehensively. At this point, the principal concern is to establish whether a relationship exists between muscle imbalance and altered neurodynamics. Therefore, one of the essential aspects in physical examination is to test the nervous and muscular systems with respect to one another.

An example of the above is to test whether a weak lower trapezius muscle is weaker in the presence of a neurodynamic test. In this case, contraction of the lower trapezius muscle would be performed whilst the upper limb is held in a neurodynamic position that is relevant to the patient problem, such as shoulder pain with serving at tennis. Whilst the shoulder is held in the serving position nominated by the patient,

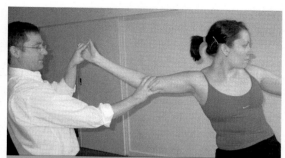

Figure 4.4 Addition of a neurodynamic test to a functional movement for the purposes of differentiation. A throwing action position is held prior to addition of wrist extension with the option of applying contralateral lateral flexion of the cervical spine. Muscle function tests can then be performed in this position and the effect of the neurodynamic movements is assessed.

the elbow wrist and fingers may be straightened to the end point of the neurodynamic test for the brachial plexus. The lower trapezius muscle is then contracted actively and its function observed. If the contraction changes with application of neurodynamic positioning, a relationship with neurodynamics exists. This can be compared with the opposite side and even electromyographic readings can be taken. In addition, relaxation of the upper trapezius muscle could also be performed to see if this has an impact on the response to the neurodynamic test. Contralateral lateral flexion could also be added to sensitize the neural component (Fig. 4.4).

Clearly, many options are available for assessment and treatment of motor control problems when they interact with abnormalities in neurodynamics.

C. Localized hyperactivity dysfunction – alias trigger point

Although it does not always, I believe that the localized trigger point dysfunction can at times occur as a result of neuropathodynamics, as explained in Chapter 3. When this is the case, the key goal is to establish if a match exists in the location of the muscle in which the trigger point is affected with the neural structure that innervates the muscle. For instance, a trigger point might be present in the rectus capitus

muscles in the case of headache. For the localized hyperactivity dysfunction to be present, this trigger point must relate to tenderness in the greater occipital nerve and possibly abnormality in the upper cervical slump test (see Chapter 9). Another example would be the presence of a trigger point in the calf muscle in the presence of an S1 radiculopathy. Patients in whom a trigger point interacts with a neurodynamic problem will at times need simultaneous treatment of the neural and muscle components.

D. Muscle hypoactivity

Muscle hypoactivity can have a number of causes. It could be driven by central motor control changes in the presence of pain. In this case, the problem would fit in the muscle imbalance dysfunction category. Another cause is neurological deficit from neuropathology, treatment of which is not covered in this book.

A particularly relevant type of muscle hypoactivity is that caused by transient abnormalities in neurodynamics. In some of these cases, it may be necessary to sensitize the system by performing a neurodynamic test immediately prior to muscle testing. In the event that this reveals a muscle hypoactivity, it may be appropriate to treat through neurodynamics, on the proviso that the basis for the hypoactivity is well understood by the therapist and it is safe to do so.

2. Inflammation dysfunction

A. Increased inflammation
Symptoms and their behaviour
The symptoms of increased inflammation consist of pain and swelling in the region of the problem. Inflammatory changes follow the distribution of the neural structure, i.e. a region, rather than being localized to a specific musculoskeletal structure. Hence, inflammatory changes that do not follow a specific structure, and are rather vague and diffuse in distribution, should raise suspicion that neurogenic inflammation is a factor. Another feature of neurogenic inflammation is that sometimes the patient experiences loss of sensation in the inflamed area. This indicates a neural dysfunction that produces reduced conduction whilst also creating increased efferent

activity to produce the inflammation. The pains of neurogenic inflammation are provoked by application of mechanical forces to the site of inflammation, as would occur with any inflammatory event. Pins and needles and numbness can also be experienced in the area of inflammation. For a case history of diagnosis and treatment of inflammation in a musculoskeletal structure, e.g. plantar fasciitis, see Shacklock (1995).

History

Sometimes there is a history of previous or current neural problems, such as radiculopathy or a nerve tunnel syndrome. Disorders that predispose nerves to neuropathy, such as diabetes and thyroid disturbances, can coexist and may be significant predisposing factors.

Physical examination

Active movements

Active movements can reproduce the patient's pain and will show many of the features that would normally be present in an inflammatory problem. Sometimes the patient can nominate an active movement that reproduces their symptoms but this movement may not actually apply mechanical stress to the tissues in which the pain is experienced. Instead, this movement loads the nervous system. In the case mentioned above (Shacklock 1995) a patient with heel pain and swelling could reproduce her pain with what she called a hamstring stretch. At the point of pain onset, no force was applied to the heel. The movement she had performed turned out to be a self-administered neurodynamic test for the posterior tibial nerve, i.e. straight leg raise with dorsiflexion/eversion.

Neurodynamic tests

Responses to neurodynamic testing can range from being normal to being grossly abnormal, depending on neural sensitivity, and, ultimately, the whole clinical picture is weighed up before coming to a diagnosis of neurogenic inflammation.

Neurological examination

Reduced conduction can occur with this problem but it does not predict the presence of neurogenic inflammation. However, research in which sophisticated neurological and inflammation measurement

techniques have been used shows relationships between neuropathy and altered inflammation, as mentioned in Chapter 3. It is possible that certain kinds of fibre involvement, such as small fibres, is one of the key variables in whether neurological changes predict the onset of neurogenic inflammation.

Palpation

Palpation of the nerves related to the inflamed structure, particularly at their tunnels, is important. Changes such as swelling in and around the nerve can be detected and the nerve can show abnormal sensitivity by producing local pain and sometimes reproducing the patient's symptoms in the inflamed area. Frequently, pain at the site of the inflammation can be produced by palpation of that area and swelling can also be visible in some cases.

Evaluation of the inflammatory response

As mentioned in Chapter 3, the clinician can come to some idea of whether the inflammatory response is altered by firmly running the back of the fingernails over the skin, approximately half a dozen times in quick succession. Symmetry can, and should, be tested for and the extent, rate and severity of development of redness should be observed. In the increased inflammation dysfunction, the redness can be more prolific and develops more rapidly in the problem area than in unaffected sites.

B. Reduced inflammation

Symptoms that accompany reduced inflammation tend more towards loss of neural function such as numbness, muscular weakness and decreased sensitivity of the neural structure. This is probably because nervous system conduction has been so severely impaired that its efferent capacity to produce inflammation are reduced. Neuropathies associated with this dysfunction can produce poor nutrition and reduced healing of the tissues.

The development of redness with the skin scratch test, as mentioned above, can be more sluggish and less prolific than normal. However it is important to test both sides at exactly the same time to prevent time-based discrepancies in the behaviour of the inflammation.

References

Boissonnault W 1994 Examination in Physical Therapy Practice: screening for medical disease, 2nd ed. Churchill Livingstone, New York

Denny-Brown D, Doherty M 1945 Effects of transient stretching of peripheral nerve. Archives of Neurology and Psychiatry 54(1): 116–129

Elvey R 1998 Treatment of arm pain associated with abnormal brachial plexus tension. Commentary: Adverse neural tension reconsidered. Australian Journal of Physiotherapy Monograph 3: 13–17

Maitland G 1986 Vertebral Manipulation 5th edition. Butterworth Heinemann, London

Shacklock M 1995 Clinical application of neurodynamics. In: Shacklock M (ed) Moving in on Pain. Butterworth-Heinemann, Sydney: 123–131

Shacklock M 1996 Positive upper limb tension test is a case of surgically proven neuropathy: analysis and validity. Manual Therapy 1: 154–161

Sunderland S 1981 Stretch-compression neuropathy. Clinical and Experimental Neurology 18: 1–13

Diagnosis with neurodynamic tests

5

Sensitizing movements, differentiating movements

Neuropathodynamics in a balanced context – central nervous system mechanisms and the biopsychosocial model of pain and disability

Interpretation of neurodynamic tests

Diagnostic efficacy

A systematic classification of neurodynamic tests responses – musculoskeletal and neurodynamic (normal, abnormal, overt, covert)

Relationship of responses to the clinical problem – relevant, irrelevant, subclinical, anomalous, atypical

Clinical examples

NEURODYNAMIC TESTS

Neurodynamic tests move and deliver a mechanical stimulus to the tested neural structures. Hence, the tests are used to gain an impression of their mechanical function in relation to their state of sensitivity. As such, neurodynamic tests are a probe that is used to simultaneously explore aspects of mechanics and physiology. However, before presenting the tests directly, it is necessary to discuss some essential points.

Sensitizing movements

Definition

Sensitizing movements are those that increase forces in the neural structures in addition to those movements employed in standard test. However, they are *not* differentiating movements.

Sensitizing movements can be useful in loading or moving the nervous system in the form of sensitizing neurodynamic tests. However, since they also move musculoskeletal structures, they are not as effective as differentiating movements in determining the existence of a neurodynamic mechanism. This is why they are called *sensitizing* movements rather than *differentiating* movements.

The sensitizing movements for the upper quarter consist of contralateral lateral flexion of the cervical spine, scapular depression, glenohumeral horizontal extension and sometimes external rotation. Radial deviation can be used to sensitize the ulnar neurodynamic test. The movements for the neurodynamic tests of specific peripheral nerves are part of the standard tests and have therefore not been included as sensitizing movements.

The sensitizing movements for the lower quarter consist of contralateral lateral flexion of the spine, internal rotation of the hip and possibly hip adduction.

Differentiating movements

Definition

Differentiating movements emphasize the nervous system. They do this by producing

movement in the neural structures in the area in question rather than moving the musculoskeletal structures in this area. Hence, differentiating movements are used to establish whether a neurodynamic mechanism takes part in symptom production.

The method of application of differentiating movements is discussed in more detail in Chapter 6 but, generally, a movement that is remote from the offending problem is used to move the neural structures in the problem site in preference to musculoskeletal structures. If a change in symptoms occurs simultaneously with the differentiation movements, a neurodynamic mechanism may be implicated. For instance, dorsiflexion of the ankle with the straight leg raise for low back pain is a such a manoeuvre.

Neuropathodynamics in a balanced context

Central nervous system mechanisms

As mentioned, central pain mechanisms are a great clinical challenge because they provide the potential for such large disparities in pain and motor responses with mechanical tests. It is therefore crucial that performance and interpretation of neurodynamic tests be placed in the context of central pain mechanisms (Zusman 1992, 1994; Shacklock 1996, 1999a, 1999b; Gifford & Butler 1997; Butler 2000).

An important aspect of applying the diagnostic categories presented in the previous chapter is that the clinical features of each dysfunction are reasonably specific, localized and reproducible. For instance, the reproduction of a patient's symptoms with a closing movement will be consistent. In many patients, the yielding of such localizing signs is not possible. It could be that many components of pathodynamics coexist or central mechanisms may be more relevant. In which case, careful analysis of the problem in terms of pain mechanisms (peripheral and central) will be necessary in which the mechanisms are balanced with the whole clinical problem.

Biopsychosocial model of pain

It is important for the reader to understand that, like any physical manoeuvre that is applied to the body, neurodynamic tests, palpation and neurological examination are actually psychophysical tests that can house significant psychosocial aspects. For instance, motor reflexes and muscle activity can be modified significantly by thoughts (Stam et al 1989) and imagining the performance of a task can produce significant subliminal changes in muscle tone and electromyographic activity in a fashion that is specific to those thoughts (Jacobson 1930a, 1930b). Naturally, the clinician will place the procedures presented in this book correctly in the context of the pain sciences. This incorporates the biopsychosocial model of pain and disability, including all relevant contextual factors.

INTERPRETATION OF NEURODYNAMIC TESTS – DIAGNOSTIC CATEGORIES

If neurodynamic tests were to reflect directly the mechanical function of the nervous system, it would seem that the question of their validity in diagnosis would be redundant. This is because the corollary is that whatever occurs clinically in terms of observed movement would reflect the mechanical events related to the patient problem, making diagnosis perfect. Unfortunately, this leap of faith is far from the truth. Neurodynamic tests vary greatly between individuals, normal or otherwise. Such variations occur in the parameters of type of symptom response, range of motion, effect of structural differentiation and many others. For instance, the range of motion of elbow extension in the median neurodynamic test 1 varies in normal subjects between full elbow extension to −60° (Pullos 1986). Hence, in isolation, range of elbow extension is usually of no value in establishing whether a test is normal or abnormal. But when compared with the contralateral test, asymmetry in range of motion may be a highly relevant component of the analysis and could implicate neurodynamic mechanisms. This further depends on the result of structural differentiation. If the range of elbow extension does not change with contralateral lateral flexion of the neck, the importance of the nervous system reduces. If contralateral lateral flexion produces a change in elbow movement, as the patient's pain is reproduced, the nervous system may be a factor. Also, nerve movement itself varies between individuals (Kleinrensink 1997; Erel et al 2003) which will naturally be reflected in variations in the related neurodynamic tests. This leads us to the following key point.

> **Key point**
> The way neurodynamic tests are interpreted is a key aspect of diagnosis.

Diagnostic efficacy

Background

If the therapist is to achieve effective diagnosis through neurodynamic tests, it is essential to understand the basic principles of diagnosis. Diagnostic efficacy asks the question – how effective is a test in diagnosis? This is a particularly important aspect of understanding clinical neurodynamics because, as mentioned above, neurodynamic tests in the conscious human are influenced by many variables that can give rise to variation and leave therapists in a difficult position. It is possible for tests to produce false positives and false negatives which necessitates that the clinician understand two key aspects of diagnostic efficacy, sensitivity and specificity.

Sensitivity

Sensitivity is the frequency at which a clinical test shows abnormalities in the presence of disease. For instance, if a neuropathic problem is present in 100 subjects and the relevant neurodynamic test is abnormal in 90 of them, the sensitivity rating is 90%. Conversely, if the test shows abnormalities in the absence of disease, it produces a false positive result, which is clearly undesirable.

Specificity

Specificity is the frequency at which a clinical test is normal in the absence of disease. Once again, if the relevant neurodynamic test shows a normal response in 90 of 100 subjects who have no problem, the specificity rating would also be 90%. If a test is normal in the presence of disease, it produces a false negative result and is also undesirable. Therapists must therefore be acutely aware of two categories of responses, namely false positives and false negatives.

Clearly, the better diagnostic efficacy of a neurodynamic test, the higher its sensitivity and specificity ratings will be. In assessing the sensitivity and specificity ratings of neurodynamic tests in clinical disorders, not much research can be called upon. However, what has been shown with a test such as the standard median neurodynamic test 1 is that it can be excellent in diagnosis. In carpal tunnel syndrome sufferers, our research group showed that the test produced sensitivity of 82%, specificity of 75% and a positive predictive power of 93% (Coveney et al 1997). Similar results have also been shown by Selvaratnam et al (1997). This is good news from a clinical neurodynamics standpoint, however, much more work must be done before global acceptance of these techniques will occur.

A systematic classification of neurodynamic test responses

The two diagnostic icons and categories of neuro-dynamic test responses, positive and negative, must be critically appraised if neurodynamic tests are to be used appropriately. Several reasons for this statement are as follows.

Neurodynamic tests are normally positive because they evoke neurogenic symptoms in asymptomatic subjects (Kenneally et al 1988). If you pull hard enough on a nerve it will hurt, and this correlates with the research on mechanosensitivity in Chapter 3. Hence, a positive test does not necessarily mean that the nervous system is abnormal. To judge a test as positive in this situation is technically correct but the response could be a *normal positive* one. To judge it as abnormal merely because it produces neurogenic symptoms would be an error and could produce a false positive result. Hence, the first milestone in evaluating neurodynamic test responses is through a positive/negative distinction in response to a differentiating manoeuvre. If the response is negative, that is, remains constant during structural differentiation, it is likely that the symptoms arose from musculoskeletal or other tissues. If the response is positive to structural differentiation, i.e. neurodynamic, the next milestone is then to establish whether the response is a normal or abnormal neurodynamic one.

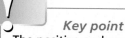

Key point

The positive and negative classifications in isolation during neurodynamic testing are only likely to help determine whether the responses to the tests are neurodynamic or musculoskeletal. At this early stage in testing, this offers no information on whether the test is normal or abnormal. Hence, the distinction of positive/negative is earmarked for *structural differentiation only*.

Negative structural differentiation – musculoskeletal response

Structural differentiation is negative when the symptoms, range of motion or resistance to movement stay constant with a differentiating manoeuvre. Hence, the nervous system is eliminated and the response is deemed musculoskeletal in origin.

Positive structural differentiation – neurodynamic response

Structural differentiation is positive and may implicate the nervous system when the symptoms, range of motion or resistance to movement change with a differentiating manoeuvre.

Once a positive response to structural differentiation has occurred, the next step is to establish whether the nervous system currently behaves normally or abnormally by further classifying the response.

Based on the above, a suggested classification of responses to neurodynamic test responses is as follows.

1. Musculoskeletal response

As mentioned, the symptoms evoked by the neuro-dynamic test are established with structural differentiation to be musculoskeletal. An example of the musculoskeletal response is hand symptoms evoked by the median neurodynamic test *not* changing with contralateral lateral flexion of the neck. Another illustration would be low back pain with the straight leg raise remaining constant with the addition of ankle dorsiflexion.

2. Neurodynamic response
Effect of structural differentiation
Restating, the key diagnostic criterion for a neurody-namic response is that at least one of the parameters consisting of symptoms, range of motion or palpable

resistance, change with the differentiating manoeuvre. An increase or decrease marks such a response. However, at this point, whether the response is normal or abnormal is *not* established and further analysis is necessary.

2a. Normal neurodynamic response

The normal neurodynamic response is *positive* to structural differentiation and the events fit within what has been reported in the literature on normative responses and are presented under standard neurodynamic testing (Chapter 7).

2b. Abnormal neurodynamic response – neuropathodynamic

In this kind of response, the symptoms, resistance pattern or range of motion show a positive response to structural differentiation *and* differ from those that occur in normal subjects. With a unilateral problem, there is frequently significant asymmetry in the above parameters. For instance, reduced range of motion compared with the asymptomatic side in a pattern that protects the relevant nerve structures is common.

Problems located in the midline can present symmetrically, which reduces the value of asymmetry in diagnosis. The therapist must then rely on clinical experience and relate the disorder to known neurodynamics with even greater precision than if the problem were unilateral. Bilateral techniques can be used.

At this point, it is important to distinguish between different types of abnormal (neuropathodynamic) responses that present in some patients. Two types can occur, the overt and covert.

2bi. Overt Abnormal Response (OAR)

In this category of response, the two essential features are *reproduction* of the patient's symptoms and *differentiation* of those symptoms is positive. Reproduction refers to the exact same symptom that the patient experiences, or part thereof. Abnormalities of movement may also occur but they do not specifically indicate an overt abnormal response. The term 'overt' is used to show that it is obvious that something is wrong with the nervous system by the reproduction of the patient's symptoms with a neural movement. It is important to state that the cause of the

> **Key point**
>
> The overt abnormal response is the 'smoking gun' for neurodynamic tests. It involves reproduction of the patient's clinical symptoms and positive structural differentiation.

abnormal response is not yet established and diagnosis is completed with the use of information gained from the rest of the clinical examination.

2bii. Covert Abnormal Response (CAR)

In this category, responses to neurodynamics tests may differ in one or some parameters from the known normal response. Also, even though something about the test is abnormal, the patient's pain is *not* reproduced. The abnormality might consist of significant asymmetry of symptoms, symptoms in an abnormal location, loss of range of motion or a difference in palpable resistance to movement. It might also manifest as a difference in the quality of symptoms compared with the normal side. For instance, the patient might report an ache in their anterior forearm with the standard median neurodynamic test 1 which is differentiated to be positive (implicating a neurodynamic mechanism) but the pain they experience with daily arm movements is actually sharp and severe. The ache with the neurodynamic test is accompanied by reduced range of wrist extension which increases with release of contralateral lateral flexion of the neck. This is a covert abnormal response because it does not reproduce the patient's clinical pain but it does show covert or hidden neuropathodynamics that later may be deemed relevant, given more detailed analysis. Naturally, in all cases of the covert abnormal response, the test response is by definition positive to structural differentiation. Another example of a covert abnormal response is that which produces a small compensatory movement whereby the pronator teres muscle contracts more on the symptomatic side than on the unaffected with median neurodynamic testing. More supination occurs with release of contralateral lateral flexion. Pronation protects the median nerve and the presence of this type of physical sign may therefore justify further inquiry.

Key point

The covert abnormal response is the 'circumstantial evidence' for neurodynamic tests. Even though it shows a neurodynamic abnormality that may be considered a comparable sign, it does *not* reproduce the patient's symptoms.

There are three reasons for presenting this category of test response. First, it addresses the issue of lack of sensitivity in some patients who may have a problem that is difficult to detect because standard testing does not make use of specific sensitizing manoeuvres and the patient's symptoms can not be easily evoked. In these patients, the danger of producing a false negative result can be reduced by intricate application and interpretation. If a therapist were to miss this response, the neurodynamic component to the problem would remain undetected and therefore untreated. This category of response also challenges the notion that if a test does not actually reproduce the patient's symptoms then the nervous system is normal. Many patients fall into this category and this kind of problem is often missed.

The second reason for presenting the covert abnormal response is that it provides a stimulus to, when clinically appropriate, investigate neurodynamics in more detail than with a standard examination. Higher and more intricate levels and types of examination may be needed for this type of problem and are discussed in Chapter 6.

The third reason for having the covert abnormal response is that, I have observed many times, patient's who start off with an overt abnormal response often retreat through the covert before becoming normal. This suggests that the covert is a transitional zone of abnormality that is located between the normal and the frankly abnormal (Fig. 5.1).

Clinical example

An example of the covert abnormal response is the patient who experiences pain and cramping in the calf after jogging for

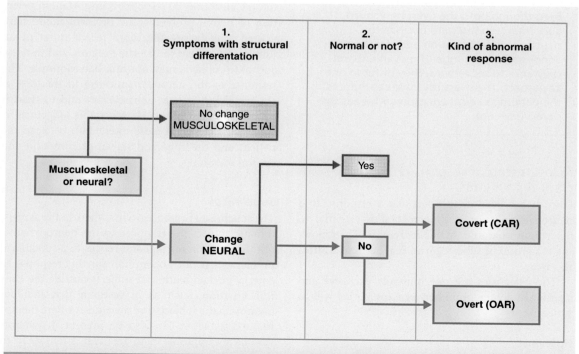

Figure 5.1   Flow chart for diagnosis (classification) of neurodynamic responses.

20 minutes. There is a history of low back pain and a laminectomy several years earlier for sciatica on this side. The ipsilateral straight leg raise with dorsiflexion added is normal. However, when the sequence of movements is reversed, that is, the dorsiflexion is performed first, followed by the straight leg raise, an aching stretch is produced in the calf and the dorsiflexion is tighter than on the contralateral side. This is not the pain experienced whilst running, but it is in the correct area. The pain increases with hip flexion and the calf muscle tightens during this manoeuvre. Muscle length testing separately reveals normal and symmetrical calf muscles. Clearly something about the neural system could be abnormal, even though reproduction of the patient's clinical pain does not occur. The neural component to this problem would have remained undetected had the therapist not looked beyond the standard straight leg raise.

Key point
Even though both the overt and covert abnormal responses are positive to structural differentiation and can show abnormalities in range of movement and resistance to movement, they differ in one key aspect. The overt response reproduces the patient's clinical symptoms whereas the covert does not.

Relationship of responses to the clinical problem
Once it has been established that a response to a neurodynamic test is abnormal, it is essential to determine what exactly this represents. The following is a group of subcategories that helps to address this issue.

The categories are not mutually exclusive and significant interactions between categories will at times occur.

Relevant
The relevant abnormal neurogenic response is one that is causally linked to the disorder in question.

The most obvious example of this type of response is the overt abnormal one that matches localizing signs of a disorder, such as a local pathology or specific mechanical or physiological dysfunction. Alternatively, in the patient whose problem produces a covert abnormal test response, the problem could be a subtle one that needs treatment. A patient who experiences unilateral buttock pain with activities that involve lumbar flexion is a good example. The slump test may not reproduce the patient's pain but the knee extension component of the test might be stiffer than that of the asymptomatic side and movement of this component improves when neck flexion is released. In addition, some stretching in the ipsilateral buttock occurs with the test and this also reduces with releasing neck flexion. The symptom response is in the same region as the patient's clinical pain but the clinical pain is *not* reproduced. This response could be relevant and to treat it with neurodynamic techniques mobilization may be appropriate.

Irrelevant
An irrelevant abnormal neurodynamic response occurs when the neuropathodynamics are not causally related to the current clinical problem. Even though an abnormal response is important in detection of neural problems, the problem might have existed long before the more recent onset of an unrelated problem in the same region, and the new and old problems may not link behaviourally. The response to the neurodynamic test in this case is abnormal but it may be irrelevant and to treat it could be inappropriate. However, this judgement is very much based on close interaction between the patient and therapist and skilled examination and clinical reasoning.

Subclinical
The subclinical response occurs when, in the asymptomatic subject the response to the neurodynamic test differs from normal and relates to a subclinical problem. It is not uncommon for this response to emerge in examination of subjects outside the clinical situation, such as in research that includes asymptomatic subjects and on courses where therapists are tested. It can also be present in patients who have symptoms in an area that is remote from the tested structures. Since the neurodynamic test is abnormal in a region in which symptoms are not

experienced, a subclinical problem may yet become symptomatic.

Anomalous

Some people experience atypical responses to neurodynamic testing in the absence of clinical symptoms. In addition to the response being a subclinical type (as above), it could also be a manifestation of anomalous anatomy. For instance, the presence of medial elbow symptoms during the median neurodynamic test 1 through an arc of 60°–120° elbow extension is not uncommon and could represent anomalous anatomy or function of the median or ulnar nerve. Also a burning pain at the fibular head with the straight leg raise could be another example of an anomaly. I have seen in cadavers that some have a small band of connective tissue that tethers the common peroneal nerve to the neck of the fibula.

Atypical but normal for that person

Some people simply have a system that behaves differently from that in the general population. Short hamstrings due to a tight nervous system or a greatly restricted elbow extension component of the median neurodynamic test 1 are such examples. These people often say that they have always been like that. The response is possibly normal for that individual and may not require treatment. The therapist will then have to establish its relationship, or lack thereof, to the current patient problem.

References

Butler D 2000 The sensitive nervous system. NOI Press, Adelaide

Coveney B, Trott P, Grimmer K, Bell A, Hall R, Shacklock M 1997 The upper limb tension test in a group of subjects with a clinical presentation of carpal tunnel syndrome. In: Proceedings of the Manipulative Physiotherapists' Association of Australia, Melbourne: 31–33

Erel E, Dilley J, Greening J, Morris V, Cohen B, Lynn B 2003 Longitudinal sliding of the median nerve in patients with carpal tunnel syndrome. Journal of Hand Surgery 28B(5): 439–443

Gifford L, Butler D 1997 The integration of pain sciences into clinical practice. Journal of Hand Therapy 10: 86–95

Jacobson J 1930a Electrical measurements of neuromuscular states during mental activities. II Imagination and recollection of various muscular acts. American Journal of Physiology 4: 22–34

Jacobson E 1930b Electrical measurements of neuromuscular states during mental activities. IV Evidence of contraction of specific muscles during imagination. American Journal of Physiology 95: 703–712

Kenneally M, Rubenach H, Elvey R 1988 The upper limb tension test: the SLR test of the arm. In: Grant R (ed) Physical Therapy of the Cervical and Thoracic Spine. Clinics in Physical Therapy 17. Churchill Livingstone, Edinburgh

Kleinrensink G 1997 Influence of movement and posture on peripheral nerve tension. Anatomical, biomechanical and clinical aspects. PhD Dissertation, Chapter 4, upper limb tension tests as tools in the diagnosis of nerve and plexus lesions: 41–51

Mauhart D 1989 The effect of chronic ankle inversion sprain on the plantarflexion/inversion straight leg raise. Graduate Diploma thesis, University of South Australia

Pullos J 1986 The upper limb tension test. Australian Journal of Physiotherapy 32: 258–259

Selvaratnam P, Cook S, Matyas T 1997 Transmission of mechanical stimulation to the median nerve at the wrist during the upper limb tension test. In: Proceedings of the Manipulative Physiotherapists' Association of Australia, Melbourne: 182–188

Shacklock M 1996 Positive upper limb tension test is a case of surgically proven neuropathy: analysis and validity. Manual Therapy 1: 154–161

Shacklock M 1999a Central pain mechanisms; a new horizon in manual therapy. Australian Journal of Physiotherapy 45: 83–92

Shacklock M 1999b The clinical application of central pain mechanisms in manual therapy. Australian Journal of Physiotherapy 45: 215–221

Stam J, Speelman H, van Crevel H 1989 Tendon reflex asymmetry by voluntary mental effort in healthy subjects. Archives of Neurology 46: 70–73

Zusman M 1992 Central nervous system contribution to mechanically evoked responses. Australian Journal of Physiotherapy 38: 245–255

Zusman M 1994 The meaning of mechanically produced responses. Australian Journal of Physiotherapy 40: 35–39

Planning the physical examination

6

What to observe – changes in movement, movement diagram

Planning the examination – how extensive should it be?

Level zero (contraindicated), 1 (limited), 2 (standard) and level/type 3a, b, c and d

Description, indications, method of examination

Modified structural differentiation

General points on technique

WHAT TO OBSERVE

In the course of neurodynamic testing, the therapist concentrates on several key variables. The location, extent, quality and behaviour of the patient's symptoms are the principal subjective aspects and the resistance pattern to movement, range of motion and compensatory movements are the main physical ones. Other more subtle non-verbal cues such as quality of breathing, tone of voice, facial expression, protective muscle tone and avoidance behaviour are also taken into account. Effectively, a mental movement diagram involving these variables is performed in the mind of the therapist so that responses can be used to construct diagnosis and treatment. Sensitivity and skill are the essential ingredients.

Feeling for changes in movement

The movement diagram – Maitland's legacy

The reason for including the movement diagram in neurodynamic testing is to emphasize the importance of manual skill. It is this ability that enables the therapist to make the transition from only being able to perform a cursory examination, with the potential for false positives and negatives, to making an accurate diagnosis. Maitland (1991) has provided an excellent tool, the movement diagram, for the purpose of developing such skill and I encourage all therapists dealing with the nervous system to become au fait with it.

An exercise in the use of the movement diagram in testing neurodynamics can be applied to the median neurodynamic test 1. It should be performed slowly and gently and on an asymptomatic individual. Two therapists are needed. If the reader is unfamiliar with the test it is presented in detail in the following chapter.

1. Therapist A performs the median neurodynamic test 1 to the point of evoking a moderate stretch. The range of elbow extension at the point of onset of resistance (R1) and the behaviour of resistance are noted. The position should only be held for a short time to prevent undue production of symptoms and necessitates clear communication with the subject.
2. Therapist A then returns the limb to a satisfactory rest position and draws a movement diagram on

the elbow extension movement based on their observations of symptoms, range of motion and onset and behaviour of the resistance.
3. Therapist B then performs a firm contralateral transverse glide on the lower cervical spine and holds that position *perfectly* stationary whilst stage 4 is executed.
4. Therapist A then performs the neurodynamic test again and draws the same parameters on the diagram as in the first instance. Comparisons can then be made.

It will often be noted that the available range of elbow extension reduces and/or the resistance commences earlier in the range and rises more steeply to the limit of movement.

As seen above, the benefit of the movement diagram is to highlight specific variables of movement and pain with neurodynamic techniques. Another benefit is that the diagram provides the user with the opportunity to document and analyse therapeutic movements, such as grades, amplitudes and ranges of motion. Mental movement diagrams are made during all neurodynamic testing.

Planning the examination – how extensive should it be?

General points

Judgement on the extensiveness and type of neurodynamic testing is one of the most important aspects of clinical neurodynamics because it addresses the issue of provocation of symptoms. Provocation has been the single most common reason for therapists omitting a neural approach in treatment of musculoskeletal disorders. A great deal of confusion exists in relation to decisions on selection of tests and how to apply them. Of particular importance are how strongly a test should be performed, how far into a movement should a test be taken, what particular variations in testing might be more appropriate for each patient and how decisions on these variations are made. There is currently a lack of understanding of these aspects and this section seeks to solve this issue.

Some patients' symptoms are severe and easily provoked, or their problem might require particular caution. In this case, the most gentle and refined of examinations will be performed and the therapist must decide on factors such as which neurodynamic sequence to use, how far to move the nervous system, how much resistance should be encountered and to what extent symptoms should, or should not, be evoked. At the other end of the spectrum, the standard examination of the patient whose symptoms are infrequent, and whose problem is difficult to detect, will not be sufficient and a more extensive investigation will be warranted. In this event, the techniques used will be more specific and will focus on specificity in examination through variations in neurodynamic sequencing.

Decisions on the extent of examination are influenced by many clinical factors that need clarification. In my opinion, a system of deciding on the nature and extent of examination should be applied. This system should take into account the relevant neuropathodynamics and the patient's clinical presentation. Specifically, levels and types, of examination can be applied to different patient problems.

Below is a tiered system of deciding on the extent and kind of examination in the planning of neurodynamic testing. Naturally, not all criteria will occur simultaneously in the same patient and it is the role of the practitioner to choose the most appropriate elements.

Level zero – neurodynamic testing is contraindicated

It seems odd to place a level zero in the context of physical examination. However, this is an important aspect of management of the person with neuropathodynamics because, sometimes, physical examination is simply inappropriate for either physical or psychosocial reasons. A case in point follows.

Clinical case

A young woman who came to see me after being involved in a rear-end vehicle accident. She experienced neck and upper thoracic pain. The patient had been treated by a colleague for twelve weeks, who, at this point, referred the patient to me '... with the view to cervical manipulation'. At the first consultation, the patient was tearful and could hardly speak of her difficulties.

It became clear that a physical examination would be inappropriate until the patient could communicate clearly about them and become more involved in the decision making process. If provocative physical tests were performed at this time, and her symptoms were to worsen as a result, ethical and medicolegal problems would arise because the patient was in no state to offer informed consent. I told her that I was not prepared to examine her until she could communicate more effectively and suggested that she return when she had gathered her thoughts sufficiently. I also suggested that, if it was so difficult to articulate her experiences, she was free to write them down, which I could read at the next consultation. She returned a week later with a large document. One of her concerns was the frustration that she had attended physiotherapy for such a lengthy time, without effect. Interestingly, it was not for several consultations and some discussion that she started to appreciate her responsibility in the problem solving process. Physical examination could only be performed after four sessions, at which time, it only comprised observation of the patient's active cervical and thoracic movement, a limited median neurodynamic test, neurological examination and gentle palpation of the relevant areas. Little in the way of physical dysfunction could be matched with symptomatology and history. Hence, it was decided that a cognitive and activity based pacing program would be the best approach. Seeing the patient once per week, how her pain was occurring and what she could do to alter it was explained. After six weeks, she was markedly improved in pain and was able to function normally in her social life and at work as a clerical officer when, previously, these aspects were compromised. She was discharged with the knowledge that the problem was, for all practical purposes, cured and, if she was not happy with her situation, she could return for further help. This is a case of *not* performing neurodynamic tests on the first consultation and, in any case, to treat with them would have been inappropriate.

Another example that leads to neurodynamic tests being inappropriate is severe pain in which an examination would be too intrusive and provoke the patient's symptoms unnecessarily. Also, it may be inappropriate to perform neurodynamic tests in cases where there is a heavy bias toward psychosocial issues. Any contraindication that exists for manual therapy generally also applies to neurodynamic testing.

Level 1 – limited examination

Description

The level 1 (limited) examination is performed when care not to provoke symptoms is the primary concern. Some of the components of a neurodynamic test may be omitted so that only minimal forces are applied to the nervous system. It may also be necessary to modify the sequence of movements to achieve the desired goals. In the level 1 examination, the full neurodynamic tests are not completed. However, sufficient neural movements are performed so as to gain the information necessary to make a diagnosis and plan treatment, whether treatment be with or without neurodynamic tests. This level of examination is designed to open new and safer avenues for assessment and treatment of the patient with irritable symptoms or pathology. Previously, in this situation, 'neural tension' tests were omitted, partly because of the way they were performed. But now, with increased refinement and using the tests neurodynamically (rather than with respect to tension), the tests can be performed much more safely and deftly than before. Hence, more information can be obtained and gentle treatment can be administered in cases that were previously considered to be futile.

Indications

Level 1 tests are performed

- When symptoms are easily provoked and take a long time to settle after movement. This relates to Maitland's concept of irritability in which irritable problems are treated more gently and with greater caution than non-irritable problems (Maitland 1986).
- When severe pain is present, a complete neurodynamic assessment may not be appropriate for ethical and safety reasons.

- Latent pain – when the patient's symptoms develop some time after physical testing. Latency carries risk because adequate warning of an imminent increase in symptoms does not occur at the time of testing.
- When pathology is present either in the nervous system or the mechanical interface. An example of this would be a severe disc bulge or stenosed lateral recess in which pressure on the nerve root might be elevated and the excursion of a sensitized nerve root may be limited, or its sensitivity increased.
- The presence of a neurological deficit may necessitate a level 1 examination so as not to produce neural irritation.
- When a lasting increase in neurological symptoms is possible.
- When the problem shows a progressive worsening prior to physical examination. This is common in nerve root problems of recent onset.
- Testing of the nervous system should be limited to a level 1 examination, or even not be performed at all, in any cases where it is uncertain that the nervous system will tolerate testing. If performance of a level 1 examination is found to be safe and does not reveal sufficient information, the therapist may then progress carefully toward a level 2 examination, if further information is required.

Method

In the level 1 examination, the therapist performs neurodynamic tests and mechanical tests for the musculoskeletal structures separately. This means that testing is not deliberately biased toward simultaneous testing of the nervous system, interface and innervated tissues at the same time. In keeping with the name 'limited', this kind of examination is restricted to evoking minimal symptoms and generally approaches only the first onset of symptoms (P1) once only. Full range of motion is not achieved. However, this level 1 examination may provide sufficient information about the problem, particularly whether a neural component exists. Structural differentiation can still be performed, however, it takes a modified form.

Modified structural differentiation

In modified structural differentiation, a differentiating tension movement that does not evoke symptoms is usually performed prior to the application of some of the other test movements. The rest of the level 1 test is performed so that, at the first onset of symptoms, the differentiating movement is *released* to produce a *reduction* in symptoms. The differentiating movement then becomes an 'off switch' rather than an 'on switch'. This is instead of performing a differentiating movement that increases tension at the end of the neurodynamic test and so prevents provocation of symptoms.

> ### Clinical example
> As an illustration of the level 1 (limited) examination, contralateral lateral flexion of the neck could be performed as the first test movement for an irritable problem in the median nerve at the wrist. This first movement is not likely to evoke excessive neural tension at the wrist but can be used later in the test for differentiation. The nerves are then taken to the initial onset of symptoms using a remote sequence of movements, then tension in the nerves is reduced by returning the differentiating movement (contralateral lateral flexion) to the neutral position. This way, the changes in symptoms may not only be attributable to the nervous system, but the differentiating movement does not provoke symptoms. Also, wrist and finger movements will be omitted and the key movement could be elbow extension.
>   Hence, the neurodynamic sequence for the above case is as follows:
>
> - Contralateral lateral flexion
> - Glenohumeral abduction/external rotation
> - Elbow extension to the first onset of symptoms
> - Release contralateral lateral flexion – reduce symptoms

Key aspects of the level 1 (limited) examination

- Start in a position of greatest comfort for the patient and/or lowest force on the nervous system
- Perform the technique slowly and carefully

- Only move to first onset of symptoms once
- The technique may not achieve full range of motion
- The therapist may need to alter the sequence of movements to protect the nervous system e.g. start remotely
- The therapist may need to prevent unwanted loading of the mechanical interface and innervated tissues by positioning them accordingly
- Modified structural differentiation is performed (off switch is used)
- To avoid provocation, the nervous and musculoskeletal systems are examined separately

Level 2 – standard examination
Description
This examination consists of use of the standard tests for musculoskeletal and neural structures and, as in the level 1 examination, tests the three key components (interface, neural, innervated tissue) separately. The neurodynamic tests are performed to a comfortable production of symptoms. If sufficient information has been gathered without much in the way of symptoms, all the better. It is not necessary that the tests be taken to their end range but it is permissible, as long as this is clinically appropriate. The neurodynamic position is only held for a matter of seconds.

Indications and contraindications
- The problem is not especially easily provoked and the symptoms are not severe.
- Neurological symptoms are absent, or are only a minor part of the condition, and these neurological symptoms are intermittent, not easily provoked and are stable.
- The problem is stable and is certainly not deteriorating rapidly.
- The pain is not severe at the time of examination, neither is there latency in terms of symptom provocation.
- The level 2 examination is contraindicated when the problem is unstable, hypersensitive, irritable, or when a pathology or pathophysiology that is likely to be provoked by testing is present.

Method
In the level 2 examination, the nervous system is effectively put through its normal paces, but without sensitization movements or specifically combining

neural tests with musculoskeletal ones. The test movements should not evoke excessive pain, neurological symptoms or go into a great deal of resistance.

- Standard neurodynamic sequences are used (outlined in Chapter 7).
- Neural and musculoskeletal structures are examined separately. For instance, a problem with the median nerve at the elbow would involve a test of the median nerve but it would not involve contraction of the pronator teres muscle during performance of the neurodynamic test. Contraction of pronator teres would instead be tested in isolation.
- Movement into some symptoms is acceptable, as long as they are not severe and they settle down immediately after the test.
- A degree of resistance may be encountered. However, it should not be strong.
- Full range of movement may be reached but this is not essential.

Introduction to higher levels of examination

The term 'sensitization' refers to making testing of the nervous system more able to detect changes in nervous system function. Hence, even though sensitization is a generic term that applies to all levels of examination above standard testing (level 2), specific features apply to higher levels that are reflected in the following. Furthermore, it is at level 3 that specific 'types' of examination are applied and these are based on the method of sensitization and the causal mechanisms. Sensitization of neurodynamic tests can be achieved in several ways:

1. Increased magnitude of force applied to the nervous system – in this way, the test under consideration simply applies more tension to the nervous system than the level 2 examination so that detection of some problems may be more effective. The progression from standard testing (level 2) to testing of this level is one of increased magnitude rather than being mechanistically different from the level 2 examination. This higher level of testing is termed the level 3a examination (sensitized neurodynamically). Execution of examination at this level involves adding the known sensitization manoeuvres to standard tests. When compared with the level 2 (standard) examination, the level

3a examination is essentially a more-of-the-same technique.

2. Greater localization of forces is the second progression or type of neurodynamic testing – here, in addition to the forces of standard tests being exerted on the nervous system, they are made more specific and are therefore more localized to the problem site than only applying greater force. This is termed the level 3b (localized) examination and is sensitized by neurodynamic sequencing with the use of a sequence that starts locally. Of course, the forces on the nervous system with examination at this level will not be purely localized to the nervous system, but they may be more localized than with standard (level 2) examinations.

3. Making the forces applied to the nervous system more multistructural – the forces on the nervous system seize the causative mechanisms in many domains. Examination at this level involves the simultaneous testing of the mechanical interface, neural and innervated tissues in varying combinations. As such, it is termed the level 3c (multistructural) examination.

4. In this method of sensitization, the patient's symptomatic position or movement are utilized whilst neurodynamic movements are added to sensitize or differentiate the neural aspects of the technique. This is a level/type 3d examination technique.

It is not always necessary to pass through each type 3 technique (i.e. 3a, b, c and d) because this is where the causal mechanisms are examined more specifically. Sometimes it is acceptable to pass from a level 3a examination to a type 3c or d, as long as this decision matches the clinical features.

Indications and contraindications
- The level 2 examination test is normal, or does not reveal sufficient useful information, and the clinician wishes to investigate the problem more extensively.
- The symptoms are not severe or easily provoked.
- The problem is stable.
- When there is no evidence of pathology that might adversely affect the nervous system.
- In any patient in whom sufficient information has been gained by a level 1 or 2 examination, the

level 3 examination is unnecessary and, I believe, contraindicated.

- The remaining contraindications for the level 3 examination are the same as those of the level 2 examination.

Level/type 3a – neurodynamically sensitized

Description

As mentioned above, the key feature of the type 3a (neurodynamically sensitized) examination is that more neural tension is added to the standard neurodynamic test. A 'more-of-the-same' test is applied through the addition of sensitizing movements to a standard test. For instance, the straight leg raise is sensitized by internal rotation of the hip, which adds tension in the nerves to that which has already occurred with the straight leg raise. Recapitulating, the difference between a level 2 (standard) test and the level 3a examination is one of magnitude.

Method

The level 2 (standard) examination is performed prior to executing one at level 3a. This is to be sure that the nervous system can cope with such testing. The movements applied in addition to the standard tests are those that are known to sensitize the test in question. These are described in the chapter on standard neurodynamic tests.

The sensitizing movements are performed gently in which particular attention is paid to the symptom responses, resistance and range of motion of all the relevant component movements. This is where the mental movement diagram is crucial because subtle changes are usual for this type of examination. It is worthwhile having a good knowledge of all the sensitizing movements for each test so that the clinician can easily move along the spectrum of testing to the most appropriate level of examination.

Level/type 3b – sensitized by neurodynamic sequencing – localized technique

Description

Testing at the type 3b (localized) examination is qualitatively different from previous levels. This is because, rather than attempting to simply add further tension to the nervous system in a 'more-of-the-same'

fashion, the modifications are designed to make testing more specific and localized. As such, testing at this level is a deliberate deviation from the standard sequence. An illustration of this type of sensitization is the straight leg raise in which the patient experiences pain in the posterior buttock. In the event that a standard test does not reveal sufficient information, the sequence of the leg raise can be altered to start with flexion/adduction and internal rotation of the hip. The rest of the test can then be completed with knee extension and possibly dorsiflexion of the foot. Alterations in neurodynamic sequencing are the key feature of the level 3b examination.

Indications and contraindications

The indications and contraindications for the level/type 3b examination are the same as for all level/type 3 assessments (presented in level 3a). The main reasons for testing at level 3b is that level 3a testing did not reveal sufficient information or the nature of the problem suggests that localization of forces to a specific site, with some degree of tension increase, is warranted. For instance a minor carpal tunnel syndrome might be more easily detected with a type 3b test than a type 3a one because the forces of the level 3b testing are more localized to the wrist.

Method

The neurodynamic sequence is modified in such a way as to localize forces on the nervous system and is executed the following way:

Focusing the sequence of movements at the site of the problem (starting locally) – e.g. a minor carpal tunnel problem might require a sequence that commences with wrist and finger extension, followed by the remaining component movements of the median neurodynamic test. Another variable in this area is the firmness of the technique. My research showed that the more firmly the first movement was performed, the more likely the test was to evoke local neurogenic symptoms (Shacklock 1989).

Level/type 3c – multistructural

Description

The type 3c (multistructural) examination is designed to capture the causative mechanisms in multiple domains simultaneously. It is also supposed to be as specific as possible. As such, the key aspect that distinguishes it from the other types of examination is that structures of different *types* are tested at the same time and their influence on the nervous system is assessed. It is true that testing at all the previous levels will also test multiple structures simultaneously but, with this level of testing, the multistructural approach will be more effective because of its design.

The indications and contraindications for testing at level 3c are the same as the other level/type 3 examinations.

Type 3c (multistructural) examinations are particularly used in the person with high expectations in which minor mechanical problems will produce symptoms more easily than in patients whose needs are less extensive. Such patients with advanced needs consist of athletes, sports people and persons who work in occupational settings where high demands are a feature of their activities. However, the type 3c examination is not localized to these people and it may be necessary to take an elderly person with a stiff interface into this level of testing to be sure that all possibilities have been explored.

Method

Type 3c testing is effected in the following way. Combinations of manoeuvres are performed that include simultaneous testing of the interface, neural and innervated tissue structures. In this manner, the dynamics of the nervous system are assessed *in relation to* the interface and innervated tissues, rather than being tested without focus as in the previous levels of examination. For example, the radial neurodynamic test could be applied whilst the supinator muscle is contracted (mechanical interface pushing on the posterior interosseous nerve) and the common extensor tendons and muscles are also stretched (innervated tissues). This type of examination is likely to be more sensitive than testing each structure separately and assesses integrated multistructure dynamics. It is common to also alter the sequence so as to start locally at the site of the problem. Hence, testing at type 3c can also involve the characteristics of type 3b of testing. Skill and specificity, rather than force, are the key aspects of the level 3c examination. Another example is the calf problem in which testing

at level 3b is unsuccessful, such as performing the dorsiflexion straight leg raise without production of an abnormal response. Addition of resisted static plantarflexion to the dorsiflexion straight leg raise can be more effective. This is a case of adding testing to the innervated tissue with the dorsiflexion/straight leg raise whose sequence is altered in favour of the calf muscles.

Level/type 3d – symptomatic position or movement

The type 3d method of sensitizing neurodynamic testing is to perform neurodynamic movements at the same time as the patient adopts or performs their symptomatic posture or movement. It can be nominated by the patient and is analysed in terms of interactions between the interface, innervated tissues and nervous system.

Clinical example – level/type 3d examination

A young man consulted me for treatment of his right-sided low back pain. It was intermittent and mild and the only time it occurred was whilst he drove his car and turned his body to the right to look in his blind spot. The straight leg raise and slump tests at level 2 were completely normal and so were all his spinal movements. Palpation revealed a tender spot over his ipsilateral lumbosacral posterior intervertebral joint. Testing his symptomatic movement revealed a great deal of information. In the bilateral long sitting position, thoracic rotation to the right reproduced his back pain. In this rotated position, dorsiflexion of the ankle and neck flexion increased the pain. This is an illustration of the value of analysing neurodynamics in terms of what is relevant to the patient. Treatment consisted of lumbar rotations with the patient laying on his contralateral side combined with the straight leg raise. The mobilizations reproduced his pain very slightly but it subsided progressively with repeated oscillations. Both retesting the symptomatic movement and driving became asymptomatic after several treatments. The diagnosis in terms of specific dysfunction

> was a reduced closing interface dysfunction with a neural tension component and treatment was directed at both components simultaneously. Treatment at lower levels of extensiveness may have been less effective.

For summary of the progressional system see Figure 6.1.

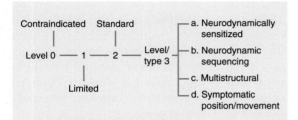

Figure 6.1   Summary of the progressional system for determining the extensiveness and type of technique in physical examination and treatment of neurodynamic disorders.

Standard neurodynamic tests

General points

A set of standard neurodynamic tests should be available for clinical use. These tests ought to occupy the middle ground of testing in terms of extensiveness. Hence, they will be easy and appropriate to perform in all asymptomatic subjects and many patients. The tests that follow from this point are those that I would consider standard ones and occupy the level 2 examination category. What should be borne in mind is that the standard tests can not be performed on all patients but, in the context of learning the essential points in testing, they serve our purposes.

Sequence of movements

The sequences of movements for standard neurodynamic tests vary significantly between authors (Bragard 1929; Chavany 1934; Von Lanz Wachsmuth 1959; Elvey 1979; Kenneally et al 1988; Butler 1991, 2000; Selvaratnam et al 1997). In fact, the best sequence for the standard tests has not actually been established and what follows is largely a result of convention that has emerged over the years. Any preferred sequence will vary according to situational

requirements. For instance, a test that evokes maximum tension at a certain site in the nervous system will be different from one in which the intention is to produce sliding of a nerve relative to a specific interfacing structure. The specific sequences of the standard tests that follow have been derived from cadaveric, clinical and biomechanical observations and materialized for reasons that finally balance simplicity and safety with accuracy and effectiveness. Hence, they tend to be a result of compromises that provide good general application. However, because of this, standard (level 2) tests will not be as specific as neurodynamic sequences that are directed at producing distinct effects in the nervous system.

Level of testing

The standard tests that have been presented in the literature (Elvey 1979; Kenneally et al 1988; Butler 1991, 2000) occupy the level 2 category. This is because they are taken generally toward their end range and all their component movements are applied. In this respect, many of the standard tests in this book are similar to those in the past. However, it is clear that to test all patients at level 2 will not be entirely appropriate. In some cases, the level 2 examination will be too severe and, in others, it will not be sufficiently specific or extensive to detect a subtle problem.

At no stage in this book is it implied that the level 2 examination is the preferred one. However, for learning purposes, it is the best starting point for two reasons. First, the research into normal responses to neurodynamic testing has been performed on young, asymptomatic subjects and was taken to level 2. This means that the known normal responses and ranges of motion have really only been established at level 2, so it is all the clinician has in terms of understanding test responses. The second reason the level 2 examination is the best starting point is that therapists usually learn to perform neurodynamic tests on their colleagues who tolerate level 2 testing quite well.

General points on technique

Explanation to the patient

An explanation of the procedure about to be performed should be offered to the patient prior to testing. This introduces the patient to what is about to happen so they can relax and cooperate fully. If the patient is unsure about the upcoming events, there will be a higher risk of a fearful and protective response, which will contaminate the test. Hence, I suggest that a brief, simple and reassuring introduction be given in such a way as to elicit cooperation. However, it is preferable to omit instruction on the purpose of the test. This is because expectation influences pain and motor control and these aspects should be as neutral as possible prior to, and during, testing. The following instructions are the kind that I would recommend for a standard test.

Clinical example

'If it is alright with you, I'd like to perform some movements on your arm. This helps me evaluate the problem and may or may not produce some mild symptoms. It doesn't matter either way, but I need to know precisely what happens, as it happens. So, without moving your body, please tell me verbally what happens. Do you understand? Now, are you comfortable and relaxed?'

The above instructions contain several essential ingredients; informing the patient what will happen, the gaining of the patient's consent, reassurance and as neutral an approach as possible so that patient's expectations or concerns are not aroused. It is also important that the test evokes mild or moderate symptoms only. This is so that trust in the therapist is maintained and fear not does not enter the test the next time it is performed.

Bilateral comparison

Bilateral comparison of responses to neurodynamic testing is crucial in diagnosis. This provides the opportunity for the therapist to detect subtle changes in neurodynamic tests and establish baseline responses for detection of abnormality. In bilateral conditions, or ones in which the problem is in the midline, the therapist will have to rely on a good understanding of the norm for each test.

Test the unaffected side first

In order to reassure the patient that the neurodynamic testing about to be performed is acceptable to them, the contralateral side can be tested prior to

testing the affected side. This measure also provides the therapist with baseline information to which the responses to testing the affected side can be compared. The particular benefit of this is also realized when it comes to making the diagnosis of the covert abnormal response. By nature, this response is a subtle one such that bilateral comparisons can easily contrast small changes in test responses.

Maintain each movement precisely

As each movement of a neurodynamic test is completed, it must be held stationary whilst the remaining movements are added. It is common for therapists to 'lose a movement' once it has been completed. This reduces the tension in the nervous system, alters the neurodynamic sequence, and is a source of inaccuracy. Hence, unless modifications are performed for specific and deliberate reasons, once a movement is applied, it is normally held stationary for the duration of the test, except when it is a differentiating movement.

Be gentle and do not hurry

It is absolutely essential that the technique is gentle and is not hurried. This helps the therapist perform the test without provoking symptoms and allows the therapist to feel abnormalities in movement more easily, not to mention enhancing trust and cooperation. It also gives the patient an experience of security during the test and offers the opportunity for patients to protect themselves.

Evoke versus provoke

At this point, it is important to make a distinction between the words 'provoke' and 'evoke'. 'Provoke' has a more negative aspect to it and suggests that the consequent pain is more severe and lasts longer than in the latter case. 'Evoke' simply means to produce an effect which only happens to be a short lived creation of symptoms and is a less noxious term. Hence, I often use the word 'evoke' in discussion of tests to emphasize the fact that provocation of symptoms is not the aim of the test. Instead, the aim is to 'evoke' symptoms as part of assessing the response.

Short duration of testing

The technique should not be sustained for long. It is impossible to be absolutely specific about the time tests should take because this variable is influenced by many factors. I would suggest that, at level 2, a test be held at its final point (not necessarily at the end range) for no more than 10 seconds. This would only be to satisfy the test requirements and not for the purpose of sustaining stretch on a neural structure. However, at level 1, holding a test in the provoking position for 10 seconds could be excessive. If sufficient information has not been obtained at this point, it will be necessary to release the test and discuss the events with the patient retrospectively. After discussion, the patient can often be more definite about what happens. In any case, it is better to explain the procedure well prior to its performance so that the patient can participate more effectively and excessive testing is avoided.

Observe the site and quality of symptoms

It is imperative that both the site and quality of symptoms are observed during the performance of neurodynamic tests. The site can be used to determine whether the distribution of symptoms is normal and the quality of symptoms assists in differentiating kinds of normal or abnormal responses. For instance, in abnormal cases, an ache in the lower calf region evoked by the straight leg raise test might not have the same quality as the patient's clinical pain but it might occupy the same location. This is not a normal site for symptoms with the straight leg raise test, so it would, in some cases, constitute a clue as to neural involvement in the form of the covert abnormal response (see Chapter 5).

Perform structural differentiation

Structural differentiation is always performed in diagnosis with neurodynamic tests. For without this procedure, evidence of a neurodynamic mechanism does not exist and testing could produce false positives or false negatives, which would then lead to inappropriate treatment or lack thereof. It is essential also that the technique of structural differentiation be performed with precision.

Use movement diagrams

The use of mental movement diagrams during testing is a key part of manual therapy in general and is absolutely essential in detecting subtle variations in responses to neurodynamic tests. It is even possible that the movement diagram might reveal the only detectable abnormality. For instance, the patient whose supination tightens up more than normal during the standard median neurodynamic test 1 (and this changes with contralateral lateral flexion of the neck) may not report any abnormal symptoms with the test. This is actually quite common. The restriction in supination may be a dynamic shortening in the pronator muscle. Such a dysfunction could constitute a physical abnormality in the test in the absence of any subjective ones and might indicate the need for more specific testing.

Watch for antalgic movements

Antalgic movements are an important part of neurodynamic testing. It is common for patients to perform involuntarily small movements that reduce forces in the nervous system. Ipsilateral lateral flexion is a common one for a tension problem in the nervous system and elevation of the scapula during upper limb neurodynamic testing is another. Other more subtle ones consist of pronation when testing the median nerve or external rotation and hitching of the hip with the straight leg raise test. It is important to be aware of these adaptations and correct for them during testing. For instance, if pronation occurs with median nerve testing, manual correction of the pronation can expose a problem in neurodynamics that could otherwise pass unnoticed. The same applies to testing of the mechanical interface. For instance, in the spine, it is common for a reduced closing dysfunction to show itself by producing contralateral lateral flexion during extension of the spine. The contralateral lateral flexion reduces pressure on the nervous system and, if not corrected manually, may not expose the neural relationships. It is common for patients' peripheral symptoms to be reproduced more readily when such corrections are made. Reproduction of symptoms with manual correction of such deviations confirms the relevance of the compensatory movement.

Qualitative changes in technique produce quantum changes in diagnosis

This statement means that small variations in technique can lead to completely different diagnoses. For instance, if the performance of the structural differentiation component of a test is incomplete, the diagnosis could be that the test response is musculoskeletal. Performing the structural differentiation fully and precisely can result in a change in the response to a neurodynamic one. Another example would be not detecting a small compensatory movement that reduces tension in the nervous system. Prevention of this movement manually will test the neural structures more effectively and can produce a transition from a normal neural response to a covert or even overt abnormal one.

References

Bragard 1929 Die nervendehnung als diagnostisches prinzip ergibt eine reihe neuer nervenphänomene. Münchener Medizinische Wochenschrift 76: 1999–2003

Butler D 1991 Mobilisation of the Nervous System. Churchill Livingstone, Melbourne

Butler D 2000 The Sensitive Nervous System. NOI Press, Adelaide

Chavany J 1934 A propos des neuralgies cervico-brachiales. Bulletin Medicine 48: 335–339. Cited by Frykholm R 1951 Cervical nerve root compression resulting from disc degeneration and root sleeve fibrosis: a clinical investigation. Acta Chirurgica Scandinavica Supplement 160: 70

Elvey 1979 Brachial plexus tension tests and the pathoanatomical origin of arm pain. In: Idczak R (ed) Aspects of Manipulative Therapy. Lincoln Institute of Health Sciences, Melbourne: 105–110

Kenneally M, Rubenach H, Elvey R 1988 The upper limb tension test: the SLR test of the arm. In: Grant R (ed) Physical therapy of the cervical and thoracic spine. Clinics in physical therapy 17. Churchill Livingstone, Edinburgh

Maitland G 1986 Vertebral Manipulation, 5th edition. Butterworth-Heinemann, London

Maitland G 1991 Peripheral Manipulation, 3rd edition. Butterworth-Heinemann, London

Selvaratnam P, Cook S, Matyas T 1997 Mechanical stimulation to the median nerve at the wrist during the upper limb tension test. In: Proceedings of the 10th Biennial Conference of the Manipulative Physiotherapists' Association of Australia, Melbourne: 182–188

Shacklock M 1989 The plantarflexion/inversion straight leg raise. Master of Applied Science Thesis. University of South Australia

Von Lanz T, Wachsmuth W 1959 Praktische Anatomie. Ein lehr und Hilfsbuch der Anatomischen Grundlagen Ärztlichen Handelns. Springer-Verlag, Berlin

Standard neurodynamic testing

7

Standard neurodynamic tests – passive neck flexion, median 1 and 2, ulnar, radial, axillary and radial sensory neurodynamic tests

Unilateral and bilateral straight leg raise, tibial, peroneal and sural neurodynamic tests, slump, prone knee bend test, saphenous, lateral femoral cutaneous and femoral slump, obturator neurodynamic test

Indications, preparation, patient and therapist position, movements, common problems with technique, modified techniques

Sensitizing and structural differentiation movements

Normal responses

TERMINOLOGY FOR DESCRIPTIONS OF TECHNIQUES

Rather than presenting the techniques for neurodynamic testing for the left or right side, terminology that enables the clinician to perform the tests on either side of the body is used. This assists in a smooth transfer of techniques from side to side and enables left handed users to learn their way at first.

The terms 'far' and 'near' are used to denote which limb the therapist uses to perform a technique. Far means the therapist's limbs that are further from the patient and near relates to the therapist's limbs that are closer to the patient. Distal and proximal generally relate to the therapist's hand positions on the patient.

Facing cephalad means that the therapist faces in the direction of the patient's head. Facing caudad means that the therapist faces in the direction of the patient's feet.

PASSIVE NECK FLEXION

Introduction

Passive neck flexion applies tension to the spinal cord on account of the spinal cord being located posterior to the axes of rotation of the cervical spinal motion segments. In doing so, the cervical canal elongates, the canal and intervertebral foraminae open and the neural tissues in the neck are tensioned and slide relative to their interface. The pattern of sliding is not at all simple. In the upper cervical region, the neural tissues slide in a caudad direction and, in the lower cervical spine, they slide in a cephalad direction. Also, the brain is pulled downward toward the foramen magnum. In the thoracic spine, the neural tissues are moved in a cephalad direction and this appears to be similar in the lumbar spine, even though the magnitudes of movement are different in each region. In the lumbar spine, the key effects are an increase in tension and a cephalad displacement in the neural structures (reviewed in Shacklock et al 1994).

Preparation

The patient lies supine with their head on a low pillow and in the midline. The therapist faces the patient side on and places their cephalad hand underneath the patient's occiput, using their palm as the main support. The other hand applies pressure over the upper part of the sternum so that the thoracic spine is prevented from moving during the test. The fingers of this hand are spread out so the contact point is as wide and as comfortable as possible.

Movements

The movement is simply passive cervical flexion to the point to which the therapist has decided to advance. Even though this test is easy in comparison to others, it is important to emphasize good technique. The movement should be precisely in the coronal plane.

Common problems with technique

Deviating from the coronal plane.

Not holding the thorax properly – this allows generalized movement of the cervical and thoracic spines instead of being localized to passive neck flexion.

Pushing too hard or taking the movement into too strong a stretch.

Normal response

The normal response to the passive neck flexion test is pulling in the upper thoracic region at the end of range. It is not normal to experience low back pain, referred pain into the arms or for headache to occur. It is also abnormal for lower limb symptoms to occur with this test. For instance, if pins and needles occur in the feet, the clinician should suspect a lesion in the cervical cord and further neurological evaluation is essential. This would include testing of Babinski's sign, clonus, deep tendon reflexes and sensory and motor function for the central nervous system. Also, medical referral may be necessary.

MEDIAN NEURODYNAMIC TEST 1 (MNT1)

Introduction

The standard upper limb neurodynamic test 1 or, median neurodynamic test 1 (MNT1), moves almost all the nerves between the neck and hand, including the median, radial and ulnar nerves, brachial plexus, spinal nerves and cervical nerve roots. In normal subjects, it evokes symptoms in the distribution of the median nerve (Kenneally et al 1988) because the forces generated by the test are biased toward this structure.

Indications

The MNT1 should be performed when there is a suspicion that a neural component to upper quarter pain or other symptoms is present or when the clinician plans to exclude a neural component. This is particularly relevant in cases where symptoms are localized to the median nerve.

Preparation

Patient position – supine, arms by the side, shoulder flush with the edge of the couch, no pillow if permissible, body straight.

Therapist's position – stride standing, facing cephalad and parallel to the patient with the near hip approximating the bed. The near foot is placed forward.

Hand holds – the therapist's near hand presses on the bed above the patient's shoulder, using the knuckles as a fulcrum. The therapist's fingers then cup gently under the scapula but they are held straight and lie on the bed. At this point, the therapist does *not* apply caudad pressure on the superior aspect of the shoulder. Instead, the therapist focuses on leaning firmly on their knuckles with a straight elbow. This is to create friction between the knuckles and plinth so that prevention of scapular elevation is provided by natural resistance of the therapist's contact on the plinth rather than the therapist having to actively perform scapular depression on the patient. This technique saves energy and increases precision. The therapist may then perform small adjustments in scapular depression with the use of wrist flexion/extension movements (Fig. 7.1).

The therapist's distal hand holds the patient's hand with a pistol grip with the patient's thumb extended to apply tension to the motor branch of the median nerve. The therapist's fingers wrap around the patient's fingers, distal to the patient's metacarpophalangeal joints (Figs 7.2 and 7.3).

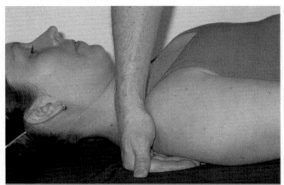

Figure 7.1 Position of the therapist's proximal hand in preparation of the median neurodynamic test 1.

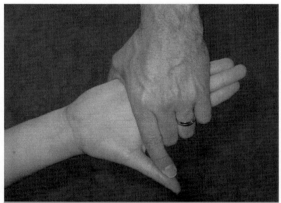

Figure 7.2 Position of the therapist's distal hand in preparation of the median neurodynamic test 1.

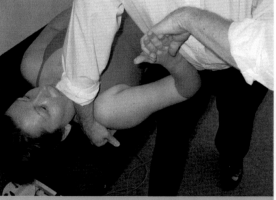

Figure 7.3 Starting position for the median neurodynamic test 1.

Movements

1. Glenohumeral abduction – if permissible, up to 90–110° in the frontal plane. Early forms of this test employed an extension component in which the limb passed posterior to the frontal plane, but this is no longer recommended because this movement is a source of inconsistency and is not actually necessary in order to produce neural symptoms. The scapula is simply prevented from elevating.
2. Glenohumeral external rotation – to available range. This movement is generally ceased at 90° if the patient is very mobile. The reason for performing external rotation immediately after abduction is that all the shoulder movements are completed at the same time.
3. Forearm supination and wrist and finger extension.
4. Elbow extension – the therapist makes sure that this movement does not result in glenohumeral adduction. This is achieved in part by the therapist supporting the patient's arm on their near thigh whilst their knee and hip are slightly flexed.
5. Structural differentiation – selection of the correct movement for structural differentiation is based on where the symptoms are located. If proximal symptoms are to be differentiated, the wrist is released from its extended position. If distal symptoms are to be differentiated, the neck is moved into contralateral lateral flexion. Unfortunately, patients are universally bad at performing contralateral lateral flexion, even when given practice.

Hence, it is often necessary to place the neck in contralateral lateral flexion prior to testing, then ask the patient to return their head to the midline at the final stage of the test. Generally, ipsilateral lateral flexion is not used because of its capacity to produce false negatives in differentiation, since it does not always produce sufficient change in neural tension (Figs 7.4, 7.5, 7.6 and 7.7).

Common problems with technique

The heel of the near (proximal) hand that stabilizes the scapula often pushes in a posterior direction on the front of the shoulder. This should not happen because the therapist's wrist joint should be straight so that the

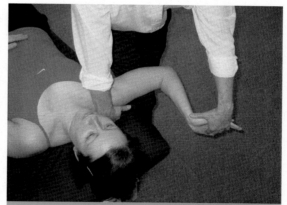

Figure 7.5   Forearm supination and wrist and finger extension during the median neurodynamic test 1.

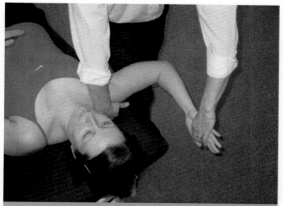

Figure 7.4   Glenohumeral abduction and external rotation during the median neurodynamic test 1.

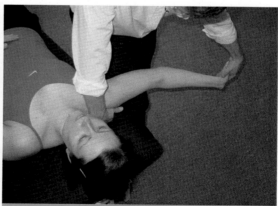

Figure 7.6   Elbow extension during the median neurodynamic test 1.

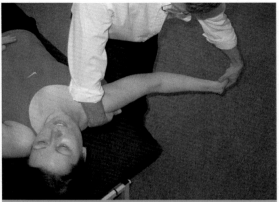

Figure 7.7   Differentiation of distal symptoms with contralateral lateral flexion during the median neurodynamic test 1. In the event that proximal symptoms are to be differentiated, release of wrist extension would be performed.

downward force passing along the therapist's arm produces friction on the bed, thus preventing scapular elevation. Scapular depression is not performed.

Not preventing scapular elevation properly. As mentioned, it is vitally important that the therapist's knuckles bear down on the couch firmly through a straight elbow so that the ensuing friction of the knuckles on the bed is sufficient to stop the therapist's stabilizing hand sliding in a cephalad direction. If sufficient pressure on the couch does not occur, the therapist will be forced to apply a scapular depression force actively which makes the test more demanding and less accurate and often leads to the therapist shaking and becoming tense. It also makes the therapist feel as if they are wrestling with the patient.

Not maintaining the glenohumeral abduction during the more distal components of the test. During performance of elbow extension, the therapist often lets the patient's arm adduct because of lack of support from the therapist's near thigh.

Not controlling the external rotation component during performance of elbow extension – this alters the test and is controlled for by the therapist making sure that elbow extension is performed exactly in the plane of the movement relative to the humerus.

Pulling the patient's hand into ulnar deviation. The therapist must raise their own elbow high enough so

as to make it easy to perform wrist extension in the proper plane as the subject's elbow is extended. Also, lack of elevation of the therapist's elbow tends to move the patient's upper limb into internal rotation, which reduces the effectiveness of the test. The therapist must have in mind the axes and planes of movement for each movement to ensure that the test movements are performed accurately.

Normal response

Symptoms – pulling in the front of the elbow, extending to the first three digits. Sometimes pins and needles occur in the median nerve distribution. These symptoms generally increase with contralateral lateral flexion and less commonly reduce with ipsilateral lateral flexion of the cervical spine (Kenneally et al 1988). Occasionally, a stretching feeling in the anterior aspect of the shoulder can occur (Fig. 7.8).

Range of movement – between −60° and full elbow extension (Pullos 1986).

Modified technique – supported MNT1

In some cases in which more support for the upper limb is needed, it is useful to modify the technique for the standard MNT1. In this procedure, the therapist supports the patient's arm with their own proximal hand by replacing the 'knuckles-on-the-bed' technique with leaning on the bed with the elbow. The therapist's proximal forearm can then support the patient's elbow and upper arm. This may be performed in cases of shoulder instability, severe pain in which control of the technique is important, or if the patient is particularly concerned about pain provocation (Fig. 7.9).

ULNAR NEURODYNAMIC TEST (UNT)

Introduction

The ulnar neurodynamic test (UNT) may be the most difficult of the standard neurodynamic tests to perform and the reason for presenting this test immediately after the MNT1 is that, from the standpoint of the therapist, the UNT follows on more naturally than the other upper limb tests. The UNT

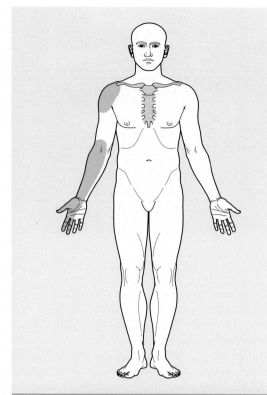

Figure 7.8 Normal distribution of symptoms with the median neurodynamic test 1 (adapted from Kenneally M, Rubenach H, Elvey R 1988. Grant ER (ed) Physical Therapy of the Cervical and Thoracic Spines. Churchill Livingstone Edinburgh). Stretch feelings in the upper limb as indicated occur and pins and needles can eventuate in the first three digits.

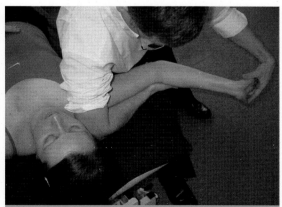

Figure 7.9 Technique of the supported median neurodynamic test 1.

produces a significant bias to the ulnar nerve in addition to testing the brachial plexus and cervical nerve roots. I am not convinced that it differentiates precisely the C8 nerve root from the others. However, it might produce an increase in stress in the lower trunks of the brachial plexus and possibly the more caudally associated nerve roots.

Indications

The UNT is used when symptoms occur in the field of the ulnar nerve, lower trunk of the brachial plexus or the C8-T1 spinal nerves or nerve roots. The corresponding region passes from the anteroinferior part of the posterior fossa, anterior shoulder, axilla, along the medial surface of the arm and elbow to the hypothenar eminence and 4th and 5th digits. Conditions that commonly warrant performance of this test are C8 radiculopathy, thoracic outlet syndrome, cubital tunnel syndrome and ulnar neuropathy at Guyon's canal.

Preparation

Patient position – supine, shoulder flush with the edge of the couch, no pillow.

Therapist position – stride standing facing cephalad, with the near foot forward and the hip next to the patient. The therapist's near hip is positioned against the edge of the couch and is sometimes used as a weight bearing point by the therapist. The proximal hand is cupped under the scapula in a fashion similar to the MNT1. It is imperative that the position adopted by the near arm is maintained. The next step is to take the patient's hand toward the therapist's lateral thigh in a fashion that simulates a 'low five' action in which the therapist's forearm is supinated. This produces a position in which the patient starts the test in elbow extension. The therapist starts in a supinated position with their hand on their thigh with their palm facing outward and clasping the patient's hand. The therapist's fingers are spread out over the patient's fingers and the therapist's thumb is located behind the patient's metacarpophalangeal joints. The reason for starting with this position is that it gets easier as the test nears completion. Other grips are possible but, once the therapist has become familiar with it, I find this the most satisfactory.

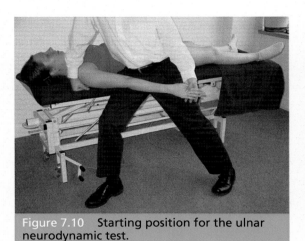

Figure 7.10   Starting position for the ulnar neurodynamic test.

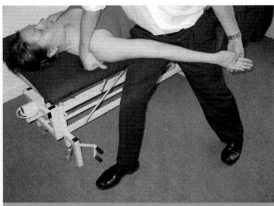

Figure 7.11   Scapular depression during the early stages of the ulnar neurodynamic test.

Joint positions – the patient's arm is straight and abducted as little as possible, and is held in the frontal plane. The patient's forearm is somewhat pronated and the wrist and hand in the neutral position. The patient's limb rests comfortably on the therapist's thigh to stop the arm from falling below the frontal plane (Fig. 7.10).

Movements

1. Shoulder depression – taking up the slack in the nerves and muscles (not stretching)
2. Wrist and finger extension/forearm pronation
3. Elbow flexion
4. Glenohumeral external rotation – at this point, the balance of the technique changes from being mainly initiated by movements of the therapist's distal hand, and the rest of the body being relatively motionless, to the therapist's whole body, particularly the legs, becoming more involved. It is necessary in the preparation of this movement that the therapist take the weight of the patient's arm on the therapist's near thigh so that the arm can be rotated by both the therapist's thigh and distal hand. This will necessitate the therapist standing with their near foot on their tip toes and rocking their thigh about their foot whilst the therapist's distal hand combines to guide the movement. It is useful at this point to practise the rocking movement to produce pure glenohumeral external rotation.

5. Glenohumeral abduction – the therapist will have to alter their position so that a walking action around the patient's shoulder with the therapist's proximal hand as the fulcrum occurs. A shuffle of the feet will naturally occur in which the therapist's back foot takes a small step forward as the therapist's body pivots around the patient's shoulder joint as the subject's arm moves into the abducted position. With practice, stages 4 and 5 can be performed deftly to the point of being a very smooth part of the test. However, it does take practice. This step must be performed smoothly with consideration for the patient. Being the final stage of the test, symptoms can be encountered quite suddenly, so extra care is needed.
6. Structural differentiation – release a small amount of pressure from the scapular depression with a small flexion movement of the therapist's proximal wrist (Figs 7.11, 7.12, 7.13, 7.14 and 7.15).

Sensitizing movements – (a) contralateral lateral flexion of the cervical spine, (b) radial deviation – our recent observations show that a significant amount of proximal movement of the ulnar nerve at the elbow can occur.

Common problems with technique

Not maintaining the scapular depression – this is the most common fault in technique for the UNT. If

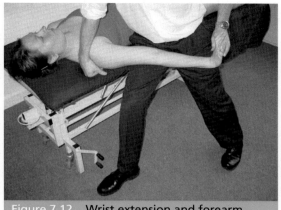

Figure 7.12 Wrist extension and forearm pronation during the ulnar neurodynamic test.

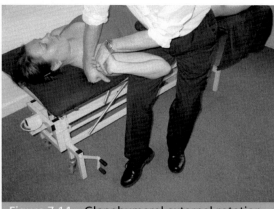

Figure 7.14 Glenohumeral external rotation during the ulnar neurodynamic test.

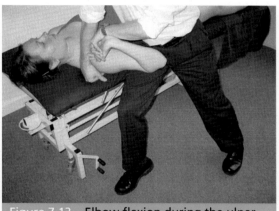

Figure 7.13 Elbow flexion during the ulnar neurodynamic test.

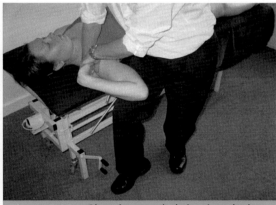

Figure 7.15 Glenohumeral abduction during the ulnar neurodynamic test.

scapular depression is lost, the arm will abduct excessively and symptoms will not be evoked. If insufficient symptoms occur with abduction, it will be necessary to revisit the scapular depression. This may necessitate recommencing the test from the beginning. The problem is usually caused by not being able to maintain the weight on the stabilizing hand (at the scapula) during the abduction phase. This is in turn caused by the therapist not adopting the correct position from the outset.

Performing the abduction component too suddenly – because this is a transitional and difficult part of the test, performance of abduction by the therapist is often coarse. Practising this part of the test slowly, emphasizing the correct starting and finishing positions, is the solution.

Strong symptoms in the hypothenar eminence – this can mean that too much force has been applied to the wrist and finger extension components and, often, radial deviation/pronation of the hand on the forearm are factors. In this case, these movements must be eliminated and the little finger may also need to be released slightly. This releases local neural tension and allows the rest of the test to be completed more evenly.

Normal response

Symptoms – stretch sensations can occur in almost any region of the upper limb, however

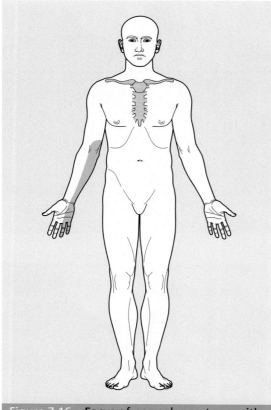

Figure 7.16 Focus of normal symptoms with the ulnar neurodynamic test.

they tend to focus in the field of the ulnar nerve. Pins and needles and burning can also occur. The elbow and wrist symptoms usually change with releasing scapular depression (Flanagan 1993) (Fig. 7.16).

Range of movement – the range of motion of glenohumeral abduction with the UNT varies considerably. With six kilograms of weight on the scapula to produce depression to the first onset of symptoms, the range averages 65° and, at maximum symptom tolerance, the limit can range between 91°–120° (Flanagan 1993). I have observed that generally the normal movement can range from 30° to approximately 90°, however, this is usually at a range short of maximum symptom tolerance.

MEDIAN NEURODYNAMIC TEST 2 (MNT2)

Introduction

Like the MNT1, this version of the MNT2 examines the lower cervical nerve roots, related spinal nerves, brachial plexus and median nerve. The symptoms that arise from this test are from the median nerve also.

Indications

The MNT2 test should be performed when symptoms occur in the distribution of the median nerve, and more particularly when the patient's symptoms are provoked by depression movements of the scapula. This is because scapular depression is a significant part of the test and is likely to emulate the provoking situation. The test can also be used in preference to the MNT1 to protect the shoulder joint by reducing the amount of abduction with the test. The test can also be indicated in cases of recent surgery in the shoulder region (e.g. arthroplasty or mastectomy) in which the intention is to evaluate the nervous system without performing glenohumeral abduction. The test may also be indicated in conditions in which abduction is either contraindicated or impossible (e.g. recent dislocation or instability or capsulitis). It can also be indicated when the aim is to test a specific provoking movement more effectively than with the MNT1.

Preparation

Patient position – supine, shoulder over the edge of the couch, if possible, no pillow. Sometimes the patient must lie diagonally on the couch but be sure to position the head so that it is as close to the midline as possible.

Therapist position – stride standing with the *near* leg forward and facing caudad. Some therapists reverse the foot position, but I find this unsatisfactory because it removes the opportunity for the therapist to support the patient's posterior shoulder region with their near thigh. Also later, this position is better for mobilizing the elbow and wrist with neurodynamic techniques. The anterior surface of

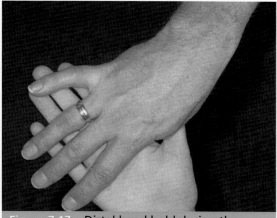

Figure 7.17   Distal hand hold during the median neurodynamic test 1.

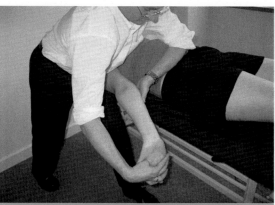

Figure 7.18   Glenohumeral abduction during the median neurodynamic test 2.

the therapist's near hip is positioned against the superior aspect of the patient's shoulder. Caudad pressure on the scapula is *not* applied at this point.

Hand holds – the therapist leans over the patient's arm. The therapist's near hand supports the patient's elbow whilst the therapist's forearm passes over the patient's abdomen (without leaning on the abdomen). The therapist's far hand holds the patient's hand by hooking the thumb behind the patient's metacarpophalangeal joints. The therapist's fingers then spread out over the palmar aspect of the patient's fingers. This hold is crucial to performing the test well because it allows the patient's wrist, fingers and thumb to be extended together (Fig. 7.17).

Joint positions – the patient's arm is down by their side, elbow at 90°, neutral wrist and finger position.

To make sure that the test will work properly, I suggest that, whilst in the starting position, the reader rehearse the following on a colleague:

- gently rock forward and backward, only a few millimetres, to produce scapular depression and reversal
- flex and extend the patient's wrist and fingers and make sure that it occurs well, is controlled and is comfortable for both parties
- the therapist should be able to hold the weight of the patient's upper limb with their distal hand and the therapist's far elbow should be held high so that flexion/extension movements of the wrist

and elbow are in the correct plane. Failure to raise the elbow will produce radial deviation at the patient's wrist joint and is incorrect. Once this has been achieved, the therapist's other (proximal) hand actually does most of the supporting of the patient's upper limb under the patient's elbow.

Movements

1. Scapular depression – gently taking up the slack in the nerves and muscles.
2. Elbow extension to available range.
3. External rotation/supination to horizontal (frontal plane) if permissible. The reason for only taking these movements to the frontal plane is that there is great variation in range of motion of them between individuals, which can be a source of inconsistency between test applications. Taking this measure helps to standardize the test. Furthermore, neural responses are still easily evoked without performing these movements beyond the frontal plane.
4. Wrist and finger extension.
5. Glenohumeral abduction if need be – if the patient's symptoms are positive to structural differentiation at this point, and sufficient information has been obtained, it may not be necessary to carry out abduction. The movement can be particularly uncomfortable, even in asymptomatic individuals (Fig. 7.18).

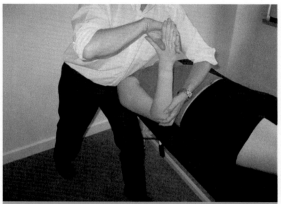

Figure 7.19   Scapular depression during the median neurodynamic test 2.

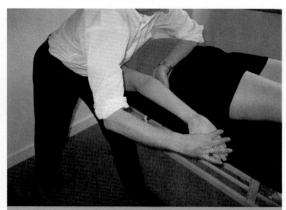

Figure 7.21   Glenohumeral external rotation and forearm supination during the median neurodynamic test 2.

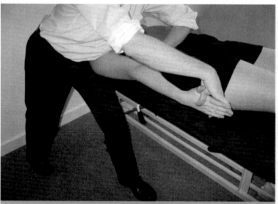

Figure 7.20   Elbow extension during the median neurodynamic test 2.

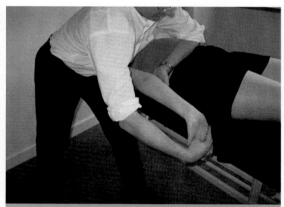

Figure 7.22   Wrist and finger extension during the median neurodynamic test 2.

6. Structural differentiation – the therapist releases a *small* amount of pressure from the scapular depression, *without moving anything else.* The scapula should only move a few millimetres at the most because usually this is sufficient to produce a change in the distal symptom response (Figs 7.19, 7.20, 7.21, 7.22 and 7.23).

   6a. Distal symptoms – use the scapular movements.

   6b. Proximal symptoms – use the wrist and fingers.

Common problems with technique

Not controlling scapular depression. This results in a large amount of glenohumeral abduction being

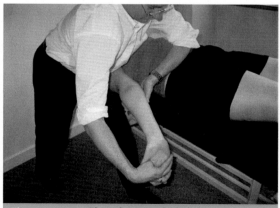

Figure 7.23   Glenohumeral abduction if necessary.

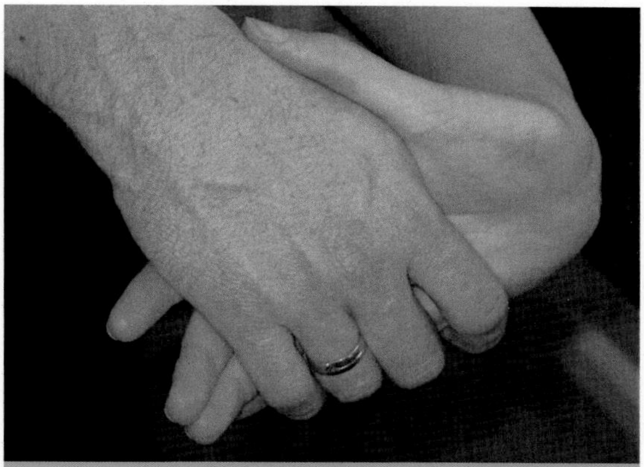

Figure 7.24 Incorrect hand hold during the median neurodynamic test 2.

permissible before the onset of symptoms. If plenty of abduction occurs, the therapist should revisit the scapular depression.

Too much release of scapular depression, creating an excessively gross movement. This is more likely to produce false positives with differentiation.

The therapist does not hold their far elbow high enough so as to perform elbow and wrist extension properly. This predisposes to radial deviation of the patient's wrist.

Not holding the patient's hand properly. Usually therapists place their own hand too far into the patient's. This impairs the therapist's ability to place their thumb behind the patient's metacarpophalangeal joints and spread their fingers over the patient's fingers. It then ends up being a hand-shake grip on the therapist's part rather than a therapeutic one (Fig. 7.24).

Normal response

The normal symptom response to the MNT2 is similar to that of the MNT1. Sometimes pins and needles in the hand and fingers occur. All symptoms typically reduce with the release of scapular depression.

Range of movement – usually full elbow extension and anything between 0° to 50° abduction.

Sensitizing movements – contralateral lateral flexion of the cervical spine.

RADIAL NEURODYNAMIC TEST (RNT)

Introduction

The radial neurodynamic test (RNT) applies mechanical forces to the cervical nerve roots and associated spinal nerves and brachial plexus with the scapular depression component and it is likely that the internal rotation component movement applies further stress to the radial nerve as it spirals around the humerus. The pronation and wrist and finger movements will apply stress to the distal part of the radial nerve. Hence, the resultant effect is a bias of stresses to the radial nerve in the distal regions. It is not currently known whether the RNT differentiates between nerve roots when compared with the effects of the MNT1.

Indications

The RNT is indicated when symptoms in the upper quarter are located in the field of the radial nerve or C6 nerve root. Such problems consist of posterior shoulder pain, lateral elbow pain, dorsal forearm pain related to occupational overuse, supinator tunnel syndrome and de Quervain's disease.

Preparation

Patient position – supine and positioned diagonally, shoulder over the edge of the couch, no pillow. The patient's head should be as close to the patient's midline as possible.

Therapist position – facing caudad, stride standing with the near leg forward, anterior surface of therapist's *near* hip positioned against superior aspect of the patient's shoulder. No caudad pressure is applied at this time.

Hand holds – leaning over the patient's arm (swap hands from the MNT2). The therapist's proximal (far) hand supports the patient's elbow. The therapist's other (distal) hand covers the back of the patient's hand and fingers ready to perform elbow extension and wrist and finger flexion.

Joint position – patient's arm down by side, elbow at 90°, neutral wrist and finger position.

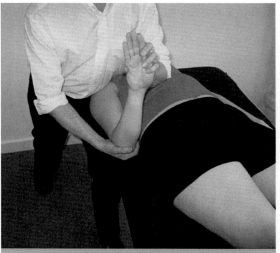

Figure 7.25   Scapular depression during the radial neurodynamic test.

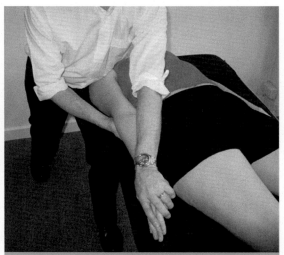

Figure 7.26   Elbow extension during the radial neurodynamic test.

Movements

1. Scapular depression – taking up the slack in the nerves and muscles (not stretching).
2. Elbow extension.
3. Glenohumeral internal rotation/forearm pronation.
4. Wrist and finger flexion.
5. Glenohumeral abduction.
6. Structural differentiation.
    6a. Proximal symptoms – release wrist flexion.
    6b. Distal symptoms – release a small amount of pressure from the scapular depression (Figs 7.25, 7.26, 7.27, 7.28 and 7.29).

Common problems with technique

Failure to maintain scapular depression – as with the MNT2, this will allow more of movement of the other component movements, particularly abduction. It will therefore be necessary to revisit the scapular depression.

Too large a movement during the release of scapular depression – this will predispose to false positive results.

Excessive pressure on the wrist flexion, producing a bias of stress to the wrist joint and associated musculoskeletal structures, and local nerves.

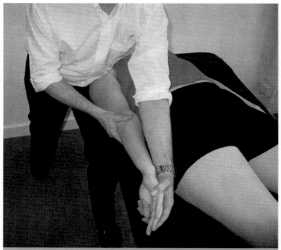

Figure 7.27   Glenohumeral internal rotation and pronation during the radial neurodynamic test.

Using the wrong hand to perform the wrist and finger extension. This produces a bow-stringing effect whereby the far (incorrect) hand bypasses the wrist joint and just pulls the fingers into flexion.

Normal response

Symptoms – pulling in the lateral elbow region, extending into the forearm. Sometimes a stretch in

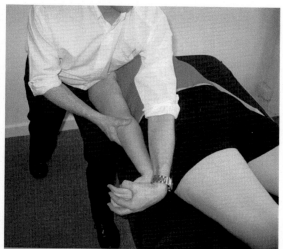

Figure 7.28   Wrist and finger flexion during the radial neurodynamic test.

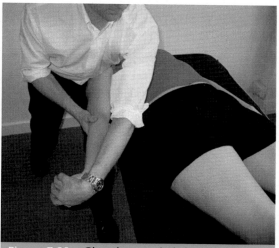

Figure 7.29   Glenohumeral abduction during the radial neurodynamic test.

the back of the wrist occurs. The elbow symptoms almost always change with releasing scapular depression and the wrist symptoms sometimes change with releasing scapular depression.

Range of movement – Yaxley and Jull (1991) found that the mean range of glenohumeral abduction in normal subjects was 40°–45°. However, this can vary considerably in individuals, in my experience, between almost no abduction to 50°.

Sensitizing movements – contralateral lateral flexion of the cervical spine.

AXILLARY NEURODYNAMIC TEST (ANT)

Introduction

The axillary neurodynamic test can place the axillary nerve under significant tension but, in my opinion, the test is often not very specific to the nerve itself. In addition to the possibility that the symptom response in normal subjects may arise from the nerve, it may also be evoked from the local musculoskeletal structures, particularly those that are located around the posterior aspect of the glenohumeral joint. This is because a prominent movement in the test is internal rotation, whereby the movement is taken to the end range in an attempt to make use of the spiral course of the axillary nerve around the posterior aspect of the humerus. Frequently, the muscles of the quadrilateral space show tenderness and thickening in the presence of problems around the posterior shoulder, including those that affect the nerve.

Indications

The ANT can be used to assess symptoms in the posterior and lateral shoulder region when they are suspected to arise from the axillary nerve. The nerve as it passes through the quadrilateral space is the target point of the test because this is where the nerve may become irritated or compressed. Problems with this nerve can develop in activities such as swimming and repetitive throwing actions. Contraction of the muscles that form the quadrilateral space is sometimes the basis for the problem.

Preparation

Patient position – supine, lying diagonally on the couch with the shoulder off the edge, no pillow, as for the RNT.

Therapist position – as for the RNT. With their proximal (far) hand, the therapist holds the patient's arm immediately proximal to the elbow. Their distal hand then holds the patient's distal forearm.

Joint positions – the patient's elbow remains flexed to approximately 30°. This is so that, at the end point of the test, elbow extension can not apply forces to the posterior interosseous nerve which would undesirably bias the test toward this nerve rather than the proximal part of the radial nerve tract. To start with, the glenohumeral joint is abducted as little as possible. The patient's wrist and fingers are left to adopt a neutral position.

Movements

1. Contralateral lateral flexion of the cervical spine.
2. Scapular depression.
3. Glenohumeral internal rotation to the end of available range.
4. Glenohumeral abduction if step 3 does not evoke symptoms.
5. Structural differentiation – release a small amount of contralateral lateral flexion (Fig. 7.30).

The level/type 3c neurodynamic test for the ANT includes resisted contraction of the muscles of the quadrilateral space.

Common problems with technique

Not achieving sufficient glenohumeral internal rotation.

Allowing too much elbow extension. This biases the test to the more distal parts of the radial nerve tract.

Losing the contralateral lateral flexion. If the patient slides on the bed during the scapular depression phase and loses the neck position, it may be necessary to ask them to hold the neck position with their contralateral hand.

Normal response

Symptoms – pulling in the posterolateral shoulder and upper arm region. Not all persons display a response.

Range of movement – approximately 45–90° abduction.

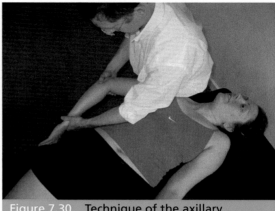

Figure 7.30   Technique of the axillary neurodynamic test.

Sensitizing movements – contralateral lateral flexion of the cervical spine.

RADIAL SENSORY NEURODYNAMIC TEST (RSNT)

Introduction

The RSNT test is a good example of using the innervated tissue to apply tension to a particular nerve and can be very useful in detection of erroneous diagnosis of de Quervain's disease. I have personally encountered a number of patients with this diagnosis who demonstrated evidence of a disorder of the radial sensory nerve. In one such patient, he happened to appear at my clinic on the spur of the moment, immediately after his doctor had anaesthetized the extensor pollicis brevis and abductor pollicis longus tendons in conjunction with injecting steroids. Local numbness was present and no pain could be produced with strong palpation of the tendons. The RSNT reproduced the patient's symptoms and scapular movements altered the response. The possibility of false diagnosis of de Quervain's disease has been reported in which the radial sensory nerve was the cause of the symptoms in the thumb (Saplys et al 1987).

Indications

The RSNT is indicated when symptoms are present in the radial sensory nerve distribution, and more so

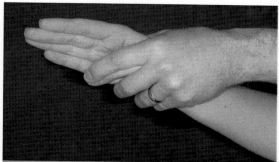

Figure 7.31   Distal hand hold for the radial sensory neurodynamic test.

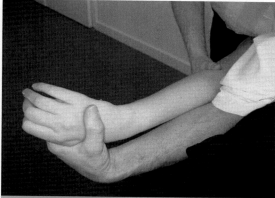

Figure 7.32   Technique of the radial sensory neurodynamic test.

when the symptoms are localized to this region in the absence of proximal symptoms.

Preparation

In relation to the proximal component movements of the RSNT, the preparation is the same as for the RNT. However, the distal components that apply to the wrist and hand are different. They are modified to incorporate flexion/adduction of the thumb and ulnar deviation of the wrist so that tension can be applied to the radial sensory nerve through movement of the extensor pollicis brevis and abductor pollicis longus tendons. Effectively, this combines Finkelstein's test with the RNT. Importantly, wrist flexion is omitted because it does not apply tension to the nerve and will tend to contaminate the specificity of the test because the extensor digitorum muscles will be stretched in addition to the tendons related to de Quervain's disease (Fig. 7.31).

Movements

The movements of the RSNT consist of the following:

1. Scapular depression.
2. Glenohumeral internal rotation/elbow extension/forearm pronation.
3. Thumb flexion/adduction.
4. Wrist ulnar deviation.
5. Structural differentiation – release scapular depression a *small* amount (Fig. 7.32).

Common problems with technique

The most common problem in technique is not taking up the slack in the wrist and thumb movements fully. This does not mean pull hard on the wrist and thumb, but it does necessitate having a good feel for when these structures arrive gently at the end of their available range.

Normal response – the normal response to the RSNT is sometimes an intense pulling, stretching feeling in the region of the distal two-thirds of the radial forearm that spreads into the thumb and sometimes into the web space and into the base of the second digit. The most concentrated part of the symptoms is in the thumb along the line of the tendons that are under tension and sometimes this is the only region of symptoms. The question of whether this is a neurodynamic response is supported by structural differentiation.

Sensitizing movement – contralateral lateral flexion of the cervical spine.

STRAIGHT LEG RAISE (SLR) TEST

Introduction

The straight leg raise test is used to test the movement and mechanical sensitivity of the lumbosacral neural structures and their distal extensions which consist of the lumbosacral trunk and plexus in the pelvis, sciatic and tibial nerves and their distal extensions in the leg and foot.

Indications

The SLR is generally applied in cases of pain and other symptoms in the posterior and lateral aspect of the lower quarter but its use can also be warranted in examination of the thoracic spine because of its potential to produce symptoms in the lower limbs with pathologies such as the thoracic disc protrusion. Heel pain also warrants performance of the SLR.

Preparation

The patient is positioned in supine and their body is aligned symmetrically. In its purest form, the test is performed without a pillow under the patient's head for reasons of consistency. In practice, however, this is often unfulfilled by clinicians because it is impractical. Consequently, if the clinician prefers to use a pillow, I would advocate use of a thin one whose behaviour is highly consistent. In patients who find it difficult to lie supine, clearly, the starting position and technique may be modified.

Movements

The SLR test consists simply of hip flexion with a straight knee. It is important to prevent any variation of the movements in the frontal and transverse planes, namely adduction/abduction and internal and external rotation of the hip. This is because all these movements sensitize the test (for review, see Chapter 3).

The therapist adopts a stride standing position, facing the patient so that the therapist's weight and direction can adapt to the needs of the movement during the technique. Some limbs are heavier and more awkward to handle than others and this position helps the therapist change the technique as necessary.

The therapist's distal hand gently clasps the posterior aspect of the leg, immediately proximal to the ankle. The reason for choosing this position is that some patients experience ankle discomfort if the calcaneum is used at the contact point because the manoeuvre tends to draw the talus anteriorly under the tibia.

The therapist's proximal hand is then placed over the anterior aspect of the knee, either immediately distal to the patella over the tibial plateau, or immediately proximal to the patella over the distal insertion of the quadriceps tendon. These hand positions are chosen to avoid patellofemoral compression and subsequent discomfort.

The limb is gently raised and the symptoms and physical responses are monitored closely. During the actual movement, it is crucial that the therapist prevent any knee flexion because small changes in knee position will produce significant changes in the response and range of motion. Movements of the hip in the transverse and frontal planes are also controlled precisely.

Structural differentiation

Structural differentiation is applied in the following manner:

Proximal symptoms – use dorsiflexion. At this point, the therapist is in a difficult position because no hand is free to move the ankle. Hence, a change in grip is necessary. The therapist turns to face in a cephalad direction, places their near knee on the couch and lays the patient's leg on their shoulder, making sure that the knee remains straight. The therapist's distal hand then moves around the medial aspect of the patient's limb and the other hand holds the foot so as to produce the dorsiflexion.

It is at this point essential to prevent proximal compression of the limb. This is because such a movement produces a rolling motion of the pelvis and moves the lumbopelvic musculoskeletal structures which, in terms of differentiation, is undesirable. Hence, the therapist's proximal hand and arm clutch the patient's limb so as to oppose the proximal forces produced by the dorsiflexion, ensuring accurate differentiation (Figs 7.33 and 7.34).

Distal symptoms – they are probably already differentiated by the event of hip flexion producing distal symptoms. For instance, if the patient reports heel or foot pain with the hip flexion component of the test whilst the foot is held stationary on the leg, the proximal movement has already produced a change in the distal symptoms. Hence, further differentiation is not necessary.

Active cervical flexion

Structural differentiation of the SLR is often attempted by the therapist asking the patient to perform active neck flexion. Unfortunately, this is entirely flawed and can produce a wide variety of false

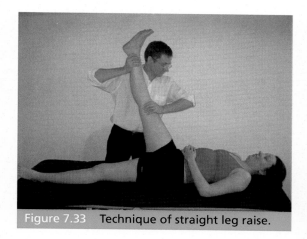

Figure 7.33   Technique of straight leg raise.

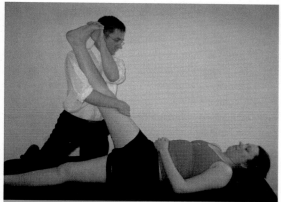

Figure 7.34   Technique of structural differentiation of spinal symptoms with dorsiflexion of the ankle.

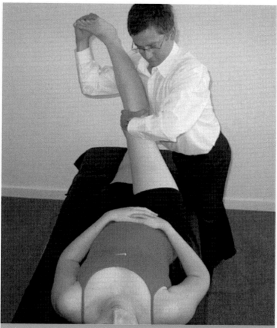

Figure 7.35   Sensitization of the straight leg raise with internal rotation and adduction of the hip joint.

results. The inadequacy of this method is by virtue of the abdominal muscles contracting during the head raise, causing the pelvis to rotate posteriorly. This reduces the hip flexion angle and often reduces the symptoms because of a lowering of the SLR by the mechanism of reversed origin. Conversely, some patients activate their hip flexors which produces an increase in SLR angle by rotating the pelvis anteriorly. On account of the above, active neck flexion in the differentiation of the SLR test is not recommended.

Sensitizing movements

Sensitizing movements for the SLR consist of internal rotation and adduction of the hip. The distal movements that are used to sensitize the SLR make use of

the foot. In these manoeuvres, the foot can be moved into dorsiflexion/eversion (tibial nerve bias), dorsiflexion/inversion (sural nerve bias) and plantarflexion/inversion (peroneal nerve bias). It is not clear whether these tests differentiate specific nerve roots. However, as commented on earlier, this principle may hold benefits for a small number of patients. My clinical experience has been that, very occasionally, patients with a specific radiologically demonstrated nerve root problem can find their symptoms more easily reproduced when the SLR is combined with a specific peripheral nerve test that corresponds with the specific nerve root (Fig. 7.35).

Common problems with technique

Not holding the knee in full extension – note that the technique of holding the knee does not force the knee into extension. It merely stops the joint from flexing. Hence, even though some force can be required, it should not produce pain from knee extension.

Not controlling movements of the hip in the transverse and frontal planes – this produces alterations in sensitization of the test.

Normal response

The normal response to the SLR is pulling and stretching in the posterior thigh that spreads into the posterior knee and sometimes into the upper third of the calf. The range of motion varies between 50° and 120° (Lew & Puentedura 1985; Slater 1988) (Fig. 7.36).

BILATERAL STRAIGHT LEG RAISE (BSLR) TEST

Introduction

The bilateral straight leg raise (BSLR) is an excellent test for producing movement of the spinal cord in the thoracic and cervical regions. This is because forces on both sides of the neural system combine along the cord to produce the movement. Movement of the cord at the level of the thoracic and cervical regions is in a caudad direction and it is likely that, with a BSLR, the tension forces produced in the cord at the higher levels are quite low. It is when the spine is flexed that the forces would increase. Hence, the BSLR is well suited to movement of the middle and upper cord segments, rather than the production of tension in these structures.

Indications

The BSLR is indicated in symmetrical or centrally located spinal conditions, those in the spinal canal and higher up the spinal column, such as the thoracic and cervical spines. A particular focus of the test is to produce caudad movement in the spinal cord. Hence, another indication would be when it is suspected that neuropathodynamics exist in the neural structures in the spinal canal.

Preparation

The patient is positioned symmetrically, in supine and near the edge of the treatment couch. The therapist stands near the patient's ankles and faces across the patient. The therapist places their distal hand under the lower calf region of both legs in preparation for the movement. It is important that the therapist bends their legs so as to get under the patient's legs with their hands to make the lift as easy as

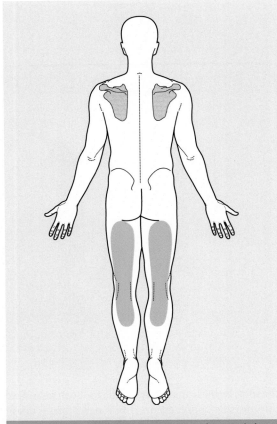

Figure 7.36   Normal response to the straight leg raise test.

Not being able to make the transition from the beginning of the SLR to the end in which the therapist's standing position changes at the middle part of the test. This will necessitate the therapist paying particular attention to altering the weight on their feet and direction of their own body smoothly.

Stopping hip flexion at the first movement of the pelvis – this has been a popular technique in structural differentiation. The idea is that, if the pelvis has not moved, neither has the lumbar spine. Therefore, if low back pain is reproduced, the problem must have a neural aspect to it. Even though the logic for the use of this approach is reasonable, it houses problems. Since the hip flexion angle never reaches full range, the neural structures are also not moved through their full range. This procedure will therefore be prone to producing false negatives.

possible. The legs are then raised only enough for the therapist to place their near knee on the bed under the patient's legs so that the therapist will have enough support and leverage to complete the movement. At this point, the therapist places their other (proximal) hand over the knees of the patient in such a way as to prevent knee extension.

Movement

The movement of the BSLR is simply hip flexion. Because the lower limbs are held together during the test, a bracing mechanism between the two legs occurs which means that the necessity to control internal rotation and adduction of the hips is less than in the unilateral leg raise.

Hip flexion is performed by the therapist arching their body in a cephalad direction around the patient's hip joint and lifting the legs, using their leg that is placed on the bed for support. As the movement progresses, the therapist may have to adjust their foot position to accommodate the change in forces produced by the manoeuvre.

An important idiosyncracy with this test is that it is common for the patient's body to creep surreptitiously in a cephalad direction on the bed. This produces a slight extension of the cervical spine as the patient's occiput sticks on the bed. Hence, it is important to control this sliding by the therapist moving their proximal hand to the patient's mid-thigh region and pressing in a distal direction, particularly toward the end of the test.

Structural differentiation

Bilateral dorsiflexion is the movement of choice for differentiation of spinal symptoms because this movement is a great distance from the more proximal structures. Active neck flexion should not be used for the reasons described in the section on the unilateral straight leg raise test. Also, the trouble with releasing knee extension in differentiation is that the consequent changes in hamstring tension are likely to produce movement in the pelvis and alter the position of the musculoskeletal structures in the region of the spinal canal. Hence, I do not recommend this movement. If dorsiflexion is used, the therapist will have to alter their hand positions accordingly to perform the movement passively and may even have to kneel on

the bed with both knees to support the patient's limbs. As with the unilateral SLR, proximal forces are minimized to make sure that structural differentiation with dorsiflexion is effective.

Normal response

The normal response to the BSLR is commonly pulling/stretching in the posterior thighs. My observation is that the range of available motion of hip flexion is sometimes larger than its unilateral counterpart in the same individual because of the bilateral effects mentioned in the chapter on specific neurodynamics, that is, the dispersion of forces over neural structures on both sides (Figs 7.37 and 7.38).

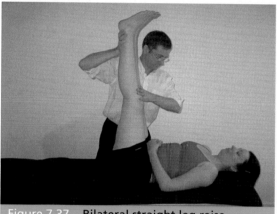

Figure 7.37   Bilateral straight leg raise.

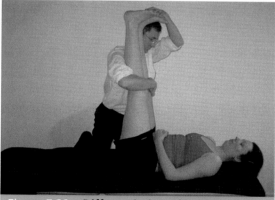

Figure 7.38   Differentiation of lumbar symptoms during the bilateral straight leg raise with the use of dorsiflexion of the feet.

Common problems with technique

Not performing the test precisely in the patient's sagittal plane – frequently, the tendency is to produce lateral flexion of the lumbar spine because the therapist does not move around the patient well enough. The test is actually quite difficult to perform well.

Not controlling the slide of the patient's body in a cephalad direction.

TIBIAL NEURODYNAMIC TEST (TNT)

Introduction

The tibial neurodynamic test is a variation on the straight leg raise in which the forces on the nervous system are biased toward the tibial nerve. Based on the distal course of the nerve in the lower limb, the movements of the TNT consist of the straight leg raise and dorsiflexion/eversion of the ankle and foot. This applies direct tension to the nerve as it passes around the posteromedial surface of the ankle joint and enters the foot through the posterior tarsal tunnel as the posterior tibial nerve (biomechanics reviewed in Chapter 3).

Indications

The TNT is indicated in patients whose symptoms are located in the distribution of the tibial nerve and its extensions, which consist of the posterior tibial nerve (at the ankle), medial calcaneal nerve and the plantar and digital nerves. Hence, calf pain, heel pain (including plantar fasciitis) and pain in the plantar aspect of the foot are cases in which the test would be indicated.

Preparation

The patient is positioned as in the straight leg raise test. Facing caudad, the therapist stands with their feet wide apart so that, when the transfer of weight from their distal foot to their proximal foot occurs, the therapist will be able to complete the test without having to walk toward the final stage.

The therapist's distal hand reaches around the lateral surface of the foot, under the sole so that the fingers pass as far as possible around to the medial and dorsal surface of the foot. The thumb trails by holding the lateral side of the foot. This ensures a clasping action for ease of movement later in the technique and encourages the therapist to initially lean their whole body in a distal direction. If this leaning action does not occur, it will be difficult to execute all the movements without making significant changes in foot position toward the latter part of the technique, which produces an undesirable jump in the manoeuvre. This is a good example of starting in a difficult position so that the therapist can finish in an easy one (Fig. 7.39).

The therapist's proximal hand controls the knee movement in the same way as in the straight leg raise.

Movements

The first movements of the TNT (dorsiflexion/eversion) are executed at the foot, followed by the straight leg raise. The leg raise is produced as the therapist straightens their body and uses their distal arm to produce the movement. Generally, little movement of the therapist's hands should occur on the patient's skin. If undue slipping occurs, it will be necessary to modify the technique to prevent this. The key here is to make sure that the distal hand has a good hold on the foot so that this hand can initiate and control the straight leg raise movement. For it is this hand that does most of the work, both in the patient's foot and hip movements. As the proximal hand prevents the knee flexion, it will tend to compete with the distal

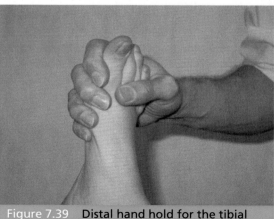

Figure 7.39   Distal hand hold for the tibial neurodynamic test.

hand, so good technique and efficiency on the therapist's part are important (Figs 7.40 and 7.41).

Common problems with technique

Not standing with the legs far enough apart – this reduces the therapist's ability to transfer their weight from foot to foot. It also creates more work for the therapist and impedes their ability to follow the patient's natural movement patterns.

Not holding the patient's foot correctly – the foot hold is actually quite difficult because much of the limb's weight is carried through this hand. Hence, it

is worthwhile practising the grip so that it is both comfortable for the patient and clinically effective.

Not holding the knee in extension properly – with the difficulty of holding the foot, it is common for therapists to release the knee extension, simply due to loss of concentration.

Normal response

My observation is that the normal response for the TNT is stretching in the calf region and this often extends into the medial aspect of the ankle and plantar surface of the foot, also behind the knee. It is often more distally focused than with the straight leg raise. The range of straight leg raise is usually between 45° and 80°. When performed effectively, the leg often can not be raised as much as the standard straight leg raise test in the same individual (Fig. 7.42).

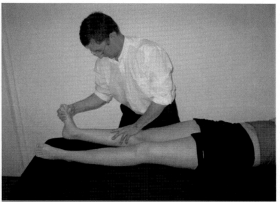

Figure 7.40   Starting position for the tibial neurodynamic test.

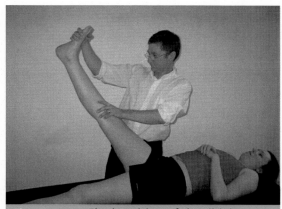

Figure 7.41   Final position of the tibial neurodynamic test. Note that the therapist has simply leaned backwards and hinged their body around the patient's hip joint.

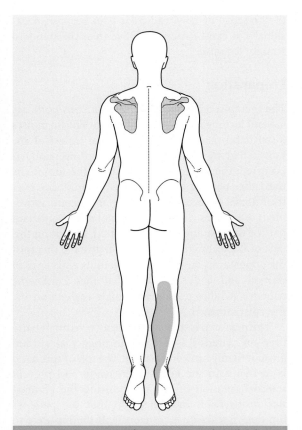

Figure 7.42   Normal response to the tibial neurodynamic test.

PERONEAL NEURODYNAMIC TEST (PNT)

Introduction

The PNT is used to examine the mechanical function and sensitivity of the peroneal part of the nervous system. It focuses primarily on the common peroneal and superficial peroneal nerves because they pass anterolaterally along the leg and ankle joint and are therefore loaded with the PNT. The test focuses less on the deep peroneal nerve because this nerve does not extend far laterally over the ankle joint and is more likely to be loaded with straight plantarflexion with the straight leg raise.

Indications

The PNT is indicated in conditions that affect the anterolateral leg and ankle and dorsal foot areas. The therapist should also be willing to use this test in the presence of L4–5 radicular pain because, occasionally, it can be more sensitive than the standard straight leg raise.

Preparation

The therapist adopts a stride standing position, facing and leaning in a caudad direction. The therapist's distal hand passes under the plantar aspect of the foot so that, by the time plantarflexion/inversion has occurred, the fingers can come over the top of the toes, after passing distally and wrapping back over their dorsal surface. This is important because movement of the toes (innervated tissue) is an important part of the test and is often omitted. Executing this part of the technique properly will give the therapist the opportunity to take the nerve to its end range of motion and will necessitate that they cradle the patient's Achilles tendon and ankle regions on the therapist's forearm.

The next step is to place the near (proximal) hand over the anterior aspect of the tibial plateau and grasp it firmly but comfortably. The job of this hand is to maintain the knee in extension and prevent internal rotation of the tibia during the plantarflexion/inversion movement so that the patient's hip does not rotate extraneously. If the hip were to rotate inwards, the accuracy of the test would be compromised (Fig. 7.43).

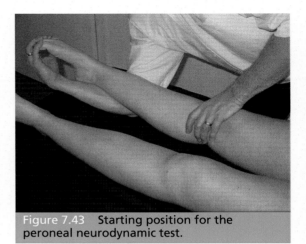

Figure 7.43   Starting position for the peroneal neurodynamic test.

Movements

The movements of the PNT consist of plantarflexion/inversion of the ankle, foot, and toes, followed by the straight leg raise. Generally, the foot movements are often completed in the preparation of the technique because of the way the hand holds work. Remembering that this is a standard test that takes the nerves and musculoskeletal structures to their end range, it may alternatively be necessary to limit the test on patients with sensitive problems. In this case, the technique will be modified accordingly.

The leg raise component movement is performed by the therapist's distal arm, such that the main weight-bearing surface is the therapist's distal forearm. This means that the therapist will have to transfer their weight from their front (distal) foot toward their back (proximal) foot so that the movement hinges around the patient's hip joint during the straight leg raise movement.

Common problems with technique

Not holding the foot correctly – in this case, the movements of the foot will be insufficient in amplitude or they may deviate into too much plantarflexion relative to the inversion.

Not using the distal forearm to produce the straight leg raise (hip flexion) component – this will make it difficult to raise the leg without losing control of the foot movements.

Not fixating the tibia on the femur – this results in internal rotation of the entire lower limb, which, although it may be used to sensitize the test, is an extraneous movement for the standard one.

Normal response

The normal response to the PNT is stretching/pulling in the anterolateral leg and ankle and dorsum of the foot. When it does not extend the whole length of this area, it can occupy patches that are within the distribution of the peroneal nerve (Slater 1988; Mauhart 1989; Shacklock 1989) (Fig. 7.44).

Sensitizing movements – contralateral lateral flexion of the lumbar spine, addition of the slump test, internal rotation and adduction of the hip joint.

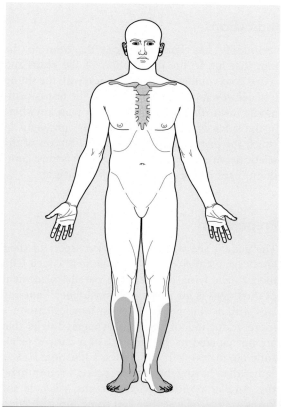

Figure 7.44   Normal response to the peroneal neurodynamic test.

SURAL NEURODYNAMIC TEST (SNT)

Introduction

The sural neurodynamic test (SNT) is used to examine for mechanical dysfunction and mechanosensitivity of the sural nerve. Since this nerve passes along the posterolateral aspect of the leg, foot and ankle, it is tensioned by dorsiflexion/inversion, followed by the straight leg raise. It can be involved in sprained ankle, especially when the injury is severe.

Indications

The SNT is indicated when symptoms appear in the posterolateral leg, ankle and foot. Conditions in which this is particularly relevant consist of sprained ankle, S1 radiculopathy, cuboid syndrome and peroneal tendonitis.

Preparation

The hand holds for the SNT test are opposite to the PNT in that the therapist's distal and proximal hands are swapped over. Facing the patient transversely, the therapist stands with their legs wide apart and leans in a distal direction. This is so that the hand that controls the foot (near hand) can clasp the foot around the medial aspect of the foot as the fingers pass underneath to its lateral aspect around the fifth metatarsal and cuboid regions (Fig. 7.45).

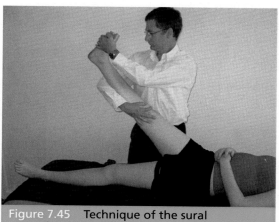

Figure 7.45   Technique of the sural neurodynamic test.

Simultaneously, the other hand cradles the patient's leg as the therapist's upper limb wraps under the calf and their hand passes proximally and medially around the patient's leg to clasp the knee on the anterior aspect of the tibial tuberosity. This is a reaching and spiralling action, much like the radial nerve around the shaft of the humerus. In this fashion, the therapist is in a position to fix the knee in extension by applying pressure over the tibial plateau in a posterior direction. The therapist's arms cross over during the establishment of this hold.

Movements

The first movement is dorsiflexion/inversion. When the slack in this movement has been taken up, the foot is held still on the leg whilst the straight leg raise movement is produced by the therapist straightening their trunk from the leaning position and moving their body around the patient's hip joint. Completion of the test involves wide amplitude of movement on the therapist's part in which their weight is transferred from their distal foot toward their proximal foot.

Common problems with technique

Not holding the knee properly – this enables the knee to flex slightly, which compromises the sequence of movements and reduces the effectiveness of the test.

Not moving around the patient's hip joint – this means that the limb will tend to abduct and, again, the effectiveness of the test is reduced. To correct this, it is essential to start by standing with the legs wide apart, leaning around the patient and being prepared to transfer weight from foot to foot.

Normal response

The normal response to the SNT is a pulling/stretch in the posterolateral ankle region and sometimes this spreads into the posterolateral aspect of the calf (Molesworth 1992). My observation is that the range of motion of hip flexion with this test in normal subjects is slightly smaller than the standard straight leg raise and is usually between 30°–60° (Fig. 7.46).

Sensitizing movements – contralateral lateral flexion of the lumbar spine, addition of the slump test, internal rotation and adduction of the hip joint.

SLUMP TEST

Introduction

The slump test is used to evaluate the dynamics of the neural structures of the central and peripheral nervous systems from the head, along the spinal cord and sciatic nerve tract and its extensions in the foot. It is a complex test and is often over simplified, misunderstood and misinterpreted. In the past, the general technique has been to lower the head and straighten the leg whilst the patient is in the sitting position. If the patient's pain is reproduced, the test is abnormal. The problem with this is that it does not take into account subtleties that should be applied in order to gain the most from the test and offer the patient an accurate diagnosis. By this, it is meant that sensitivity and attention to detail in both technique and interpretation are crucial in effective application of the test.

Indications

Technically, any symptom from the head to the foot that lies in the distribution of the brain and spinal cord could warrant evaluation with the slump test! However, conditions in which the test is commonly justified consist of headache, pain anywhere in the spine or pelvis and lower limb problems in which the pain is located in the distribution of the sciatic nerve and its extensions. The test is most commonly used in assessment of the lumbar spine.

Preparation

The patient sits with the posterior aspect of their knees against the edge of the treatment couch with their thighs lying parallel. The parallel placement of the thighs is for reasons of consistency. Tapering legs with a wide pelvis (often in females) produce more adduction of the hips, whereas thighs that are not tapered in the presence of a narrow pelvis (often in males) will produce less adduction. Hence, rather than having the knees apposed, I recommend the parallel position of the thighs. Also, if the knees are placed together and some hip adduction occurs, the test will have been sensitized somewhat (Sutton 1979).

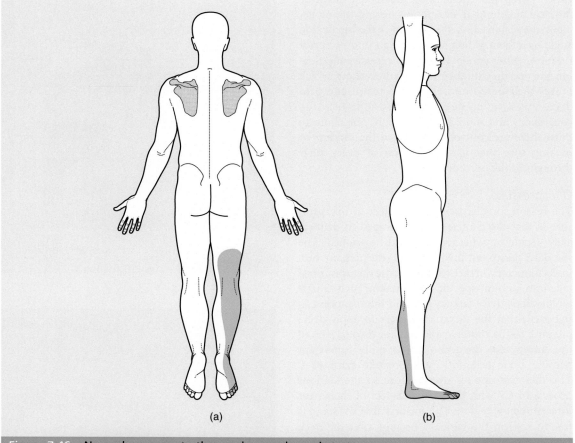

(a)   (b)

Figure 7.46   Normal response to the sural neurodynamic test.

Movements

1. Thoracic and lumbar flexion (slump component)

Thoracic and lumbar flexion are performed by the patient as a slump manoeuvre. Manual over-pressure during this component of the test is in the direction of thoracic and lumbar flexion and is applied between the C7 spinous process and the hip joint. This is to reduce the vertical distance between these two points in a bow-string fashion.

A question at this point is whether the therapist kneels on the couch. It is entirely optional, however, I prefer not to because the test movements can be controlled better with two feet on the ground. This will also offer the therapist the ability to guide the patient's foot movements with more precision which is especially important when treating the tall patient or when the therapist is particularly short. I am a short person and have easily treated a basketball player the height of 7 foot 2 inches with the slump test. Nevertheless, it is worthwhile practising the slump test with both approaches so that the contrast between kneeling on the bed and not doing so can be appreciated. If the therapist wants to get closer to the patient and still control limb movements optimally, they can lean their near hip on the couch and spread their own legs further apart to take account of both spinal and limb movements.

Another part of the thoracic and lumbar flexion component of the slump test is to control the angle of the pelvis relative to the femurs. Patients tend to either slump inadequately by producing too little thoracic and lumbar flexion, or, during the movement, they fall backwards and reduce the hip flexion angle by allowing their sacrum to go into posterior rotation. Other patients lean into excessive hip flexion and end up with their nose on their knees, which moves their pelvis into anterior rotation and produces excessive hip flexion. These are problems of consistency and should be dealt with. The clinician must therefore control the angle of the sacrum by making sure that it stays vertical at every stage throughout the procedure (Fig. 7.47).

Overpressure

The reason for discussing the subject of overpressure is that the clinician is encouraged to deliberately decide on whether it should be applied. The standard slump test involves mild overpressure but, in deciding on whether to apply it, the therapist must take into account specific information, such as irritability, sensitivity, latency and contraindications. In the event that the therapist decides to apply overpressure to the thoracic and lumbar flexion part of the slump test, the technique is quite important because poor technique will provoke symptoms. The therapist applies overpressure to the spinous process of C7 with the medial aspect of their near forearm/elbow region. This ensures that the hand is free to rest on the patient's occiput after the neck flexion phase. Using the medial forearm/elbow also enables the therapist to apply different amounts of pressure at C7 and the occiput, depending on the choice of technique, and to release pressure from the patient's head whilst maintaining steady pressure on C7. The direction of the overpressure is from C7 to the hip joints so as to reduce the distance between these cephalad and caudad points (Fig. 7.48).

2. Cervical flexion

Cervical flexion is performed by the patient slowly lowering their head toward their chest. So that provocation of symptoms is avoided, the therapist places their far hand on the patient's forehead and controls the speed and amplitude of neck flexion. On completion of the movement, the range of motion (determined by prior clinical reasoning) is maintained by the therapist changing their hand position so that the palm of the near hand rests gently on the patient's occiput. The hand that controlled the cervical flexion

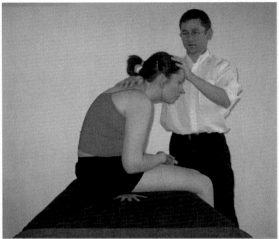

Figure 7.47   Slump test stage 1 – correct sacral position whilst in thoracic and lumbar flexion (vertical).

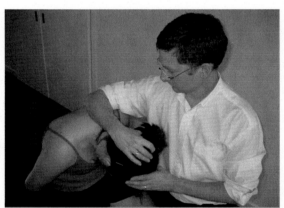

Figure 7.48   Slump test stage 2, cervical flexion with pressure exerted on the C7 spinous process with the therapist's medial proximal forearm. The therapist also gently palpates with their hand to assess the tendency of the neck to return from the flexed position.

(far hand) is thus freed to deal with the lower limbs. Importantly, the action of the hand that lies over the patient's occiput is one of *preventing release* of cervical flexion rather than applying overpressure into flexion. Usually, sufficient information can be obtained without performing overpressure. For this reason, overpressure to cervical flexion should not be part of the standard slump test (Fig. 7.48).

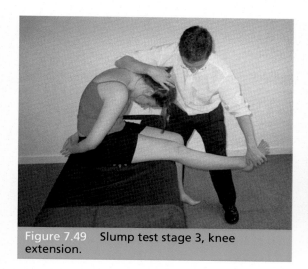

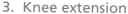

Figure 7.49   Slump test stage 3, knee extension.

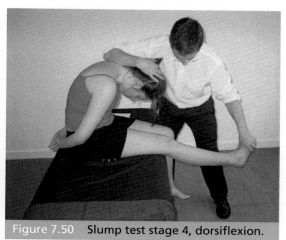

Figure 7.50   Slump test stage 4, dorsiflexion.

3. Knee extension

The knee extension phase of the slump test is performed either by the patient actively extending the knee or by the therapist producing the movement passively. Whether knee extension is performed actively or passively is at the therapist's discretion and will vary between patients. However, I suggest a combination of both. In the end, the imperative is for the therapist to have a good understanding of the relationships between each dimension.

In the performance of knee extension, the therapist holds the patient's ankle, which is the easy part. The difficult part of this manoeuvre is to hold the rest of the patient's body still so that extraneous movements do not occur. This necessitates the therapist holding their near hand and medial forearm on the patient's occiput and C7 spinous process precisely in the same position throughout the latter stages of the test (Fig. 7.49).

4. Dorsiflexion

Dorsiflexion of the ankle is the final component movement of the standard slump test and applies tension to the lumbosacral nerve roots through the sciatic and tibial nerves. It helps to establish whether the problem occurs in a distal or proximal direction, but, more importantly, it is useful in differentiation of lumbar symptoms.

The method of producing dorsiflexion is simply to reach forward and downward, hold the foot with the whole of the therapist's distal hand and make the movement. It is essential to make sure that the

movement is performed efficiently because, like the knee extension component, extraneous movements of other components of the test will occur and predispose to imprecision (Fig. 7.50).

5. Structural differentiation

If proximal symptoms (e.g. lumbar) are evoked by the slump test, the distal movements, such as release and reapplication of dorsiflexion, are used. These symptoms can also be differentiated by releasing cervical flexion.

The main point with releasing cervical flexion is that the rest of the patient's body must not move. As such, the therapist takes their hand from the patient's occiput so that cervical flexion can be released. This tempts the therapist into also altering the pressure of their medial elbow region on the patient's C7 spinous process. The pressure must stay constant because to alter it would be to alter the thoracic and lumbar flexion components and produce movement in the lumbosacral region. Naturally, this is undesirable. The movement of removing the therapist's hand from the patient's occiput is made by the therapist extending their elbow to take their hand out of the way of the rising head (Fig. 7.51).

Normal response

It must be borne in mind that the normal response to the slump test was established for the above sequence and it is likely that this response will vary with changes in the sequence.

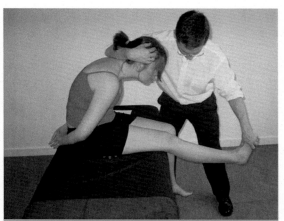

Figure 7.51   Slump test stage 5, structural differentiation with release of neck flexion. Note that the cephalad hand position is changed to permit the neck to return from flexion whilst still keeping the overpressure on C7 stable.

Seated position – no symptoms.

Thoracic and lumbar flexion – stretching in the mid-thoracic region.

Knee extension – stretching in the posterior thigh and knee regions which can extend to the upper calf. During knee extension, the stretching in the mid thoracic region can increase or decrease, or not change. The range of knee extension can be full, however it can fall short by up to 30° in normal subjects. These people are often naturally stiff and have been for a long time.

Dorsiflexion – produces an increase in the posterior thigh and knee symptoms.

Release neck flexion – this movement produces a reduction in the posterior thigh and knee symptoms and the available range of motion of knee extension and dorsiflexion increases (Maitland 1979, 1986; Butler 1985).

Sensitizing movements – contralateral lateral flexion, hip internal rotation and adduction, foot movements for each peripheral nerve.

Common problems with technique

Not being aware of the importance of maintaining a vertical position of the sacrum – this leads to inconsistency in technique between test applications, both within the same therapist and between therapists.

Pressing too hard on the cervical flexion – the aim of this part of the test is to *feel* what the neck is trying to do, rather than press on it or stretch the nervous system. Is the head trying to rise, or is the neck soft and relaxed in this position? This is particularly relevant to patients with covert abnormal responses, discussed in Chapter 5.

Not controlling sideways forces on the patient – during the performance of the test, it is easy to lose focus on the movements and positions that have already been produced. For instance, when reaching for the foot, it is common for the therapist to not adjust their posture sufficiently to prevent lateral flexion or asymmetrical pressure on the patient's buttocks. These movements are a source of inconsistency and will contaminate the test.

Too vigorous a technique – generally, as the therapist's technique improves, the need for force reduces, the patient's symptoms are not provoked and the test becomes more acceptable to the recipient.

Not isolating the release of neck flexion during structural differentiation to movement of the cervical spine. With this problem, the therapist inadvertently lets the thoracic spine, and sometimes the lumbar spine, move into extension, which makes the differentiation inaccurate by increasing the likelihood of false positive results. In extreme cases, the pelvis also moves.

Altering the amount of compression of the thoracic and lumbar spines.

PRONE KNEE BEND (PKB)

Introduction

The prone knee bend (PKB) is used to test the movement and sensitivity of the mid-lumbar nerve roots and the femoral nerve. It is a good example of making use of the innervated tissues to produce a neurodynamic test and this is achieved by applying tension to the quadriceps muscle with movement of the knee into flexion.

Indications

The PKB is indicated in cases of low back pain and symptoms that follow the course of the femoral nerve. This includes the inguinal and hip regions and cases of thigh and knee pain.

Preparation

The patient is positioned symmetrically in prone, preferably making use of a hole in the couch for the face so that cervical rotation does not occur. If a face hole is not available, the patient can place their hands under their forehead. The thighs are positioned parallel so that adduction and abduction are neutralized.

Movements

The movement in the PKB is simply passive knee flexion. Even though the clinician seeks a report of the onset, characteristics and behaviour of the symptoms during the test, other observations are made. These consist of taking note of when and how the pelvis and spine move. Frequently, the movements differ from those that occur on the asymptomatic side and relate to the clinical problem. Sometimes slight lumbar ipsilateral lateral flexion occurs but, more commonly, the point of commencement and speed of lumbopelvic movements are asymmetrical. Even though it can show physical deviations, the PKB does not always evoke any abnormal symptoms. This means that the clinician must rely on additional more sensitive testing to ascertain the significance of the findings. A key aspect of further investigation involves structural differentiation.

Structural differentiation

Differentiation of involvement of the femoral part of the nervous system can be achieved with spinal movements. However, this incorporates the slump test and is not strictly the PKB. Hence, the following illustrates differentiation of the PKB without use of spinal movements.

What is often missed about the PKB in *back pain* is that, in its usual form, it does not differentiate involvement of the nervous and musculoskeletal systems. The reason for this is that the test applies tension to the rectus femoris muscle which, through its attachment to the ilium, results in anterior rotation of the pelvis and extension of the lumbar spine. This naturally moves the intervertebral discs, posterior intervertebral joints, muscles and neural structures and, at this point, is not at all specific. Some clinicians are aware of this and take this problem into account by only moving the knee flexion to the point where movement of the pelvis and lumbar spine commence. If back pain occurs prior to commencement of pelvic movement, the test is deemed to be positive for the neural structures. Clearly, even though this approach is a good attempt to solve the problem of differentiation, it is still incomplete for two reasons. First, movement of musculoskeletal structures could pass unnoticed and produce a false positive result. Second, the knee movement up to this point may not be sufficient to move the neural structures to their end range. Hence, the approach will also be prone to producing false negatives and is likely to exhibit low sensitivity and specificity. I therefore propose that the PKB be applied in a way that addresses these issues in structural differentiation.

Step 1

Step 1 involves the knee bend component in isolation. This produces movement in all the lumbopelvic structures and does not differentiate. In the event that low or mid-lumbar back pain occurs and must be differentiated, step 2 is performed.

Step 2

The second step is to prevent pelvic movement manually whilst repeating the knee flexion. This reduces the likelihood of a skeletal source of pain because the lumbopelvic structures are held stationary, or they move less than in the previous movement at step 1. If back pain occurs with step 2, when it did not with step 1, or the pain is more severe, evidence of neural involvement is constituted. Hence, an increase in back pain with reduction of lumbopelvic movement between the two tests suggests neural involvement.

Step 3

The third step is to return the limb to the neutral position and apply the same pressure over the sacrum as in step 2 but this time in isolation. If no pain occurs with this it can be concluded that the increase in symptoms with step 2 was not due to pressure on the local musculoskeletal structures (Figs 7.52 and 7.53).

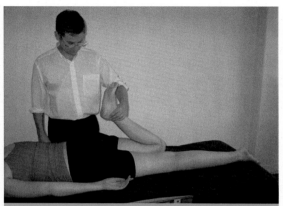

Figure 7.52   Prone knee bend, step 1. Note that no stabilisation of the pelvis is performed.

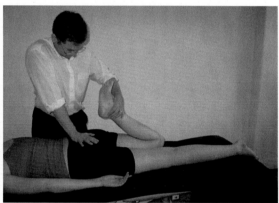

Figure 7.53   Prone knee bend, step 2 with pelvic stabilisation, producing a bias to the neural structures. Step 3 is to repeat the pressure over the pelvis with the lower limb returned to the neutral position.

Normal response

The normal response for the PKB is most commonly stretching in the anterior thigh region and the limit in range of motion of knee flexion is generally between 110°–150°. Variation in range of motion exists, highlighting the importance of bilateral comparison (Davidson 1987).

Sensitizing movements

Hip extension – this movement can be added to the PKB in sensitizing the test. This produces greater strain in the quadriceps muscle and theoretically places more force on the femoral nerve and its proximal extensions. It will therefore evoke thigh symptoms more readily than the standard test. However, it is likely that the addition of hip extension is no more specific for the nervous system than the PKB without hip extension (Davidson 1987).

Common problems with technique

Not paying careful attention to lumbopelvic movements – it is essential to observe carefully these movements because they can offer information on whether the patient is performing compensatory movements that reduce tension in the nervous system. By performing the step 2 in the test, which reduces musculoskeletal compensations, the neural component can be exposed more readily and to miss this out will predispose to inaccurate results.

Not performing steps 2 and 3 of the PKB – this deprives the therapist of the opportunity to focus on the nervous system.

Not holding the pelvis well enough – in my experience, even in the soft and supple patient, it is quite difficult to achieve complete immobilization of the pelvis. Hence, it will be necessary to apply considerable force in an anterocaudad direction over the sacrum to ensure adequate control of extraneous movements.

SAPHENOUS NEURODYNAMIC TEST (SAPHNT)

Introduction

An extension of the femoral nerve, the saphenous nerve is sensory and supplies the medial aspect of the knee, shin and anteromedial ankle regions. Its proximal component (as the femoral nerve) passes anterior to the hip joint in the neurovascular bundle and follows the course of the sartorius muscle in the thigh to pass posterior to the knee joint, through the pes anserinus. It then proceeds along the shin to the ankle. It is therefore tensioned by the movements of hip extension, knee extension and plantarflexion/eversion of the ankle. The saphenous neurodynamic test is not particularly sensitive or specific but, on occasions, it can be useful in examination of the knee, especially when the pain is located medially.

Technique

The prone position is adopted by the patient. The therapist faces the patient in stride standing and takes the patient's thigh by moving their proximal arm around the medial surface of the lower thigh to the anterior aspect of the knee and shin, so that it can both keep the knee in extension and raise the leg. The other (distal) hand holds the ankle in plantarflexion/eversion.

The test movements are hip extension and plantarflexion/eversion of the ankle. Whether internal or external rotation or adduction or abduction of the hip can be used to sensitize the test is equivocal. I suspect that internal rotation may be of value because the femoral nerve passes with the sartorius muscle which would be elongated slightly by this movement. In any case, my recommendation would be to try either, because people are individual and there may be some variation in the biomechanics of this nerve proximally that could be taken advantage of. The test may be sensitized by contralateral lateral flexion of the spine (Fig. 7.54).

Normal response

The normal response for the saphenous neurodynamic test is a stretch feeling in the anterior thigh, similar to the prone knee bend. However, usually,

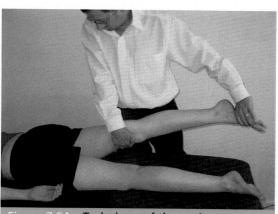

Figure 7.54   Technique of the saphenous neurodynamic test.

more hip extension occurs with this test than with the prone knee bend.

LATERAL FEMORAL CUTANEOUS NEURODYNAMIC TEST (LFCNT)

Introduction

The lateral femoral cutaneous neurodynamic test is simply the prone knee bend except the hip is taken into adduction. Like the saphenous neurodynamic test, the effect of rotation of the hip is not known. Nonetheless, it might vary according to the passage of the nerve along the anterior aspect of the hip.

Normal response

The normal response for the lateral femoral cutaneous neurodynamic test is a stretch feeling in the anterior thigh, similar to the prone knee bend.

FEMORAL SLUMP TEST (FST)

Introduction

The femoral slump test (FST) is used to assess the mechanical function and mechanical sensitivity of the femoral component of the nervous system. It includes the mid-lumbar nerve roots, the femoral nerve and their connections, not to mention all the associated musculoskeletal structures that the nerve innervates (quadriceps muscle and knee joint). The reason for using the term 'femoral slump test' as opposed to the term 'prone knee bend slump' is that the slump test combined with knee bending is not performed in prone. This distinction is important because the position of the body relative to gravity influences neurodynamic testing (reviewed in Chapter 2).

The most difficult aspect of this test is to produce sufficient tension in the nervous system through spinal flexion because the test in general is not very specific to the nervous system. This is partly because of the widespread lack of extensibility of the rectus femoris and iliopsoas muscles in the general population. Various ways of achieving sensitization have been presented and, in my experience, the way it is best accomplished varies between patients. This variation relates to how easily full spinal flexion can be obtained and the notion that there are several ways of performing the FST. Not necessarily in order of importance, the side lying femoral slump and the modified Thomas test, in which spinal flexion is added to the hip flexor stretch with knee flexion (Brukner & Kahn 2001), are the two under consideration.

Even though either test can satisfy the relevant clinical needs, a problem with the modified Thomas test is that there must be a focus on achieving full spinal flexion, and passively, whilst the patient teeters on their buttocks at the edge of the couch. If full passive flexion is not achieved, the test is likely to produce false negatives by way of insufficient spinal flexion. If the spinal flexion is performed actively, the test may suffer a similar fate to that of the straight leg raise by producing an alteration in the position of the pelvis on the spine and thigh. If full spinal flexion can be executed fully in the modified Thomas test, it is possible that this test has merits over the side lying slump test because of the vertical position of the patient which helps increase the slump component of the test.

Indications

The FST is indicated when symptoms occur in the lumbar hip, groin thigh or knee regions.

Side lying femoral slump test

Preparation

A key point with the FST is whether the tested side should be in the upward or downward position. I advocate the downward position because, like the straight leg raise, neural responses can be produced more easily than if the tested side is positioned upward (Miller 1986). This relates to the position of the neural contents in the spinal canal, as mentioned in Chapter 2.

No matter which position the tested side is placed in, it is crucial to take into account the fact the test should be repeated on the opposite side in the *same* position relative to gravity. This means that, for a right-sided test on a limb positioned on the downward side, the bilateral comparison must be to test the left limb also in the downward position.

Patient position

The first part of the side lying FST is to position the patient on the bed so that they will be in the best place for the therapist to apply the final hip extension movement. This start to the test is effectively a half-foetal position. At first, the test is quite difficult to perform. However, with practice it can become easy and effective.

The patient is positioned with the test side in the downward position, as discussed above. A pillow can be placed under the patient's head to control cervical lateral flexion. Without a pillow, the patient's head rests on the bed, which produces ipsilateral lateral flexion. The upper knee and hip (non-test side) are flexed maximally and held there with the patient's upward hand. The next step is for the patient to hold their own neck into full flexion with the downward hand. Often, the patient's face comes into contact with their knee. In which case, the patient adjusts their knee and head so that more cervical flexion can be achieved. At this point, it is important to check that the patient is in the best place on the couch for the therapist to perform hip extension with knee flexion on the test side. If not, it will be necessary to realign the patient and sometimes this can take a couple of rehearsals to obtain the best position. The patient's C7 spinous process must be close to the edge of the couch so that, as will be seen later, the therapist can use the side of the bed as a lever for the control of thoracic and lumbar flexion. At this point, the test limb has not been attended to.

Therapist position

The therapist faces the patient from behind. The therapist's cephalad hand reaches over the patient to hold the edge of the bed. Overpressure to thoracic and lumbar flexion is now essential because of the general lack of sensitivity of the test to the nervous system. Application of overpressure is achieved by the therapist using the edge of the couch to lever their forearm onto the patient's upper (non-test) side and knee. Pelvic fixation is achieved by the therapist leaning on the patient's sacrum and ilium and the patient holding their own knee to their head.

Movements

Once the proper position has been secured, the therapist flexes the patient's test (downward) knee and reaches under the patient's downward thigh to hold the anterior surface of the thigh. Hip extension is the

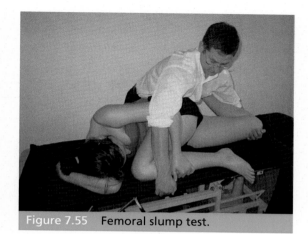

Figure 7.55   Femoral slump test.

final movement of the test. It is crucial that the spinal flexion be maintained to ensure that the test attains some degree of sensitivity. Normally, the range of available hip extension is small so, if much movement is permitted, it should be suspected that the pelvis is not fixated adequately. Even though symptoms of stretch in the thigh muscles and range of movement are two variables, an important additional variable considered by the therapist is the resistance to movement. This is because an alteration in resistance with releasing and reapplying cervical flexion may be the only aspect to vary with structural differentiation. If it does, technically a neurodynamic mechanism is supported (Fig. 7.55).

Structural differentiation

Structural differentiation is executed by the patient releasing their grasp on the head and moving their head back toward the neutral or extended position. Reapplying the cervical flexion several times whilst the therapist feels the resistance to hip extension can be the best way of establishing a neural component to the symptoms. It is imperative here that the thoracic and lumbar spines do not move, which emphasizes the value of the therapist using the couch as a fulcrum for their cephalad hand.

Common problems with technique

Not performing whole spine flexion adequately – because the FST is not very sensitive for the nervous system, this movement must be performed fully.

Not holding the thoracic and lumbar spines stationary during structural differentiation – this is likely to produce false positive results.

Normal response

The normal response for the FST is pulling or stretching in the anterior thigh and it often feels quite stiff to the therapist's hand. What is interesting about this test is that normal subjects sometimes do not show a change in the thigh symptoms with neck flexion/extension movements. However, I have found on many occasions that these can be false negatives because perfecting the technique can change the response from musculoskeletal to neurodynamic. This change in response can come in two forms.

1. The symptom response in the thigh changes more readily when the technique is perfected, particularly the spinal flexion component.
2. The end feel of the hip extension changes to be less tight on release of neck flexion – as mentioned, this means that the therapist will have to repeat the hip extension component of the test several times with and without neck flexion to sense the changes between the two neck positions. Subtle changes such as this are often missed and produce erroneous diagnosis.

OBTURATOR NEURODYNAMIC TEST (ONT)

Introduction

The obturator neurodynamic test is used to examine for altered dynamics in the obturator nerve, including mechanical function and sensitivity. It is not as commonly used as many of the other standard tests because the obturator region is not a common area for symptoms of neuromusculoskeletal origin compared with the sciatic and femoral areas. However, the inguinal region is a popular site and this is where the obturator test can be indicated. One should always be suspicious of an intrapelvic pathology with obturator problems, such as tumours (e.g. bowel cancer), uterine disorders, ovarian cysts and the like. This effectively means that, if an obturator test is abnormal, the need for further investigation rises, especially when abnormality in the test coexists with a history of intrapelvic disease.

Preparation, movements and structural differentiation

The patient is positioned in the slump position with neck flexion whilst the therapist stands opposite the

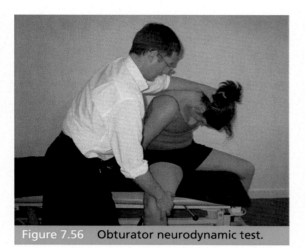

Figure 7.56   Obturator neurodynamic test.

patient's knees. This is because the test leg will be abducted to the end range, which must be catered for in the technique. Overpressure is applied to C7, as in the standard slump test. The therapist applies direct flexion overpressure to C7 with their forearm whilst their hand prevents the head from rising in two independent actions. The therapist then abducts the patient's test limb whilst holding the spine stationary (Fig. 7.56).

Structural differentiation is performed by the release of neck flexion, as with the other slump tests. The therapist will have to move their cephalad hand and forearm to allow for the neck movements.

Normal response

My observation is that the normal response to the obturator neurodynamic test is pulling in the adductor region of the thigh at the end of the abduction component movement. Whether this changes with neck movements is variable and often it does not. Hence, the test is not very sensitive for the nervous system, which highlights the importance of spinal flexion.

Another way to test the obturator nerve is to perform the prone knee bend test and, whilst at the end of the movement, the thigh is abducted. The merit of this test is that the part of the obturator nerve located in the anterior aspect of the lumbar spine can be moved. However, a shortcoming is that it does not tension the spinal cord because spinal flexion is not used. The nerve is generally not in a good position for tests to examine it specifically.

Sensitizing movements – contralateral lateral flexion of the lumbar spine.

References

Brukner P, Kahn K 2001 Clinical Sports Medicine, 2nd edition. McGraw-Hill, Sydney

Butler D 1985 The effect of age and gender on the slump test. Graduate Diploma Thesis, University of South Australia

Davidson S 1987 Prone knee bend: an investigation into the effect of cervical flexion and extension. In: Proceedings of the 5th Biennial Conference of the Manipulative Therapists' Association of Australia. Melbourne: 235–246

Flanagan M 1993 The normal response to the ulnar nerve bias upper limb tension. Master of Applied Science Thesis, University of South Australia

Kenneally M, Rubenach H, Elvey R 1988 The upper limb tension test: the SLR of the arm. In: Grant R (ed) Physical Therapy of the Cervical and Thoracic Spine, Churchill Livingstone, New York

Lew L, Puentedura E 1985 The straight-leg raise test and spinal posture (is the straight-leg raise a tension test or a hamstring length measure in normals?). In: Proceedings of the 5th Biennial Conference of the Manipulative Therapists' Association of Australia, Brisbane: 183–206

Maitland G 1979 Negative disc exploration: positive canal signs. Australian Journal of Physiotherapy 25: 129–134

Mauhart D 1989 The effect of chronic ankle inversion sprain on the plantarflexion/inversion straight leg raise. Graduate Diploma thesis, University of South Australia

Miller A 1986 The straight leg raise test. Graduate Diploma Thesis, University of South Australia

Molesworth J 1992 The effect of chronic inversion sprains on the dorsiflexion/inversion straight leg raise test and the plantarflexion/inversion straight leg raise test. Graduate Diploma Thesis, University of South Australia

Pullos J 1986 The upper limb tension test. Australian Journal of Physiotherapy 32: 258–259

Saplys R, Mackinnon S, Dellon A 1987 The relationship between nerve entrapment versus neuroma. Complications and the misdiagnosis of de Quervain's disease. Contemporary Orthopaedics 15: 51–57

Shacklock M 1989 The plantarflexion inversion straight leg raise. Master of Applied Science Thesis. University of South Australia, Adelaide

Shacklock M, Butler D, Slater H 1994 The dynamic central nervous system: structure and clinical neurobiomechanics. In: Boyling G, Palastanga N (eds)

Modern Manual Therapy of the Vertebral Column, Churchill Livingstone, Edinburgh: 21–38

Slater H 1988 The effect of foot and ankle position on the 'normal' response to the SLR test, in young, asymptomatic subjects. Master of Applied Science thesis, University of South Australia

Sutton J 1979 The straight leg raising test. Graduate Diploma in Advanced Manipulative Therapy Thesis, University of South Australia

Yaxley G, Jull G 1991 A modified upper limb tension test: an investigation of responses in normal subjects. Australian Journal of Physiotherapy 37(3): 143–152

Method of treatment: systematic progression

8

Guidelines for treatment – mechanical interface (opening and closing dysfunctions), neural dysfunctions (sliding and tension)

Sliders and tensioners – one and two-ended, when to apply

Technique and dosage

Progression through the levels

INTRODUCTION

Since this book focuses on making treatment of neuropathodynamics systematic, it is important to discuss treatment techniques in this light. A progressional system of techniques is therefore presented that covers the spectrum of relevant components, starting at the mild end of the spectrum and advancing to the more extensive. As with other aspects of clinical neurodynamics, the topic of treatment techniques is divided into general and specific. This chapter presents the general aspects of treatment techniques from which a range of other techniques is derived later in this book.

TREATMENT GUIDELINES

Mechanical interface

Openers

Interface opening techniques are those that produce an opening action around the nervous system and can consist of movements of joints, muscles and fascia. For example, a release technique for a muscle that is pressing undesirably on a neural structure is an opening technique, or a contralateral lateral flexion mobilization could be used to reduce pressure on a nerve root. There are two types of openers, static and dynamic. The static opener remains in the open position for a certain period of time. This enables blood flow to return to neural tissue so that oxygenation is improved, hence, the reason for *time* being involved in its application. The dynamic opener involves passive or active movement in the opening direction and naturally involves repeated movements.

Closers

Interface closing techniques are those that produce a closing action around the neural elements. This can be in the form of flexing or extending a joint or contracting or stretching a muscle. An example of a closing technique for a nerve root would be ipsilateral lateral flexion. It is therefore important to have a good understanding of the biomechanics of the movement complex in question in addition to the specific neurodynamics. Technically, as with the openers, there are two types of closers (static and dynamic). However, generally, static closers are not

usually the treatment of choice for the reason that maintenance of pressure on a neural structure is not usually desirable.

Treatment of conditions that affect the nervous system through the mechanical interface (opening and closing disorders) are directed at normalizing pressure dysfunction on the nervous system.

Reduced closing dysfunction
Level 1
Generally, treatment of the reduced closing dysfunction at level 1 requires the interface to be opened in order to take pressure off the neural structures. This is because, usually, the dysfunction is produced by a lesion that either houses a space occupying element or increased sensitivity due to a process such as inflammation or ischaemia in or around the neural tissues. Consqently, in the early stages of treatment, alleviative techniques will be required until the sensitivity of the involved structures decreases. In the first progression at level 1, it is therefore preferable to offer the patient an opening position that relieves their symptoms. Initially, this is performed as a trial treatment and is only maintained for approximately 30–60 seconds. This static opener sometimes offers several progressions, the selection of which is dependent on the patient's response and clinical (particularly neurological) status. Nevertheless, the static opener should never increase symptoms. If, in the first application, no change results, then it is worthwhile repeating the procedure up to several times in the same session to be sure of its effect. Frequently, the problem improves after two or three applications, probably because it takes this long to reduce venous congestion or improve arterial flow through the neural structure. If the static opener takes several applications to produce an improvement, this indicates that a degree of stability in the condition exists and justifies the patient performing this at home. If the first application of the static opener produces a dramatic improvement, it is *not* advisable to repeat it until the next visit, and the patient should not use it as a home exercise until the response is stable. The reason for making these recommendations is that the risk of symptoms increasing after a dramatic increase in blood flow through the neural structure will be minimized. In the event that the opener produces a slight improvement each time it is applied in

the first session, it is recommended that as many as several applications be performed, however without the patient performing them at home. This is so the therapist can establish the long-term effects of the technique. If, at the second session, symptoms improve nicely, then the patient may perform the opener at home. The self treatment technique should be performed at least several times per day and, if possible, once per hour. If the static opener produces no improvement in the first session or two, it is up to the clinician to decide whether or not to continue. Given a likely slow response, I am more amenable to repeating it over several treatments. However, if a quick improvement is expected, I would not dwell on the technique. If the symptoms or neurological signs increase with the opener, it should not be repeated and another direction should be taken.

The reassessment points in relation to the static opener are symptoms at rest and neurological status. Neurodynamic tests and tests for the mechanical interface can also be performed as reassessment tools but, because the static opener is often applied at level 1, these are sometimes omitted until after several repetitions of the opener for reasons of prevention of provocation. Sometimes, I do not reassess these until the next visit so that provocation is avoided.

The static opener is particularly suited to spinal conditions that house a problem in the intervertebral foramen with a preponderance of distal symptoms, particularly neurological signs and symptoms. On occasions, its effectiveness can surprise both patient and therapist and can produce resolution of sciatica or cervicobrachialgia in a very short time, sometimes without the need for direct neural mobilizations.

At high level 1, the opener becomes dynamic and is effectively a mobilization in the opening direction. The range at which the technique is performed is of course based on the patient's response but usually it is applied in the mid-range and can be progressed toward the outer range.

Level 2

At level 2, the direction of the mobilization changes to approach the pathomechanics of the problem. Gradually, the interface can be gently and sensitively closed down around the neural structures, but this is entirely on the basis that the patient responds well.

Therefore, several small movements in a closing direction are performed as a trial treatment and the patient's response is monitored closely in terms of subjective reports and physical signs, including neurological examination, neurodynamic tests and musculoskeletal findings.

Distinction between level 1 and 2

Having said the above, the distinction between high level 1 and low level 2 in terms of changing from a static to dynamic technique is somewhat arbitrary and subject to variation and overlap. Decisions on this transition are based on the patient's needs. The main reason for presenting this approach is that it helps the practitioner focus on a safe, logical and systematic means of progressing technique selection.

Reduced opening dysfunction

Treatment of the reduced opening dysfunction overlaps with the reduced closing dysfunction. At level 1, the interface can not be opened a great deal due to pain provocation. Also, there is not as much concern about the blood flow in, and pressure on, the neural tissues as there is with the reduced closing dysfunction. This is because the problem is not one of excess pressure on the neural structures. Rather, it is one of insufficient opening. Therefore, the treatment starts with mobilizations in the opening direction in much the same way that one would mobilize a painful joint. The dynamic opener is applied gently and short of the patient's symptoms.

At level 2, the distance in the range taken by the mobilization increases to be virtually full by the time the problem reaches the high end of this level. In the process, all the relevant neural and musculoskeletal signs are monitored carefully. It is common for this dysfunction to contain a neural tension dysfunction which will necessitate that the mobilization enter the end range slowly and with particular respect to the neurodynamic signs.

Excessive closing and opening dysfunctions

The excessive closing and opening dysfunctions clearly link to instability and dynamic control of the mechanical interface. Therefore treatment of these dysfunctions takes on the motor control and stability paradigms which are not the subject of this book.

Neural component

Sliders

One-ended

The one-ended slider moves the neural structures with the use of body movements at one end of the neural system. For instance, a one-ended caudad slider for a lumbar nerve root would be, in supine, knee extension with the hip flexed to 90°. The one-ended slider technique utilizes the fact that most of the sliding of a nerve occurs in the mid-range of a neurodynamic movement (reviewed in Chapter 1).

Two-ended

The two-ended slider is produced by applying tension at one end of the nervous system whilst letting it go at the other. This permits the neural tissue to slide toward the location at which the movement is initiated. An example of the two-ended caudad slider for a lumbar nerve root is knee extension/neck extension in the seated position.

When to apply sliders

Slider techniques can be excellent for neural problems in which pain is the key symptom. This is because they may milk the nerves of inflammatory exudate and produce increased venous blood flow thereby increasing oxygenation of the neural tissues. The result is thought to be improvement of the inflammation/hypoxia cycle that develops in the nerves (see Chapter 3). It could also be because movement may help control pain at a central nervous system level.

Slider techniques are also applied to conditions that involve specific neural sliding dysfunctions at low levels and serve as a primary mobilization aimed at treating the dysfunction. For this, they can be applied to the sliding dysfunctions at any level. Slider techniques are also used as a secondary mobilization for tension dysfunctions and high level combinations (e.g. 3c, see Chapter 6) so as to reduce the after-effect of mobilizations. For instance, after a tensioner or a multistructural technique at level 3c, the slider can be used to reduce any residual 'awareness' or discomfort. They can also be used as a home exercise when the patient wishes to prevent pain or reduce its likelihood after being involved in a provoking situation.

Technique and dosage

The slider technique is large in amplitude so as to ensure that the neural structure under consideration returns frequently toward its rest position and moves a great deal. This is for reasons of pain modulation and improvement of neurophysiological mechanisms, rather than forcing the neural structure toward its mechanical obstacle, at lower levels. Sliders are performed several times at first and, when a beneficial response is established, they can be repeated several more times in the same treatment session. Once a good response becomes consistent, each movement can be performed in four or five sets of as many as 5–30 repetitions in the same session, with breaks of approximately 10 seconds to several minutes between sets. If an adverse response occurs, they are not reapplied unless the technique is altered to produce a beneficial effect. Generally, the patient's clinical pain should not occur during or after these techniques. At higher levels of treatment (levels 2 and 3) sometimes, extraneous symptoms occur, such as heaviness, stretching and tight feelings. However, these are not necessarily indicators of an adverse reaction and, when appropriate, the therapist may counsel the patient to bear with these symptoms during the technique. Nevertheless, the patient's response dictates whether the sliders are useful or not. The slider should generally not reproduce the patient's symptoms and any other symptoms associated with its performance should subside rapidly afterwards.

When given as a home exercise, sliders are generally not offered the first time that they are performed in the clinic. This is because, in view of the fact that latent responses often occur, a 24-hour pattern should be established before settling on such a technique. The patient can commence sliders after the second session in which their value has been established. They can be performed as frequently as every hour or as infrequently as once per day, depending on the patient's needs. However, if the desire is to reduce the likelihood of the neural structure developing reduced mobility from scarring, my recommendation is to have them performed hourly, if symptoms permit and it is safe. Such cases are acute hamstring injury relating to the sciatic nerve or soon after carpal tunnel release, mastectomy or shoulder surgery. However, if the patient can only tolerate a small amount of movement due to pain or other symptoms, sometimes it is better to space the sliders out to once or twice per day.

Tensioners

One-ended

Just as the slider can be performed in its components to produce different effects, so can the tensioner. The therapist can take advantage of the fact that neural tension increases mostly at the outer range of neurodynamic tests (reviewed in Chapter 1). For instance, a mobilization can be performed in the outer range where the tension movement ratio in the neural tissues is high. For instance, in the median neurodynamic test 1 position, a distal tensioner for the median nerve at the elbow would consist of wrist and finger extension at the end range.

Two-ended

The tensioner can also be performed as a two-ended technique in which both ends of the nervous system are elongated from each end of the neural container. All other things being equal, the two-ended tensioner is likely to produce greater tension in the nervous system than the single-ended one. Again in the median neurodynamic test 1 position, a two-ended tensioner for the median nerve at the elbow would consist of elbow, wrist and finger extension *and* contralateral lateral flexion of the cervical spine.

When to apply tensioners

Tensioner techniques are generally more potent than sliders in terms of producing adverse reactions, as many clinicians have observed. Therefore, they are reserved for tension dysfunction problems at level 2 or higher. Commonly, the tensioner is often followed by sliders for the reasons mentioned above. It is absolutely essential that the therapist be familiar with tension progressions in order to provide safe and effective treatment of the tension dysfunction. In addition, the anti-tensioner can be applied in case of level 1 tension dysfunction so as not to provoke symptoms and indeed even reduce tension in the neural system.

Technique and dosage

Tensioners are performed as a wide amplitude movement in which the neural structure is returned to its off-loaded position. This is because the aim is to stimulate an improvement in the ability of the neural structure to respond to tension changes. The response is on two levels, reduction of its sensitivity to tension

and improvement of its viscoelastic behaviour. Hence, the aim is not to stretch the neural structure and it is on this basis that the term 'neural stretching' should be abandoned. Each movement is performed several times to start with and the patient's response is monitored closely during and after the technique. Given an improvement, it can be reapplied up to several times in the same consultation. Naturally, some symptoms will be evoked in many of the patients on whom tensioners are performed. However, care is always taken to ensure that the technique is taken only into a small amount of resistance and that all responses to the technique are small in magnitude. Hence, even though an improvement may occur with these techniques, it is preferable that this benefit is small so that an adverse latent response is prevented. In one session, I would be quite satisfied with an increase in straight leg raise of 5°–10° in a patient with lumbar and posterior thigh pain with a tension dysfunction at level 2. It is likely that further improvements will occur if the same technique is performed regularly in the near future. The reason for typically making the tensioner a wide amplitude movement is not to enter the deep part of the range of motion but to *withdraw* to a point of low tension each time the movement is repeated. Hence, it is off-loaded probably more than it is tensioned which offers a good recovery time with each movement cycle.

The procedure for offering tensioners as a home exercise is identical to that for sliders. In terms of how frequently the patient is treated, my recommendation is to see the patient almost every day or second day for the first few treatments so that the effect of neurodynamic techniques is well established. The patient is then guided through a progression of neurodynamic and musculoskeletal treatment that ultimately helps them become independent. Tensioners should not produce lasting symptoms and it is imperative that the therapist communicate closely with the patient about this. I always instruct the patient on the importance of symptoms settling completely between each single movement.

Progression through the levels

In the early stages of treatment of neuropathodynamics (e.g. level 1), treatment techniques are directed at improving the pathophysiology in the nervous system. Hence, techniques that provoke symptoms are not employed. Reiterating, the word 'provoke' is used to denote a lasting increase in symptoms in response to performance of a neurodynamic technique. This is different from 'evoking' some mild symptoms at the time of treatment. Also, in the sliding dysfunctions at level 1, the recommendation is to move the nervous system away from the offending dysfunction. For instance, a lumbar caudad sliding dysfunction at level 1 is treated with a *cephalad* slider. As the problem improves, the neural elements are progressively placed in the direction of the dysfunction (caudad), yet they are still mobilized away from it (cephalad). With the higher level mobilization, the neural elements are taken gently into the direction of the dysfunction, but not in a fully sensitized fashion. Also, the tension dysfunction at level 1 does not usually respond well to tension movements, so slider techniques can be employed and these are designed to reduce the sensitivity of the neural structures and encourage movement so that an improvement in their ability to cope with tension occurs. The anti-tensioner (neurodynamic offloader) can also be used in this situation.

It can be seen that, at low levels, therapy tends to address issues of pathophysiology through neurodynamic treatment whereas, at higher levels, mechanical function becomes the focus of attention. With this system, the neural structures are gently and sensitively moved toward the problematic mechanisms in an incremental and systematic way that attacks the causative neuropathodynamics, without provoking the problem. As a general guideline and in relation to the specific neural dysfunctions, combinations of the following progressions apply and these are illustrated in the practical parts of this book.

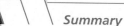

Summary

Progressions
1. position away, move away
2. position toward, move away
3. position away, move toward
4. position toward, move toward

Cervical spine

9

Radiculopathy, headache

Specific neuropathodynamics of each region

Specific dysfunctions – mechanical interface (opening closing), neural tension dysfunction, level/type 3c combination dysfunctions

Mechanical interface, neural components

Progression of physical examination and treatment through the levels

Off-loaders sliders and tensioners, contralateral and bilateral neurodynamic tests

Lower cervical and upper cervical slump tests

Combined muscle, joint and neural treatment

SPECIFIC NEUROPATHODYNAMICS

Mechanical interface

By far the most common cause of cervical radiculopathy is malfunction or pathology in the mechanical interface. The sequelae then consist of pressure on the nerve root, reduced venous return, further increases in tissue fluid pressure and hypoxia and mechanosensitivity in the nerve root. This is compounded by the motion segment sometimes showing altered movement, which may then cause further neural irritation and inflammation. Additionally, it is possible for a sudden and short-lived injury to cause long term primary neural problems. Such triggers could consist of stretch to the brachial plexus or a short-lived compression of a nerve root with an unaccustomed or traumatic closing movement such as extension or ipsilateral rotation or lateral flexion. As described in Chapter 3 (general neuropathodynamics), these aberrations should be examined for and a diagnosis on the specific neurodynamic dysfunction made.

In addition to the above, the patient's posture and habitual activities are key elements of the problem. Analysis of these aspects commonly reveals increased closing, which is often produced by the patient remaining in a seated and slouched (closed) position for sustained periods. The thoracic spine and cervicothoracic junction flex and the intervertebral foraminae in the mid- and lower cervical regions close and may deprive the nerve roots of blood flow, especially when coupled with the possibility of habitual movements to one side. Furthermore, a crucial factor is the duration of the compression on the nerve roots, which translates to the time the patient spends in the slouched position. On release of the pressure, reperfusion and inflammation in the nerve roots may occur. Hence, part of the examination involves analysis of posture and the duration it is held by the patient.

The other relevant scenario is a past history of trauma, which can produce slow and long-term changes in the tissues around the nerve root, resulting in further alterations in pressure dynamics.

In the patient with neck and arm pain, it is possible that two basic kinds of mechanical interface dysfunction exist. The first involves direct pressure on the nerve root and axons, such as that produced by a large disc bulge, and correlates with the tourniquet effect. The second is the mechanical dysfunction in which opening and closing dysfunctions such as instability, hypermobility and hypomobility may produce mechanical irritation. The end result embroils several common mechanisms, namely altered intraneural pressure, inflammation and ischaemia and hypoxia. Consequently, the treatments for different nerve root problems at level 1 often gravitate toward similar techniques that initially focus on the reduction of pressure on the root. Release of pressure in this situation may help venous return, improve resolution of the inflammatory process in the nerve root, reduce tissue fluid pressures and improve intraneural circulation. Therefore, from a clinical neurodynamics point of view, the most effective treatment at level 1 of the problem with a preponderance of distal symptoms is usually to use opening techniques to start with. This is also because inflamed and exquisitely sensitive neural tissues generally do not respond well to increases in tension or pressure.

PHYSICAL EXAMINATION

Cervical slump test

Levels 1 and 2

The cervical slump test at level 1 incorporates modification of the neurodynamic sequence for the standard slump test to accommodate the sensitivity of the problem in the cervical region. With the patient comfortable and in the seated position, they straighten their knee(s) and dorsiflex both ankle(s). The thoracic and lumbar spines are then flexed downward into the slump position, with the patient's head staying vertical. With the therapist supporting the patient's forehead or chin so as to supervise a slow descent of the head, the cervical spine can be flexed to the first point of symptoms. If and when symptoms occur, ankle dorsiflexion or knee extension is released a small amount. If the symptoms ease with release of the lower limb movements, tension and caudad aspects to the problem may exist. If the symptoms increase with release of the knee extension and ankle dorsiflexion, there may be a cephalad sliding dysfunction. If the patient can not sit easily due to symptoms, they may lie supine and the bilateral or unilateral straight leg raise tests may be used instead.

The level 2 cervical slump is simply the standard slump test, differentiated with distal movements such as knee extension/flexion or dorsiflexion of the ankles.

Level 3

The level 3 cervical slump test can be sensitized in certain ways. The level/type 3a version (neurodynamically sensitized) is simply to perform the standard slump test but to add contralateral lateral flexion of the spine (including the neck), internal rotation and adduction of the hip joint. This is more useful for unilateral problems, however, sometimes symmetrical techniques will be needed. The level/type 3b test (sensitized by neurodynamic sequencing) is somewhat more exotic. Whilst the patient is in supine lying, the therapist performs passive neck flexion first, then the remaining components of the test are added; thoracic and lumbar flexion, hip flexion, knee extension, then finalized with dorsiflexion of the ankles. This means that the patient will need to assist in sitting up during the hip flexion component movement, which may take some explaining and practice before the test is perfected. Also, it is critical that the therapist controls all the movements precisely and does not lose any components throughout the whole manoeuvre. The key movement here is cervical flexion and control of this movement will necessitate the therapist using a hand position around the head and neck that accommodates the large change in patient position from the lying to sitting positions. For differentiation, the patient's knees are flexed slightly or the ankle movements of dorsiflexion/plantar flexion are used (Figs 9.1, 9.2, 9.3 and 9.4).

The level/type 3c cervical slump test is simply performance of the level/type 3a test except that the muscles of the neck are elongated (e.g. upper trapezius) whilst at the end of the test. The test will therefore involve some degree of contralateral lateral flexion of the cervical spine. Once again, differentiation is performed with a small release of bilateral knee extension whilst the therapist retests the resistance to elongation of the trapezius muscle. Also, contraction of the upper neck muscles can be resisted to see if this alters the patient's pain, comparing any changes with and without knee extension. The same differentiation can be performed during segmental testing of the cervical spine (Fig. 9.5).

An example of the level/type 3d examination for the cervical spine is to perform a functional provoking

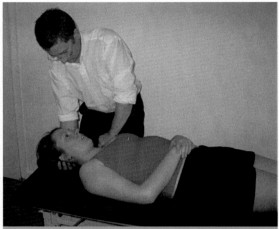

Figure 9.1   Stage 1 of the level/type 3b cervical slump test, starting position.

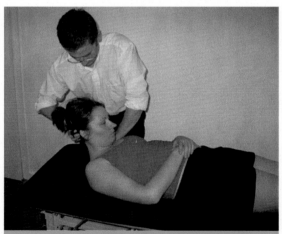

Figure 9.2   Stage 2 of the level/type 3b cervical slump test, passive neck flexion.

movement and add various cervical or upper limb movements. A valuable test is reaching downward (median neurodynamic test 2) in which the therapist can alter the neck lateral flexion position or open and close the cervical interface with various lateral flexion and rotation movements. Whilst the symptoms are present and one of the median neurodynamic tests is applied, wrist movements can be used to differentiate the proximal symptoms. Another variation is that of the median neurodynamic test 1, in which the patient performs a throwing movement. This is commonly a problem in the sporting shoulder

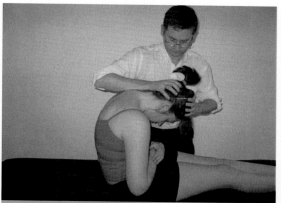

Figure 9.3   Stage 3 of the level/type 3b cervical slump test, hip flexion (sitting up).

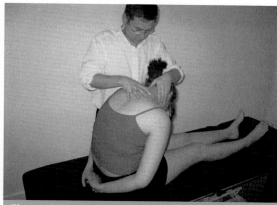

Figure 9.5   Level/type 3c cervical slump test, segmental testing at the end stage. Differentiation can be added.

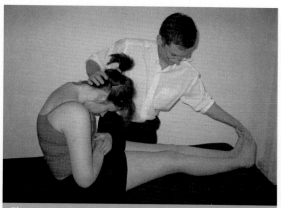

Figure 9.4   Stage 4 of the level/type 3b cervical slump test, ankle dorsiflexion if so desired.

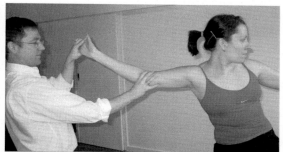

Figure 9.6   Throwing action whilst the therapist performs structural differentiation of proximal shoulder or neck symptoms using wrist and finger movements.

such as with swimming, throwing or serving at tennis. Here, the patient performs their provoking action and freezes in the position in which their symptoms arise. At this point the therapist can perform structural differentiation of the shoulder or neck symptoms using wrist and finger movements (Fig. 9.6).

Median neurodynamic test 1

Level 1

If performed correctly, the standard MNT1 for level 1 is generally a safe manoeuvre. The neurodynamic sequence is modified to take into account the method of testing at this level (Chapter 6). The key

points are that the test is only taken to the first onset of proximal symptoms once and release of the differentiating movement is performed as the last movement so as not to provoke symptoms. Therefore, wrist extension is released in the execution of modified structural differentiation of neck symptoms. The sequence of movements is as follows:

1. Patient in a comfortable position, elbow flexed to 90° – perform wrist and finger extension, forearm supination.
2. Glenohumeral abduction in the frontal plane only up to 90° if permissible (slowly and gently, carefully monitoring symptoms and patient behaviour) or to the first onset of proximal

symptoms. External rotation is optional but is often not necessary.

3. Elbow extension, to the first onset of proximal symptoms. If no symptoms then it is permissible to move to a higher level of testing, as long as the problem fits the inclusion criteria for level 2 testing (see Chapter 6 on planning the examination).
4. Release wrist extension for differentiation of proximal symptoms.

If the proximal symptoms occur very early in the range of glenohumeral abduction, it is possible that this prevents enough elbow extension to produce sufficient tension in the distal nerves to allow differentiation with wrist and finger extension. In this case, the test can be modified with the elbow extended before the abduction phase with differentiation as planned. This then starts to overlap with the MNT2. However, it should still be performed as a modified and supported MNT1.

The level 2 neurodynamic test for the cervical spine is the standard MNT1.

Level/type 3

The level/type 3a (neurodynamically sensitized) MNT1 consists of the standard neurodynamic sequence except contralateral lateral flexion of the cervical spine and depression of the scapula may be added at the end of the manoeuvre. It may be necessary to perfect the technique of lateral flexion in order to make the test effective.

The level/type 3b sensitization of the median MNT1 for neck problems is to start with contralateral lateral flexion and then perform the remaining movements in proximal-to-distal order. The overall sequence is therefore as follows:

1. Contralateral lateral flexion
2. Scapular depression
3. Shoulder abduction/external rotation
4. Forearm supination
5. Elbow extension
6. Wrist and finger extension

Reduced opening dysfunction with neural dysfunction (level/type 3c testing)

In the event that a specific dysfunction in the mechanical interface is evident, the level/type 3c MNT1 can be sensitized precisely. This is achieved by performing an opening movement, such as contralateral lateral flexion as a general technique or localized for the segment in question, combined with the remaining parts of the chosen neurodynamic test. So the overall sequence for this neurodynamic test is exactly as for level/type 3a, except the contralateral lateral flexion is performed as a focus of the technique. It will be necessary that the patient cooperate by maintaining the neurodynamic position themself. Also, the therapist will have to adjust their position so as to control the depression of the scapula. This is achieved by the therapist gently placing their knee on the plinth so that the knee prevents scapular elevation (an interpositioned towel may be necessary here). Alternatively, the scapular stabilization can be performed by use of the therapist's hand holding the scapula and the upper part of their abdomen combining with the contralateral hand to perform the segmental movement. The therapist makes sure to pivot their body so that the relevant segment is moved correctly. This will necessitate them supporting the patient's head partly with their contralateral hand and partly with their abdomen (Fig. 9.7).

Differentiation of whether a neural component to the reduced opening mechanical interface dysfunction exists is performed by the release of wrist and finger extension or a small amount of elbow extension. If release of these movements produces a palpable change in the behaviour of the segmental opening (e.g. increased range or decreased resistance) or results in a reduction in proximal symptoms, a neurodynamic component may be implicated. It is worth perfecting this technique because it is relatively common for patients to present with this dysfunction. Whilst practising, it is useful for two practitioners to perform the technique on a third asymptomatic colleague. Therapist A takes the neck and therapist B takes the subject's upper limb to a reasonably symptomatic end-point and holds it there for a short time. Whilst the neck is moved in the segmental opening direction several times, therapist B releases the wrist or elbow extension. The difference in resistance to opening with and without wrist or elbow movements on therapist A's part is often quite palpable. Clearly, bilateral comparison is essential because it is common for such effects to occur. Hence, the key aspect is whether asymmetry exists and if this relates to the patient's problem.

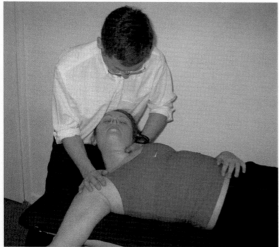

Figure 9.7 Segmental movement of the right C4–5 with neurodynamic testing. The scapula is stabilised with the therapist's ipsilateral hand whilst the segment is moved with the therapist's contralateral hand applying pressure through the opposite side and gently levering open the ipsilateral intervertebral foramen. The median neurodynamic test is also applied and differentiation is achieved with wrist movements.

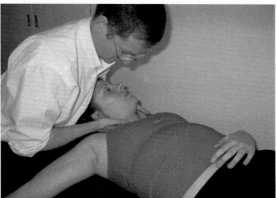

Figure 9.8 Assessment (and treatment) of the reduced closing dysfunction with a neurodynamic component. Ipsilateral lateral flexion is performed with the median neurodynamic test 1. Contralateral lateral glide can be added to enhance the closing mechanism and neurodynamic effects if so desired.

Reduced closing dysfunction with neural component (level/type 3c)

The technique for diagnosis of the reduced closing dysfunction with a neurodynamic component is to test the mechanism of closing at the same time as performing a neurodynamic movement. The following is used as an example.

Position – the patient's upper limb is placed in the MNT1 position. The therapist adopts a position so as to perform either generalized or segmental closing (ipsilateral lateral flexion) at the appropriate level.

Movements:

a. ipsilateral lateral flexion is combined with the patient performing elbow and wrist and finger extension.

b. ipsilateral lateral flexion with contralateral lateral glide – this latter movement is added in the event that movement a. does not reveal sufficient information. Clearly, these can be used as both assessment and treatment techniques.

Differentiation is performed with release of wrist extension and/or elbow extension, as previously. However, the reader should remember that, because the causative mechanism is related to closing, decisions on whether to apply this technique should be made with circumspection, are applied gently and should never provoke symptoms or signs (Fig. 9.8, Chapter 6).

TREATMENT

Mechanical interface

Reduced closing dysfunction
Level 1

As mentioned earlier, in the level 1 cervical radiculopathy, the key concern is to take pressure off the nerve root and improve its blood flow and oxygenation. This may be achieved by the application of the following techniques. For generic details on technique application, see Chapter 8.

Progression 1 – Static opener

The static opener at level 1 for the reduced closing dysfunction is a particularly useful technique for patients with cervical radiculopathy with neurological symptoms and signs. I believe that it

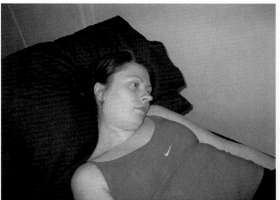

Figure 9.9   Static opener for the cervical radiculopathy, incorporating flexion, contralateral lateral flexion and contralateral rotation.

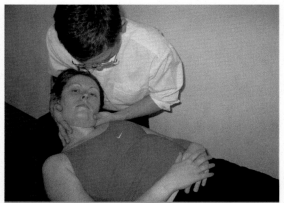

Figure 9.10   Technique of dynamic opener for the right intervertebral foramen and nerve root.

produces more significant changes in space and pressure in the intervertebral foramen than cervical traction and is especially useful for unilateral problems with distal predominance of symptoms, such as pain and neurological changes.

Position – the patient is placed with their cervical spine in flexion/contralateral lateral flexion and a small amount of contralateral rotation. The range into which these components are taken will vary between patients according to their available range and symptomatology. However, I recommend taking the neck into as far a range as possible without producing discomfort. Pillows or raising the headpiece may be needed to offer sufficient support (Fig. 9.9).

A common problem with technique here is not taking the cervical spine into enough flexion and contralateral lateral flexion.

Progression 2 – Dynamic opener

The dynamic opener is performed as a contralateral lateral flexion mobilization whilst the patient is in the supine position. The technique can either be generalized or localized, depending on the patient's needs. The reader will most likely be familiar with the technique of passive lateral flexion. However, in general, the therapist stands above the patient's head. They use their second metacarpophalangeal joint over the contralateral laminae to direct the movement and provide a

pivot point about which the neck must move. In the meantime, the other forearm supports the head, while the hand on this side supports under the patient's neck, chin and on the ipsilateral side at the levels to be moved (side to be opened). The patient's neck and head are therefore cradled in the therapist's ipsilateral arm and anterior aspect of their ipsilateral shoulder. The next manoeuvre to perform is to find the best joint position from which to start and finish the mobilization. This is achieved by the therapist adjusting the cervical flexion/extension so that the symptomatic level or region of the spine starts to open. Finally, the neck mobilization is initiated by the therapist moving their whole body from their feet upward around the pivot point in the neck about which the lateral flexion will occur. Clearly, the main objective is to open the relevant segment or segments sufficiently to reduce symptoms, physical signs or neurological changes. The practitioner adjusts the style and direction of the technique so as to maximize the opening according to the patient's response and the movement idiosyncrasies of the patient's cervical spine. The main aim is to produce lateral flexion so as to direct the mechanism toward opening of the intervertebral foramen (Fig. 9.10).

Level 2
Progression 1 – Dynamic closer – mid-range

The dynamic closer is performed exactly as the above opener except it is in the closing direction, that is, ipsilateral lateral flexion. Once, again the therapist will be able to feel which is the best movement pattern to adopt for the patient's closing mechanism to maximize effectiveness. It is critical that this technique is performed slowly, gently, sensitively and with respect to subtle changes in the patient's response. This technique is performed largely in the mid-range of the joint movement. As it enters the end range it becomes the second progression dynamic closer at level 2.

Progression 2 – dynamic closer – gentle end range

The progression 2 closer is taken toward, although not necessarily achieving, the end range of closing and is generally only selected in the absence of neurological changes. Usually, it is performed as a gentle mobilization and is best not to reproduce symptoms. Often at this level, the patient only shows covert abnormal responses with neurodynamic tests.

Reduced opening dysfunction

The reduced opening dysfunction can be treated with exactly the same techniques as those of the reduced closing dysfunction. At level 1, the same technique (dynamic opener) is performed except for different reasons. With the reduced closing dysfunction earlier, the aim is to reduce pressure on the nervous system. Whereas, with the reduced opening dysfunction, it is to improve the opening mechanism, even though the effects of the two mobilizations can overlap somewhat. At level 1, the static opener is generally not used because, in acute pain states, to sustain the motion segment in the direction of provocation would increase symptoms.

To advance the technique through the levels, the level 1 technique only passes a small amount into the desired movement and is in the form of a repeated mobilization. At low through to higher level 2, it passes into the mid-range and outer or end range.

Neural dysfunctions

Generalized two-ender slider

As mentioned before, the two-ender slider is one of the most useful techniques in the treatment of neuropathodynamics, probably because it promotes movement without generating much tension in the

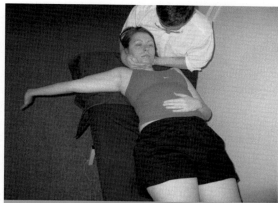

Figure 9.11   Distal slider, incorporating ipsilateral lateral glide and elbow extension with the MNT1.

nervous system. The neck is no exception to this and the technique can be used at all levels of problems, especially level 1, and before and after other techniques to provide a relieving or settling effect.

Position – the patient lies supine whilst the symptomatic upper limb is placed in the appropriate position for the relevant upper limb neurodynamic test (e.g. MNT1). The degrees of shoulder abduction and elbow extension are particularly important in deciding on the extent to which the nerves are moved and are selected judiciously. The therapist supports the patient's head and neck so as to be able to glide the patient's neck in an ipsilateral direction. It is important that the head is moved in a translatory fashion so as to maximize the gliding of the neural tissues toward the ipsilateral shoulder, rather than focusing on lateral flexion. Having had prior practice at performance of the neurodynamic test, the patient then performs elbow extension whilst the therapist glides the head in the ipsilateral direction. The chosen level of mobilization can be set up for a generalized technique or one for a specific level. This technique should not evoke any significant symptoms. It can also be reversed so the nerves are glided to the opposite side by the performance of a contralateral slide with elbow flexion rather than extension. This will necessitate the therapist changing sides to control the neck and head movements. Hence, the two techniques incorporate the following movements as shown in Figures 9.11 and 9.12.

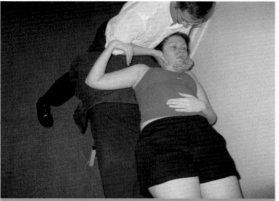

Figure 9.12 Proximal slider, incorporating contralateral lateral glide and elbow flexion with the MNT1.

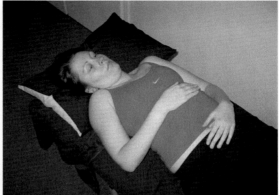

Figure 9.13 Generic off-loader for the cervical nerve roots, brachial plexus and median nerve, incorporating, ipsilateral lateral flexion, scapular elevation, elbow flexion/pronation and comfortable wrist and finger flexion.

Tension dysfunction

Low level 1 – position away/move away

At level 1, my recommendation for a good off-loaded position for the lower cervical nerve roots is as follows. The patient is positioned in supine with their scapula elevated and their arm beside their side. Some patients with an acute C5–6 nerve root problem in fact aim to achieve this by raising their arm above their head themselves which is most likely effective through achieving scapular elevation. The neck is placed in the most comfortable position possible. This is usually a slight degree of flexion to reduce pressures and tensions in the interface, ipsilateral lateral flexion and a small degree of ipsilateral rotation. Clearly this position releases forces on all the structures in the upper quarter. If this provides some relief, it is recommended that the patient adopt the position for their own pain relief (Fig. 9.13).

The second progression is to mobilize the neural tissues further into an off-loaded position, then back to the starting position. Elevation of the scapula is therefore a position and movement of choice. It can be mobilized or may remain in position whilst the therapist performs other techniques. In the event that it is mobilized, the technique is performed by the therapist supporting the whole shoulder girdle with their proximal hand and forearm whilst the other hand and forearm support the patient's elbow and hand. The movement is performed gently and slowly and with respect to the patient's symptoms.

In the event that the scapula is not mobilized to reduce tension in the neural structures, a suggested progression at level 1 is that the contralateral upper limb be placed in a neurodynamic position (e.g. MNT1 to reduce tension in the ipsilateral neural tissues, see Chapter 2) and gently mobilized. The ipsilateral straight leg raise can also substitute the contralateral MNT1, if so desired.

High level 1 – position towards/move away

Subsequent progressions at level 1 that utilize the contralateral MNT1 or leg raise involve adding a small amount of tension to the nerve roots through application of the ipsilateral MNT1, whilst they are still mobilized away from tension with the use of the contralateral MNT1. Hence, even though a small amount of tension is applied to the nerve roots with components of the ipsilateral MNT1 (position towards), they are still mobilized in a direction that reduces tension (move away). The therapist may use scapular depression, shoulder abduction or elbow extension. Furthermore, the amount of tension during the mobilization may well be less than in the anatomical position and that which is produced by the patient's daily movements.

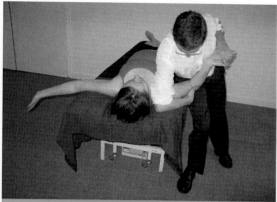

Figure 9.14 Level 2 treatment of the cervical nerve root tension dysfunction, performance of the supported MNT1 on the symptomatic side with contralateral MNT1 positioned to reduce tension in the nerve roots (position away/move toward).

Level 2 – position away/move towards

At level 2, when the problem has settled somewhat, the mobilization of choice is as follows. The patient is again positioned in supine and in the contralateral MNT1 position, however movement of the *ipsilateral* MNT1 is introduced (position away/move towards). The first progression is to perform the ipsilateral MNT1 whilst the contralateral one is positioned prior to the mobilization. This is to ensure that tension that is applied to the nerve roots commences in a tension-reduced situation and prevents an undesirable build-up of force. Generally, the technique is to perform the supported MNT1 (if necessary) and produce a gentle scapular depression movement with a degree of elbow extension already positioned or vice versa. It is optional as to whether the wrist and fingers are extended. Naturally, this is influenced by the patient's response (Fig. 9.14).

Subsequent progressions are achieved by adding more distal tension to the mobilization (ipsilateral MNT1) with the addition of shoulder abduction and the rest of the components of the MNT1, depending on the patient's response.

The final progressions at high level 2 are produced with reduction of the 'assistance' given by the contralateral MNT1. Therefore, gradually, each component is removed whilst the therapist mobilizes the ipsilateral MNT1. Reduction of the positions of

contralateral elbow extension and glenohumeral abduction would be useful progressions whilst the therapist heads toward performance of the MNT1 without any components of the contralateral test being present.

Level 3

The key aspect of level 3 treatment is sensitization. The tension dysfunction is sensitized neurodynamically (level/type 3a) with the addition of contralateral lateral flexion of the neck and/or depression of the scapula. The key points about tensioners for the neck are to perform them as two-ended tensioners, make the amplitude of movement large so that returns to the non-tension position are cyclic and not likely to provoke symptoms and perform them slowly and gently with respect to the patient's symptoms (see Chapter 8 on method of treatment).

The MNT1 is performed with the neck positioned in contralateral lateral flexion. This is achieved by the therapist placing the limb in the correct position then placing their distal hand over the superior aspect of the scapula for stabilization purposes. The other hand is then used to produce lateral contralateral flexion whilst the patient performs elbow extension and flexion. The starting position is ipsilateral lateral flexion with little pressure on the scapula, the patient's elbow flexed with the wrist and fingers extended. The mobilization involves contralateral lateral flexion, pressure on the scapula to either stabilize or depress it slightly as the patient straightens and bends their elbow through a large range of motion (Fig. 9.15).

Reduced opening dysfunction with neural tension dysfunction

The reduced opening dysfunction and tension dysfunction can be treated with quite specific techniques. Localized contralateral lateral flexion of the appropriate spinal segment can be combined with the tensioner as above. The treatment technique for this dysfunction is illustrated under level/type 3c examination for this dysfunction (p. 164). Also, mobilizations can be performed on the patient's spinal joints whilst the patient is in prone and their upper limb in the neurodynamic position of choice.

Another option with the reduced opening with neural tension dysfunction is to perform muscle

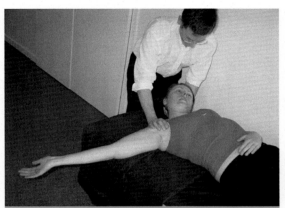

Figure 9.15   Level/type 3c tensioner, end position, however, each cycle should involve large amplitude movements that return the system to the non-tensioned position and symptoms should cease at each return.

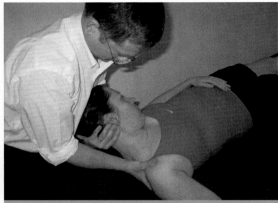

Figure 9.16   Release of the upper trapezius muscle during MNT1 (level/type 3c treatment).

release techniques in the upper limb neurodynamic position. This is particularly important because so many of our patients present with muscle dysfunctions in combination with neuropathodynamics. In the reduced opening dysfunction with a neural tension component, gentle contract-relax and other muscle release techniques can be performed manually with scapular depression and contralateral lateral flexion. It is optional as to whether the patient mobilizes their elbow into extension or performs other neurodynamic techniques. Nevertheless, the upper trapezius, myelohyoid and levator scapulae muscles are particularly relevant here (Fig. 9.16).

Reduced closing dysfunction and neural tension dysfunction

This dysfunction can be treated with the contralateral lateral glide of the cervical spine, combined with ipsilateral lateral flexion at the segment concerned. In this case, the same MNT1 technique is applied by the patient as above whilst the therapist mobilizes the cervical spine into the contralateral glide position and performs a gentle closing action at the appropriate segment. This technique is performed gently and with sensitivity with specificity focusing on the correct spinal level. It is shown in examination on page 164.

HEADACHE

Introduction

Headache is vexing for both patient and practitioner because it is a complex problem and involves many factors that can interact in the same patient. Much has been written on headache, such that it is not practicable to cover the theory of this massive subject. However, what can be said is that different categories of headache have been offered in an attempt to link causative mechanisms to the different syndromes that appear clinically (IHS 2000). Some of these categories include cluster headache, migraine (with and without aura), tension-type headache and cranial neuralgia. Unfortunately, nothing in this classification is mentioned on the potential role of adverse neurodynamics. Irrespective of this, possible mechanisms that relate to clinical neurodynamics are those in which the musculoskeletal system dynamically influences the nervous system. The reader is referred to Shacklock et al (1994) for a review of the neurodynamics of cervical spine and brainstem.

A particularly common headache that relates the musculoskeletal system to the nervous system is that caused by altered mechanics in the upper cervical and suboccipital regions. This involves combinations such as the forward head posture, hypoactive longus coli muscles, hyperactive and shortened rectus capitus posterior muscles and stiff upper cervical joints. These features are often associated with a stiff thoracic spine. It is likely that reduced movement and excessive kyphosis in the thoracic spine will impart altered forces on the cervical region because the neck must move differently to compensate for the stiffness in the thoracic region. The position of high brain stem tension is one of upper cervical flexion. Interestingly, a particularly common postural imperfection in this region is the forward head posture in which the upper cervical region is *extended*. The holding of this position by the patient is likely to produce two consequences for the nervous system: a. a reduction in tension in the brain stem and b. an increase in pressure on the occipital nerves as they pass through the rectus capitus muscles on their way to the head. In short, an imbalance may exist which consists of decreased movement and tension in the brain stem tissues and increased pressure on the occipital nerves. In addition, it is possible that an increase in neural tension in the thoracic cord and dura could be a product of excessive thoracic kyphosis or insufficient periodic reduction of tension with daily movements.

Clinically, the above mentioned problem may manifest itself as an abnormal upper cervical slump test, the testing for which follows.

Upper cervical slump test (UCST)

Mechanical interface

Relevant structures in the mechanical interface in relation to cervicogenic headache are the upper cervical joints and muscles. These must be tested individually as a routine part of examination as a means of coming to an understanding of their possible relationship to the nervous system. Passive accessory and physiological movements and muscle function are evaluated, whereby the pattern of changes is compared with the pattern of neurodynamic tests. For instance, if contralateral lateral flexion is reduced with isolated testing of the upper cervical joints, and this restriction increases with the upper cervical slump and varies with structural differentiation, then a neurodynamic relationship to the musculoskeletal dysfunction may be supported. Upper cervical flexion is the key movement in which the muscular relationship with the nervous system is evaluated.

Level 1

Examination

In performing the level 1 upper cervical slump test, the patient is seated on the couch, as in the starting position for the standard slump test. The main difference between this and the standard general test is that the cervical component is performed last (starting remotely). An option is to perform the movements in a sequence that combines convenience with care. In the sitting position, the movements can be performed in the following order; ankle dorsiflexion/knee extension, lumbar and thoracic flexion and lastly, cervical flexion. The movements are ceased at the first onset of symptoms and modified structural differentiation is achieved by releasing knee extension. Clearly, it is not necessary to perform all the component movements or to take them to their full range. For instance, it might be adequate to omit the dorsiflexion and only perform knee extension and lumbar and thoracic flexion. If the headache were to be reproduced with thoracic flexion, structural differentiation would also be performed by the release of knee extension or dorsiflexion. Since care is the key part of this technique, it is necessary to manually support and control the neck flexion component and to perform the movements slowly with close attention being paid to the patient's symptoms.

Treatment

Interface and innervated tissue problems can naturally be dealt with according to the tissue and method preferred by the practitioner. Since it is likely that the patient's symptoms will be easily provoked, it will be necessary to use techniques of only small force.

Neural sliders

Sliders are a valuable option in the treatment of cervicogenic headache with a neural component when the problem occupies the level 1 category. Such mobilizations can be achieved by performance of the bilateral straight leg raise (one-ended slider) whilst the neck is positioned in the most comfortable position for the patient. Often the position of choice is upper cervical neutral flexion/extension, or slightly extended, to reduce neural tension. It might also be necessary to place the upper cervical spine in relation to the mechanical diagnosis. For instance, in a reduced closing interface dysfunction at C1–2, the neck may be placed in slight localized opening (contralateral lateral flexion) prior to starting neural mobilizations. Even though head movements are not used in this particular procedure, a slider may be achieved by producing a large amplitude ipsilateral straight leg raise without producing a great deal of tension because the neural tissue in the upper neck is not elongated prior to neural movement. Hence movement, rather than tension, is the key event. An alternative to use of the straight leg raise is to gently mobilize the ipsilateral MNT1.

The same would apply for the different interface dysfunctions in which the starting position of the interface would be influenced by the dysfunction and the patient's symptomatology.

Level 2

Examination

The level 2 upper cervical slump examination for headache is simply the standard slump test but with emphasis placed on analysis of the structures in the upper cervical region. In the slump position, upper cervical movements are palpated and moved passively and related symptoms investigated. Headache symptoms are sometimes evoked or reproduced by this level 2 test but, more commonly, it is the covert abnormal response (Chapter 5) that reveals a neural component to the problem. This is usually in the form of subtle tightness in the cervical flexion component of the test and the tightness changes with releasing knee extension. The symptoms may also be altered with contralateral lateral flexion of the neck which is often tighter than ipsilateral lateral flexion.

Treatment

Sliders

Treatment of headache at level 2 when it has neurodynamic relationships consists of neural sliders, tensioners and interface techniques. These are accomplished by the therapist and patient working together to produce the correct movements.

Sliders for the cervicogenic headache patient are executed by combining upper cervical movements with the MNT1 or leg movements (Fig. 9.17).

The above is primarily suited to a unilateral headache, however, in symmetrical problems, the

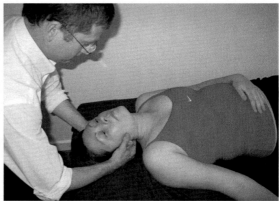

Figure 9.17   Distal slider for the upper cervical spine for headache, incorporating upper cervical extension and ipsilateral lateral flexion with the MNT1. The proximal slider makes use of upper cervical contralateral lateral flexion and elbow flexion.

movements can be modified. Instead of the MNT1, lower limb movements can be used and the neck movements will be performed in the sagittal plane i.e. flexion/extension. For instance, upper cervical extension would be performed with the straight leg raise for a distal slider and vice versa for a proximal slider.

Tensioners

At level 2, tensioners can be applied in the form of combining upper cervical flexion and contralateral lateral flexion with lower limb movements. The movements are naturally graded according to the patient's needs. These techniques can also be combined with the MNT1.

Upper cervical slump test – level/type 3a

The UCST is derived from the principles of neurodynamic sequencing as mentioned in the chapter on general neurodynamics. At level/type 3a, the standard slump test is performed and the sensitizing manoeuvres are added to the test. The main sensitizing movement consists of contralateral lateral flexion of the upper cervical spine. It will then be necessary to change the hand positions and movements to accommodate the difference in technique from that used in the standard slump test.

Upper cervical slump test – level/type 3b (localized)

Examination

Technique

My experience is that the level/type 3b examination is an essential aspect of assessment of the patient with cervicogenic headache that is not easily detected with physical examination. It is much more sensitive than testing at lower levels because it biases forces to the upper cervical region and is therefore more specific and localized.

Position – the patient lies supine on the bed with a pillow under their head. Their body is symmetrically positioned. The therapist stands facing across the patient. The therapist plans their position so as to be able to walk a couple of short paces during the technique which means that their feet should be approximately a metre apart. The therapist's more cephalad hand cups under the patient's occiput by using the palmar surface of their hand. The second hand hold is executed by the therapist placing the first web space of their other hand around the front of the patient's mandible so that upper cervical flexion can be performed by the combined action of both hands. It is imperative at this point that the therapist has in their mind the correct movement for upper cervical flexion. It is produced by rotation of the head around an axis that passes approximately through the patient's ears, as if the patient's head is a wheel rotating about its axis. The movement should not result in retraction or protraction of the patient's head on their spine. A short practice of this movement is appropriate before proceeding with the rest of the test. The next step is to check that that patient can breathe freely and is comfortable whilst their neck is in upper cervical flexion. The therapist should also ask whether the patient experiences any jaw problems, or is likely to, with this technique. If a problem exists, then it may not be possible to perform this technique, or it might be necessary to adapt to the patient's needs by altering the hand positions or not performing the upper cervical flexion as fully as desired (Fig. 9.18).

Movement – the movements of the UCST consist of upper cervical flexion, lower cervical flexion, thoracic flexion, lumbar flexion and, finally, hip flexion. In addition to this manoeuvre being more localized to the upper cervical region than the standard test, it provides the opportunity to progress easily to a

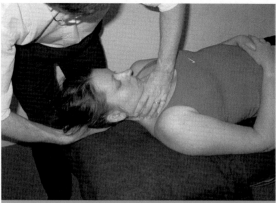

Figure 9.18 Starting position and hand holds during the upper cervical slump test.

level/type 3c (multistructural) examination, by way of patient positioning and the therapist's hand holds. Hence, it is a stepping stone between levels 3a and c. Before the application of the first movement (upper cervical flexion), it is explained to the patient that the test will involve flexion of their head toward their chest and immediately after this they will have to sit themselves up. The therapist also says that they will assist in the sitting-up action but it is imperative that the 'chin tuck' part of the test be maintained once it is applied. If the patient experiences difficulty in breathing or talking they should raise a finger, at which point, the patient is released from the position and a solution discussed. It is common for patients to not be able to speak easily so it is important to communicate accurately.

Upper cervical flexion is performed passively by the therapist, followed by lower cervical flexion. The patient then sits up by flexing their thoracic spine first, followed by lumbar and hip flexion. This is a point where the hand that cups the patient's occiput swivels on the occiput so that, by the time the final position is arrived at, the therapist's hand is in a position to hold the upper cervical flexion fully. The final position is consequently a long sitting slump with emphasis on upper cervical flexion (Fig. 9.19).

Structural differentiation

Structural differentiation is performed by the patient flexing their knees. This often produces a reduction in the patient's symptoms and tightness in the upper cervical flexion to the therapist's feel.

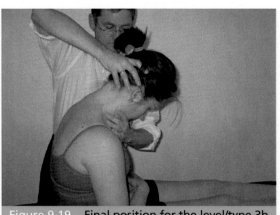

Figure 9.19   Final position for the level/type 3b upper cervical slump test for cervicogenic headache.

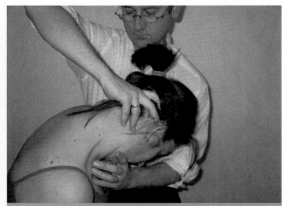

Figure 9.20   Contralateral lateral flexion of the upper cervical joints at the end stage of the upper cervical slump test for patients with cervicogenic headache (level/type 3c).

Normal response

The common response in normal subjects for the UCST is tightness in the cervical region. However, this does not always occur. Some people feel nothing but stretching in the thoracic region. In the clinical context, the key aspect is to establish whether changes in the cervical region are adverse to the therapist's feel which takes much practice and performance of the test on many people. However, with experience, the therapist will quickly be able to establish whether the test behaves in a 'desirable' way. The changes that would suggest otherwise are pain, tightness and stiffness in the cervical region or head. These alter with structural differentiation and occur on the same side as the patient's headache.

Upper cervical slump test – level/type 3c

The main extension that this level and type of testing provides over the level/type 3b UCST is that the interface and innervated tissue structures can be tested simultaneously. This involves opening and closing mechanisms at the upper cervical joints and contraction of the musculature in the area.

Technique

The technique for the UCST at level/type 3c is to perform the test at level/type 3b, as described above, with the addition of variations in lateral flexion and rotation, particularly in the contralateral direction. By far the most common movement to be abnormal

is contralateral lateral flexion, such that specific elaboration on this aspect is necessary.

Once the patient has reached the end range upper cervical slump position, the therapist performs contralateral lateral flexion of the upper cervical joints. The therapist must be familiar with the axes of rotation for the specific joints in this region so that localization of stresses to these sites can be specific. Generally, because these joints do not provide much lateral flexion, the movement should only occur over a small range of motion. If a large amount of lateral flexion results, the movement is probably not sufficiently localized to the correct joints and must be revisited. The therapist will have to make small adjustments to their hand positions to achieve localization to the right location. Generally, the therapist's fingers of the hand that holds the patient's occiput will need to spread further apart and move closer to the upper cervical joints so that forces can be directed toward this site. All it takes to produce lateral flexion to the ipsilateral or contralateral side is reversing the direction of the movement, rather than changing the hand holds. Bilateral comparison of lateral flexion to both sides is essential. When the manoeuvre is completed, the knees are flexed and the same movements are repeated. Changes in the contralateral lateral flexion with knee extension and flexion are common and usually the manual resistance to contralateral lateral flexion increases with knee extension (Fig. 9.20).

In addition to testing the opening and closing mechanisms of the upper cervical spine with the UCST, the muscles in the area can also be tested. This is performed by the therapist resisting active upper cervical extension and ipsilateral lateral flexion. The rectus capitus muscles are thus contracted, applying force to the occipital nerves and testing the dynamic relationships between the muscular and neural components. Coaching of the patient with this manoeuvre is sometimes necessary.

During structural differentiation of the above manoeuvre, the knees are flexed. What is commonly found in the abnormal situation is that the patient's symptoms are reproduced, or a covert abnormal response occurs, more easily when the knees are extended.

Treatment of this problem involves mobilizations and muscle release techniques, including contract/relax, in the neurodynamic position, depending on which structures are involved.

References

IHS (International Headache Society) 2000. Members' Handbook. Scandinavian University Press, Oslo: 43–53

Shacklock M, Butler D, Slater H 1994. The dynamic central nervous system: structure and clinical neurobiomechanics. In: Boyling G, Palastanga N (eds), Modern Manual Therapy of the Vertebral Column, Churchill Livingstone, Edinburgh: 21–38

Upper limb

10

Diagnosis and treatment – thoracic outlet, pronator, supinator and carpal tunnel syndromes

Specific neuropathodynamics and clinical features of each problem

Specific dysfunctions – mechanical interface (opening closing), neural sliding and tension dysfunctions, level/type 3c combination dysfunctions

Progression of physical examination and treatment through the levels

Off-loaders sliders and tensioners, openers and closers

Combined muscle, joint and neural treatments

THORACIC OUTLET SYNDROME AND SHOULDER PAIN

Introduction

Problems in diagnosis and treatment

Thoracic outlet syndrome is a controversial subject because authors disagree on its existence, method of diagnosis, and treatment. These discrepancies exist for several reasons. The first is related to its definition. There are probably different kinds of thoracic outlet syndrome and different health practitioners test for their own parts of the problem. So in terms of examination, who you see is what you get. Hence, the first problem in diagnosis lies in the focus of the health practitioner. The vascular surgeon considers whether vascular changes exist. The neurologist looks for a reduction in conduction velocity. The same patient may be cleared of vascular and neurological changes, yet the treating therapist establishes that neuropathodynamics exist by performing sensitized neurodynamic testing. The problem might actually be caused by mechanical irritation of the brachial plexus without vascular or neurological conduction problems.

The second riddle is related to the method of diagnosis. The vascular surgeon examines the blood vessels, the neurologist evaluates the conduction velocity and the therapist assesses neurodynamics. Because the differences between each modality of testing are radical, and the syndrome can house components of different kinds, each method of testing fails to distinguish all the causative mechanisms. This then produces false negative results.

The third problem relates to the fact that the normal response to tests (e.g. vascular tests that make use of shoulder abduction) often overlap with abnormal responses. This then produces false positive results, which challenges the specificity and sensitivity of the tests. Conversely, an advantage that neurodynamic tests have in testing for neuropathodynamics is that they are well proven and can be highly consistent and reliable both in normal and clinical subjects (Kenneally et al 1988; Selvaratnam et al 1994; Grant et al 1995; Coveney et al 1997; Selvaratnam et al 1997; Coppieters et al 2002). This means that, in relation to neurodynamics at least, the distinction between normal and abnormal can actually be quite easy to make.

The fourth problem is that treatment is often not sensitive to the kind of thoracic outlet syndrome that could exist. This is where, no matter what background they have, the practitioner who deals with this problem must be fully aware of *all* the causative mechanisms and the practitioner's own limitations in the diagnosis and treatment of this problem and refer the patient to others, should the need arise. This naturally includes therapists whose skills are localized to the neuromusculoskeletal system.

The above discussion illustrates the point that dogmatic statements as to whether or not thoracic outlet syndrome exists generally are usually of no value in relation to the individual in whom there is potential for symptoms to arise from this region. In the end, the key factor is performance of a careful and detailed analysis of all the patient's clinical findings. The following covers the relevant neurodynamics of the problem and its treatment.

Specific neuropathodynamics of the thoracic outlet region

The neurodynamic events of the thoracic outlet region are characterized by several key events. In its course to the periphery, the brachial plexus passes inferolaterally between the first rib and clavicle in a large bundle. In doing so, the relations between the neural elements, the mechanical interface and the specific neurodynamics are pivotal. The plexus behaves like cords that can be pulled and slid from both proximal and distal ends, depending on the limb and spinal movements. Interestingly, our observations are that the plexus can also be made to bowstring in a cephalad direction over the first rib as the rib elevates under the plexus with inhalation. At a point distal to the shoulder, this produces proximal movement of the nerves at least as far as the arm and correlates with the findings of McLennan and Swash (1976). Hence, breathing and rib movement form an integral part of examination and treatment of thoracic outlet syndrome. Another important aspect of this arrangement is that the clavicle can be made to approximate the plexus from above with the use of scapular depression movements. A pincer action is thus exerted between the first rib and clavicle around the plexus and this could in some cases contribute to neuropathodynamics which could come in the form of an elevated first rib and a depressed scapula, particularly when the plexus must slide and bowstring against the bony interfaces with upper limb and spinal movements. Dynamics of the shoulder girdle therefore form an integral part of evaluation and treatment of the thoracic outlet syndrome.

From our observations, significant movement in the brachial plexus occurs at the thoracic outlet and this is particularly pronounced with lateral gliding of the cervical spine and the median neurodynamic test 1. Whilst in the position of 90° glenohumeral abduction, distal sliding of the plexus is produced by elbow, wrist and finger extension movements, combined with ipsilateral gliding of the cervical spine. Proximal sliding is produced by performance of contralateral glide and elbow, wrist and finger flexion. Tension in the plexus is generated with cervical lateral gliding in a contralateral direction and elbow, wrist and finger extension. During this manoeuvre, parts of the plexus bowstring in a cephalad direction within its bed while the amplitude of sliding is noticeably reduced with these tension movements when compared with the above sliding techniques. The diameter of the plexus can also be seen to reduce as tension is applied to it.

> Movement of the brachial plexus and interface at the thoracic outlet.

Neuropathodynamics of this region can be a cause of symptoms, as evidenced by the following case, kindly provided by the orthopaedic manual therapist, Ms Tiina Lahtinen-Suopanki of Finland.

Case history

A man received an external blow from an object falling on his posterior fossa and clavicle area. He subsequently experienced pain and restriction of movement in his shoulder region and the median neurodynamic test 1 was abnormal. The treating doctors were naturally reluctant to operate in this region. After quite some time, Ms Lahtinen-Suopanki was not satisfied with his progress so a real-time ultrasound study on the dynamics of the brachial plexus was arranged. The study showed altered movement patterns of the plexus compared with the contralateral side, which gave the surgeon sufficient clinical evidence to operate and release the nerves. The nerve was freed of scar tissue that bound it to the surrounding tissues and the patient improved rapidly to return to

his normal work and be free of his symptoms. This is an excellent example of neurodynamics being one of the most effective means of assessing thoracic outlet syndrome.

Mechanical interface dynamics

What we have recently observed in our imaging studies in relation to how much the interface changes with shoulder girdle movement is extraordinary. At the space between the first rib and clavicle, the amount of opening and closing of the interface is huge. From the fully closed to open positions, the dimensions around the brachial plexus can be increased by over 100%. This provides an excellent rationale and great potential to address the issue of opening and closing around the brachial plexus as a form of treatment.

Another aspect of the mechanical interface pertinent to the thoracic outlet syndrome is the behaviour of the scalene muscles. When they contract, pressure is exerted on the brachial plexus because it passes between the anterior and middle scalene muscles. Therefore, the dynamics of these muscles and the first rib and neck are also important.

Clinical features

Clinical features of the thoracic outlet syndrome consist of shoulder pain that is often located on the anterior and inferior aspects of the shoulder region. Even though this is not always the case, the symptoms often pass distally along the course of the ulnar nerve, through the axilla and medial surface of the arm, elbow and forearm toward the ulnar two fingers. In other patients, the symptoms can emulate a patchy brachial plexus irritation in which the symptoms can appear to occupy the territory of any of the C5–8 spinal nerves. Occasionally, posterior shoulder pain can occur. Utilization of the median neurodynamic test 1 is usually sufficient to detect the problem. However, the ulnar test can be used if the problem is biased to the ulnar aspect of the upper limb. The problem is usually provoked by repetitive upper limb activities and the clinician should pay particularly attention to the dynamics of the shoulder girdle because, as mentioned, this aspect plays a key role. The mechanical pattern tends to take one of two courses. In the first, the upper trapezius and levator scapulae muscles take a protective hyperactivity dysfunction in which the scapula becomes elevated in order to reduce forces on the brachial plexus. The second is one of hypoactivity of the upper trapezius and associated muscles, such that the neural elements are not protected sufficiently during the repeated movement. Treatment of the different problems is oriented toward normalizing the dynamics of the shoulder girdle so as to improve the neurodynamics. Also, neurodynamic techniques are utilized so as to normalize the intrinsic dynamics of the brachial plexus.

Physical examination and treatment

Mechanical interface

Evaluation of the mechanical interface for thoracic outlet syndrome consists of checking the dynamics of the whole shoulder girdle and related musculoskeletal structures, including posture and movements of the cervical spine, scapulothoracic and glenohumeral joints, first and second ribs and length and function of the scalenae, upper trapezius and levator scapulae muscles. What is particularly important is to manually feel the movement of these structures and perform their related opening and closing movements to obtain information on the relationships between these aspects and the nervous system. The relevant movements comprise the passive scapular movements of elevation, depression, protraction and retraction, length of the muscles mentioned above and, in advanced cases, combining testing of these structures with neurodynamic tests, as described later. Clearly, at level 1, testing will be circumspect, particularly with closing manoeuvres such as depression and retraction with inspiration and movements that generate tension in the nervous system such as glenohumeral abduction and elbow extension. At higher levels of examination, the clinician will be more confident with testing these movements and will make the testing and treatment more multifactorial (e.g. level/type 3c).

Interface closing dysfunction

Level 1

The level 1 treatment of the mechanical interface for thoracic outlet syndrome consists of opening the interface as much as possible. The first progression is in the form of a static opener, which the patient can perform at home, if appropriate. The patient lies on the contralateral side lying with their nervous system in the upper quarter in the off-loaded position (for the

median or ulnar nerve) with a prime emphasis on scapular elevation and protraction. These positions increase the distance between the clavicle and first rib and take pressure off the brachial plexus. The movement can be facilitated by the therapist performing it passively at first. If possible, breathing is utilized also and its effects explained to the patient. Exhaling deeply increases the distance between the clavicle and first rib and can be combined with elevation of the scapula. Exhalation also reduces bowstringing of the plexus over the first rib.

Subsequent progressions involve dynamic openers for the scapula in the direction of elevation and protraction and mobilization of the first rib in a caudad direction. This is so that the rib can be brought away from the brachial plexus, especially if the first rib is stiff or located in too elevated a position. Generally, mobilizations at level 1 are quite gentle so as not to evoke or provoke symptoms because the local soft tissues are often tender.

Level 2

The first progression of opener techniques at level 2 is simply to open the interface to a greater degree than at level 1. Hence, caudad rib mobilizations are performed more toward the end of their movement. Also, manual depression of the first rib can be performed with the patient exhaling so as to promote maximal opening of the rib around the brachial plexus. The scapula can be elevated actively at the same time.

The second progression at level 2 is to commence a small degree of closing. This is achieved by the therapist testing the manoeuvre by gently depressing the scapula whilst the patient inhales slowly. If no problems result, the technique can be continued. Note that no neurodynamic techniques are performed in conjunction with closing at this stage. The degree of closing can be increased until the near full or full range of closing is achieved.

It is important at this point to reiterate that, while mobilizations are offered in treatment, the patient is also instructed on exercises for any muscle dysfunctions, as mentioned earlier.

Level 3c

Reduced opening dysfunction with neural component

If the patient shows stiffness in caudad movement of the first rib, along with a neurodynamic component,

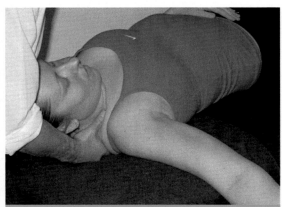

Figure 10.1   Caudad mobilization of the first rib whilst the patient performs the median neurodynamic test 1 (level/type 3c treatment).

such as tension or sliding, treatment can be directed at each of these components at the same time as mobilizing the first and/or second ribs (Fig. 10.1).

Reduced interface closing with neural sliding and tension dysfunctions
Sliding – the technique is performed by the patient producing the relevant distal and proximal sliding in the brachial plexus whilst the interface is placed in a closed position by the therapist. Hence, in the MNT1 position, the scapula is depressed whilst the patient inhales and the neural slider techniques are performed.

Tension – the movements are coordinated as an MNT1 tensioner using elbow extension and contralateral lateral flexion with inhalation as described earlier under examination.

Neurodynamics
Level 1
Neurodynamic testing for the thoracic outlet at level 1 is carried out initially with the patient in supine and the nervous system off-loaded, as in the descriptions of testing of the neural elements for the cervical spine. A key point, however, is that the scapula is elevated and the patient's first rib is not in an elevated position. This may involve the patient controlling their breathing during the examination in which full relaxation of the rib cage is performed to start with. Naturally, observation of respiration and dynamics of the rib cage is part of assessment.

Neurodynamic testing for the thoracic outlet syndrome at level 1 consists of performance of the supported median neurodynamic test 1 (see Chapter 7 on standard testing). The procedure is to perform the test slowly and carefully in the following sequence:

1. Wrist extension/supination.
2. Elbow extension gently toward the outer range to a point deemed acceptable to the patient and which gains sufficient information for the therapist.
3. Gentle and slow glenohumeral abduction to the first onset of symptoms.
4. Wrist extension is released to execute modified structural differentiation.

In the event that the technique of choice involves the ulnar neurodynamic test, the neurodynamic sequencing is as follows:

1. Wrist extension/pronation.
2. Elbow flexion.
3. Glenohumeral external rotation.
4. Glenohumeral abduction.
5. Release of wrist extension or a small amount of elbow flexion for differentiation purposes.

The level 2 neurodynamic assessment techniques for thoracic outlet syndrome are simply the standard tests for the median and ulnar nerves.

Level/type 3a – neurodynamically sensitized
Testing the thoracic outlet syndrome at level/type 3a consists of the addition of contralateral lateral flexion of the cervical spine and depression of the scapula. Hence, the sensitized median and ulnar neurodynamic tests are used and are the same as for the cervical spine.

Level/type 3b – sensitized by neurodynamic sequencing
The aim of sensitization at level/type 3b for thoracic outlet syndrome is to localize the neurodynamic forces as best possible to the thoracic outlet region through modification of the neurodynamic sequence. Hence, using the MNT1, the technique of choice is as follows:

1. Scapular depression.
2. Glenohumeral abduction and external rotation, both to approximately 90°, or what is permissible.
3. Cervical contralateral lateral flexion.
4. Elbow extension.
5. Wrist extension/supination.

The same method of sensitization can be applied to the ulnar neurodynamic test in which the following sequence applies:

1. Scapular depression.
2. Glenohumeral abduction and external rotation, both to approximately 90°, or what is permissible.
3. Cervical contralateral lateral flexion.
4. Elbow flexion.
5. Wrist extension/pronation.

Level/type 3c – multistructural

Interface closing (rib movement) and tension dysfunction

The median neurodynamic test 1 is performed, possibly with some degree of contralateral lateral flexion of the cervical spine. In the process, the scapula is depressed manually whilst the patient relaxes their upper trapezius and levator scapulae muscles. At the end point of the neurodynamic test (carefully decided on by the therapist and patient), the patient inhales deeply to elevate the first rib toward the brachial plexus. This bowstrings the plexus in a cephalad direction and applies more tension and pressure to it from its caudad (ulnar) surface from the first rib. Hence, this manoeuvre includes tension and compressive effects. The breath is held whilst structural differentiation is performed with release of wrist extension.

Reduced closing dysfunction with proximal or distal sliding dysfunctions

The test procedure for this dysfunction again utilizes inhalation and scapular depression and distal and proximal movements of the neural elements are produced whilst the interface is used to apply pressure to the brachial plexus. The median or ulnar neurodynamic test is performed. However, this time, the neck is moved into lateral flexion whilst the distal movements of the median neurodynamic test are added. Hence, for the MNT1, the sequence of movements is as follows:

1. Scapular depression.
2. Glenohumeral abduction/external rotation.
3. Wrist/finger extension, supination of forearm.
4. Inhalation.
5. Proximal slider – contralateral lateral flexion of the neck/elbow flexion, wrist and finger flexion (Fig. 10.2).

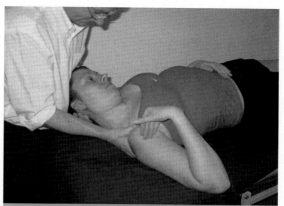

Figure 10.2   Proximal slider of the brachial plexus at the thoracic outlet with closing (scapular depression and inhalation), with the use of contralateral lateral flexion and elbow flexion.

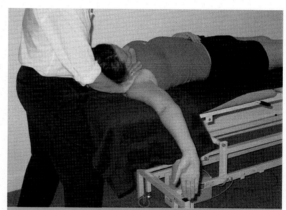

Figure 10.3   Distal slider of the brachial plexus at the thoracic outlet with closing (scapular depression and inhalation), with the use of ipsilateral lateral flexion and elbow extension.

6. Distal slider – ipsilateral lateral flexion of the neck/elbow extension, wrist and finger extension (Fig. 10.3).

PRONATOR TUNNEL SYNDROME

The pronator syndrome usually manifests as pain in the anteromedial forearm region with or without pins and needles in the distribution of the median nerve. Sometimes the pain can extend from the elbow into the ventral aspect of the forearm and wrist. The problem is often mistaken for golfer's elbow or ulnar neuritis because the symptoms are located in the medial elbow region. Generally the symptoms are provoked by repetitive activities that involve use of the pronator muscle, such as squeezing and pulling through the elbow and pronation movements. Throwing is also a possible cause.

Assessment involves neurological examination and the MNT1 and/or MNT2 tests, depending on the clinician's decision. Naturally, palpation of the median nerve at the elbow and testing of the mechanical interface is essential and is achieved with stretch and contraction of the pronator muscles in conjunction with, or separate from, the median nerve, according to the level and type of examination.

Mechanical interface
Levels 1 and 2
The causative mechanism with the pronator syndrome is generally that of excessive closing. Hence, at level 1, the static opener for the median nerve at the elbow is chosen and is performed by positioning the elbow in approximately 60°–90° flexion and the forearm into pronation. This is to reduce tension in the pronator muscle and take pressure and tension off the median nerve. The wrist and fingers are placed in neutral and the shoulder elevated, if necessary. This is offered as a rest position for pain relief, if the patient requires.

As the next progression, the dynamic opener is performed in the form of a mobilization in the direction of pronation but from a relatively neutral position.

As the patient progresses to low level 2, the closer is applied. This is performed by, in the same degree of elbow flexion/extension as above, gently moving the forearm into the supinated position to elongate the pronator teres muscle. This will apply a small amount of pressure to the nerve whereby the aim is to reduce its sensitivity to such forces and milk the nerve so that venous and arterial flow are increased. As the problem progresses toward the high end of level 2, the technique is to perform active pronation which is resisted manually, followed immediately by passive elongation of the muscle as a means of releasing the interface.

Neural component
Distal sliding dysfunction
The distal sliding dysfunction in the pronator syndrome occurs when the median nerve at the elbow shows pathodynamics in the direction of distal movement. It occurs when a movement that produces distal movement of the median nerve evokes an increase in symptoms. Hence, if, in the MNT1 position, the symptoms increase with ipsilateral lateral flexion or release of contralateral lateral flexion of the cervical spine, or the symptoms ease with contralateral lateral flexion, a distal sliding dysfunction may be implicated. In this case, the level 1 treatment is to slide the nerve proximally, away from the provoking direction (position away/move away). The technique therefore is as follows:

Patient position – for the MNT1, elbow in approximately 20°–30° flexion, forearm in a comfortable degree of pronation/supination, wrist and finger flexion to allow proximal movement of the nerve by releasing distal tension, approximately 45°–90° glenohumeral abduction (making use of the shoulder joint to draw the median nerve proximally) – the decision on the amount of abduction is, once again, judicious and depends on the patient's symptomatology. It is wise to use the treatment couch as the support for the patient's upper limb and pillows or towels can be used to enhance comfort and relaxation. The therapist then stabilizes the scapula whilst contralateral lateral flexion is performed to draw the nerve proximally (move away from the direction of the dysfunction). The technique should not evoke the patient's clinical symptoms (Fig. 10.4).

As the patient progresses toward low level 2, less shoulder abduction is used to allow more distal movement to occur during the positioning phase, whilst the neck movements remain the same. The wrist and fingers can be extended to position the nerve more distally also. At high level 2, the positions and movements are as follows:

Position – neutral lateral flexion of the cervical spine, the patient's upper limb is close to their side, scapular elevation, elbow in full comfortable range of extension.

Movements – the upper limb is supported comfortably, perform wrist and finger extension with ipsilateral lateral flexion of the cervical spine (Fig. 10.5).

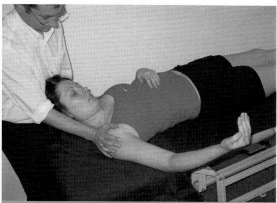

Figure 10.4   Proximal slider of the median nerve for the median nerve distal sliding dysfunction at level 1.

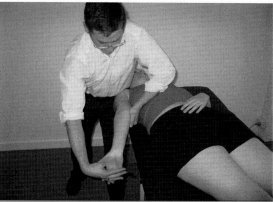

Figure 10.6   Distal slider technique at high level 2, scapular elevation and wrist extension.

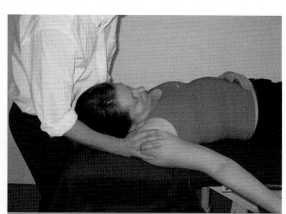

Figure 10.5   Distal slider technique at high level 2, movements – wrist and finger extension and ipsilateral lateral flexion of the cervical spine.

At high level 2, the mobilization is a more extensive distal slider and is performed as part of the median neurodynamic test 2. Scapular elevation and wrist and finger extension are performed (Fig. 10.6).

Proximal sliding dysfunction

The proximal sliding dysfunction in the pronator syndrome is illustrated by an increase in symptoms with proximal movement of the median nerve and distal movement of the nerve produces a decrease in symptoms. In the MNT1 position, symptoms will increase with contralateral lateral flexion of the cervical spine and wrist and finger *flexion*. The level 1

treatment of this dysfunction is to place the nerve in a distal position, then slide it distally in treatment (position away/move away).

Patient position – elbow in approximately 20°–30° flexion, wrist and fingers comfortably in neutral, the forearm in a comfortable degree of pronation, the patient's upper limb by their side, ipsilateral lateral flexion of the cervical spine.

Movements – extension of the wrist and fingers to draw the median nerve at the elbow distally. This technique is similar in principle to that in the later stages of the distal sliding dysfunction, except that, because it is performed at a low level, it may need to be performed more gently and modified according to the patient's needs.

As the patient progresses to low level 2, a degree of shoulder abduction and contralateral lateral flexion are added to position the median nerve at the elbow more proximally whilst wrist and finger extension are again performed (position towards/move away). Progressing through to high level 2, the positions and movements are altered, as follows:

Position – wrist and finger flexion, cervical spine in neutral, shoulder abduction up to approximately 90°, depending on the patient's capabilities.

Movements – contralateral lateral flexion of the cervical spine whilst stabilizing the scapula. This technique is similar as in the early stages of the distal sliding dysfunction, however, the glenohumeral joint is placed in more abduction to position the median

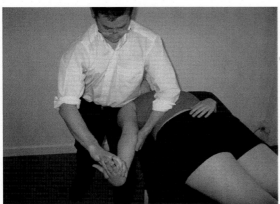

Figure 10.7 Proximal slider for the median nerve at the elbow using the median neurodynamic test 2, performance of scapular depression and wrist and finger flexion. The amount of glenohumeral abduction can be varied.

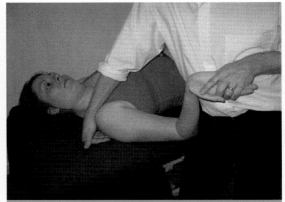

Figure 10.8 Tensioner for the median nerve at the elbow at level 1, contralateral lateral flexion and wrist extension with the elbow flexed and the scapula stabilized.

nerve at the elbow more proximally prior to the mobilization (position towards/move towards). Another way of performing this technique is to use the MNT2 slider option (Fig. 10.7).

At this point, the reader will have noticed that the treatment for the proximal sliding dysfunction at low levels is similar to the treatment for the distal sliding dysfunction at high levels. This is a common feature of all the sliding dysfunctions, is quite deliberate and is based on the progressional system presented in the chapter on Method of Treatment (Ch 8). The system allows for the treatment of the pathophysiological mechanisms early on and slowly builds up to address the pathomechanical aspects as the problems settle and will tolerate mechanical treatment better.

Tension dysfunction

The tension dysfunction in the pronator syndrome shows up as an increase in symptoms when tension in the median nerve at the elbow increases. Therefore, in either of the median neurodynamic test positions, symptoms will increase with contralateral lateral flexion of the cervical spine and wrist and finger extension. The symptoms also reduce when either of these movements is released. The treatment at level 1 is to position the nerve in an anti-tension position as for the generic off-loader for the median nerve, as shown under the section on the cervical

spine (Fig. 9.13, p. 167). Then the following mobilization or home exercise can be performed.

Patient position – elbow in approximately 90° flexion, wrist and fingers in neutral, the patient's upper limb by their side, scapula in a degree of elevation, ipsilateral lateral flexion of the cervical spine.

Movements – extension of the wrist and fingers and contralateral lateral flexion to apply a small amount tension to the median nerve from both proximal and distal ends. As the patient progresses to high level 1, more tension can be applied with the elbow being positioned into more extension and the same movements at the neck and wrist being performed (Fig. 10.8).

As the patient progresses to low level 2, the same movements are performed but, instead, the shoulder joint is abducted to a comfortable range, up to approximately 45°. At high level 2, the shoulder abduction position is taken above 45° toward 90° and the same movements are performed. Elbow extension is the movement of choice for the technique at level/type 3a, however, sensitization is added in the positioning, namely a small amount of scapular depression and contralateral lateral flexion of the cervical spine. This is effectively a series of progressions through the MNT1 (Fig. 10.9).

The level 3b neurodynamic procedure is simply to start the technique with elbow extension/supination and add the other components of the MNT1 from

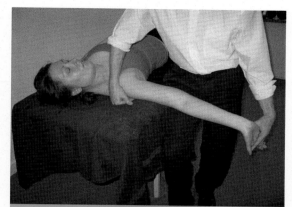

Figure 10.9   Gentle tensioner technique for the median nerve at level 3a, contralateral lateral flexion, scapular depression, glenohumeral abduction and wrist and finger extension are attained with the mobilization component being elbow extension.

just over, the pronator teres muscle. A proximal/distal slider technique is performed as the therapist maintains their thumb pressure over the nerve. This way, the nerve slides longitudinally under the therapist's thumb and a massage effect is produced. The degree of pressure applied by the thumb is arbitrary and decisions on this are influenced by the patient's needs and response. The technique operates by reversed origin. I liken this to milking a cow the wrong way round. The cow bends its knees up and down whilst the farmer holds their hands stationary around the cow's teat (Fig. 10.10).

SUPINATOR TUNNEL SYNDROME

The supinator tunnel syndrome usually expresses itself as pain in the anterolateral elbow and forearm regions and sometimes pins and needles in the distribution of the posterior interosseous nerve (radial dorsal aspect of the hand). Mysteriously, sometimes pain from this problem can be absent from the elbow and can instead localize itself in the dorsum of the wrist and it may do this in the absence of neurological symptoms. Hence, investigation of dorsal wrist pain should involve the posterior interosseous nerve at the elbow.

The disorder is often mistaken for tennis elbow, however it should not be because it does not generally cause pain solely in the common extensor origin. The symptoms are provoked by activities that involve use of the supinator muscle, such as squeezing and pulling through the elbow flexion and supination movements. As with the pronator tunnel syndrome, repetitive and postural factors almost always exist.

Because of its propensity to produce localized wrist pain, assessment, even in the absence of neurological symptoms, should involve neurological examination and the radial neurodynamic test. Naturally, palpation of the nerve and testing of the interfacing tissues are essential. These are achieved with palpation of the nerve and its environs as it passes under supinator and stretch and contraction of the supinator muscle in conjunction with, or separate from, neurodynamic testing for the posterior interosseous nerve.

The techniques for the supinator syndrome are virtually identical to those of the pronator tunnel syndrome, except that they are applied to the radial aspect of the elbow.

either end. Glenohumeral abduction is used in the mobilization. This ends up being similar to the MNT2 but is often best performed as an MNT1 because the abduction is easier to perform in this position.

Treatment at level 3c involves simultaneous treatment of the pronator muscle and other interfacing tissues whilst mobilizing the nerve. Contraction/relax of the muscle during the MNT1 is used and, during the release phase, the nerve is mobilized gently into a tension position. The technique is performed gently and only 2–3 times before returning the median nerve back to its rest position so as not to provoke symptoms. This triplet of mobilizations may then be repeated several times in the same treatment session.

Neurodynamic massage technique

This technique is directed at massaging and desensitizing the median nerve in the vicinity of the pronator muscle. It may also help improve blood flow through the nerve and squeeze away oedema within and around the nerve. It effectively slides the nerve under the practitioner's thumb whilst pressure is applied to the nerve.

Position – the position for the MNT2 neurodynamic test is adopted. Whilst stabilizing the patient's elbow in extension with the fingers, the therapist places their proximal thumb over the ventral surface of the median nerve either immediately proximal to, or

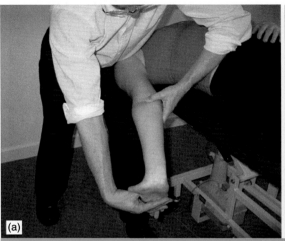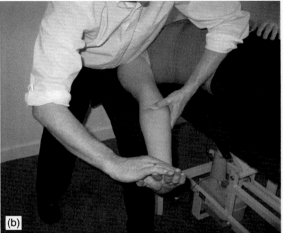

Figure 10.10   Neurodynamic massage technique for the median nerve at the elbow using the median neurodynamic test 2 and applying pressure with the therapist's thumb over the nerve. (a) Distal slider – scapular elevation, wrist and finger extension. (b) Proximal slider – scapular depression, wrist and finger flexion.

Mechanical interface

Levels 1 and 2

As with the pronator syndrome, the causative mechanism with the supinator syndrome is generally that of excessive closing. At level 1, therefore, the static opener for the posterior interosseous nerve at the elbow is performed by positioning the elbow in approximately 20°–30° short of full extension and the forearm relaxed in supination. This is to reduce tension in the supinator muscle and take pressure and tension off the nerve. The wrist and fingers are placed in neutral and the scapula elevated a little whilst the upper limb is placed near the patient's side.

If necessary, the humerus can be externally rotated to further off-load the radial nerve. If the patient requires, this rest position can be offered for pain relief at home. As the patient progresses to high level 1, the dynamic opener is performed in the form of a passive mobilization in the direction of supination from a relatively neutral position that passes toward the outer range of this movement.

At low level 2 and in the same degree of elbow flexion/extension as above, the forearm is gently moved into the pronated position to elongate the supinator muscle. As the problem progresses toward the high end of level 2, the next technique is to elongate the supinator muscle whilst it relaxes after resisted contraction and this technique is taken to the end of the comfortable range. Hence, active supination is resisted manually and this is followed immediately by passive elongation of the muscle as a means of releasing the interface.

Neural

Distal sliding dysfunction

The distal sliding dysfunction in the supinator syndrome occurs when the posterior interosseous nerve at the elbow shows pathodynamics in the direction of distal movement. Hence, if, in the radial neurodynamic test (RNT) position, the symptoms increase with ipsilateral lateral flexion of the cervical spine or release of contralateral lateral flexion, or the symptoms ease with contralateral lateral flexion, a distal sliding dysfunction may be implicated. As was the case with the pronator syndrome, the level 1 treatment for the supinator tunnel syndrome is to first position the nerve in a proximal position then slide it proximally as well, away from the provoking direction (position away/move away). Therefore the technique is as follows:

Therapist position – at the head of the patient.

Patient position – elbow in approximately 20°–30° flexion, forearm in a comfortable degree of pronation/supination, wrist and finger extension to allow

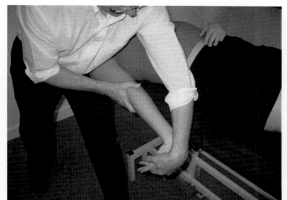

Figure 10.11   Distal slider for the posterior interosseous nerve for high level 2. Scapular elevation and wrist and finger flexion are performed. The angle of elbow flexion can be varied. Generally, the higher the patient level, the more elbow extension is used.

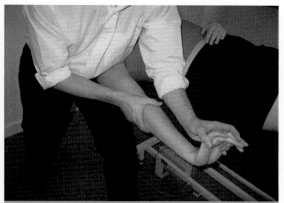

Figure 10.12   Proximal slider of the posterior interosseous nerve at low level 2 without contralateral lateral flexion of the cervical spine, movements of scapular depression/wrist extension.

proximal movement of the nerve, 30°–45° glenohumeral abduction if permissible (again making use of the shoulder joint to draw the radial nerve proximally).

Movement – the therapist stabilizes the scapula whilst contralateral lateral flexion is performed passively to draw the nerve proximally.

As the patient progresses from low to high level 1, less shoulder abduction is used to allow more distal movement to occur during the positioning phase, whilst the neck movements remain the same. The wrist and fingers are moved into the flexed to position to move the posterior interosseous nerve further in a distal direction and the forearm can be pronated (position toward/move away).

In progressing through level 2, the RNT is now used to produce the correct movements (Fig. 10.11).

Proximal sliding dysfunction
The proximal sliding dysfunction in the supinator syndrome is illustrated when proximal movement of the posterior interosseous nerve evokes an increase in symptoms. In the RNT position, symptoms will increase with contralateral lateral flexion of the cervical spine and wrist and finger *extension*. As with the pronator syndrome, the level 1 treatment is to place the nerve in a distal position, then slide it distally (position away/move away).

Patient position – arm supported on pillows if necessary, elbow in approximately 20°–30° flexion, wrist and fingers in neutral, the forearm in a comfortable degree of pronation/supination, the patient's upper limb by their side, scapula elevated, neck in neutral.

Movements – flexion of the wrist and fingers to draw the nerve distally and ipsilateral lateral flexion of the cervical spine. The neck movements can be performed by the therapist whilst the patient can move their hand.

At high level 1, glenohumeral abduction and contralateral lateral flexion are added to position the nerve more proximally whilst the wrist, finger and neck movements are repeated (position toward/move away).

At low level 2, the positions and movements are altered, as follows:

Position – for the RNT.

Movements – scapular depression, wrist and finger extension (Fig. 10.12).

At high level 2, contralateral lateral flexion of the neck is introduced prior to the mobilization. The mobilization is repeated as scapular depression and wrist and finger extension (position toward/move toward).

Tension dysfunction
The tension dysfunction in the supinator syndrome produces an increase in symptoms when tension in

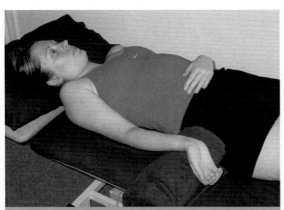

Figure 10.13 Off-loader for the posterior interosseous nerve, ipsilateral lateral flexion, scapular elevation, glenohumeral external rotation, elbow comfortably flexed and supinated with the wrist and fingers relaxed comfortably in extension.

the posterior interosseous nerve at the elbow increases. In the RNT position, the symptoms will therefore increase with contralateral lateral flexion of the cervical spine and wrist and finger flexion. The symptoms also reduce when either of these components is released.

Treatment at low level 1 is to position the nerve in an anti-tension position as for the generic off-loader for the radial nerve and offer this as a rest position for the patient (Fig. 10.13). The mobilization of choice at level 1 for the tension dysfunction is the proximo-distal slider, in both directions if possible. This is likely to soothe the nerve rather than provoke it.

At level 2, the therapist changes the technique to adopt the RNT position. The elbow remains in a relatively flexed position prior to the mobilization. The movements then consist of scapular depression and wrist and finger flexion with elbow extension as a wide amplitude technique but gentle technique. This is progressed with increases in glenohumeral abduction and wrist movements and contralateral lateral flexion positioning.

Treatment at level 3a is the same as the above but, this time, the technique can incorporate scapular depression and/or contralateral lateral flexion. Level/type 3b treatment involves performance of the same technique as in level 3a except the elbow extension is the first movement in the preparation of the technique and it is performed slightly more

firmly during the mobilization. Treatment at level 3c involves simultaneous treatment of the supinator muscle and other interfacing tissues whilst mobilizing the nerve. Hence, contract/relax of this muscle with the neurodynamic tensioner serves this purpose.

Neurodynamic massage technique

Position – the position for the RNT is adopted. Whilst stabilizing the patient's elbow in extension, the therapist places their proximal thumb over the ventral surface of the posterior interosseous nerve either immediately proximal to, or just over, the supinator muscle. A proximo-distal slider technique is performed as the therapist maintains their thumb pressure over the nerve.

Proximal slider movements – scapular depression, wrist and finger extension.

Distal slider movements – scapular elevation, wrist and finger flexion.

This technique is similar to the median nerve equivalent of milking the cow by reversed origin.

CARPAL TUNNEL SYNDROME

Introduction

I believe that the role of hands-on therapy as a conservative means of treating carpal tunnel syndrome is generally underestimated. Direct mobilizations of the median nerve and tendons for the problem have been shown to reduce the need for surgery (Rozmaryn et al 1998) and can be related to increased active grip strength and improved patient satisfaction (Akalin et al 2002). However, even with that, little has been done to link treatment techniques to what I believe to be carpal tunnel syndromes in which different dysfunctions may exist. That is, a disorder of the median nerve of the wrist could house a dominance of different mechanisms; for instance; interface, longitudinal sliding or pathophysiological (e.g. diabetic neuropathy) types and the treatment should be personalized for each problem. Hence, what follows is a breakdown of the different types of dysfunctions related to carpal tunnel syndrome and their treatments. It is also worthwhile being familiar with the chapters on General Neurodynamics and Neuropathodynamics so that the logic of technique application is clear. For the

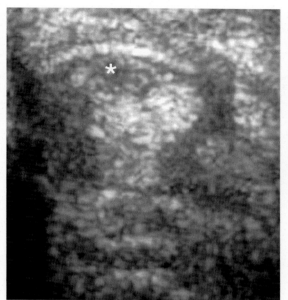

Figure 10.14   Normal median nerve at the carpal tunnel. The silvery arch at the top of the picture represents the transverse carpal ligament and the ovoid shape immediately below the ligament is the median nerve* as it adopts the shape of the tendons (lighter ovoid structures) immediately below it (Shacklock & Wilkinson 2000, unpublished observations).

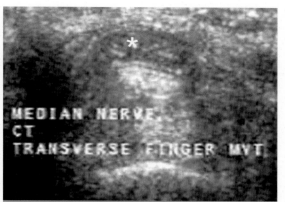

Figure 10.15   Abnormal median nerve at the carpal tunnel (patient with carpal tunnel syndrome). The nerve* is considerably darker than normal, swollen and adopts a bean-like shape as it is not as capable of adopting the shape of neighbouring structures. It is also much larger compared with the size of the adjacent tendon and, in dynamic studies, can be observed to have a tendency to rub against the adjacent tendon during hand movements (Shacklock & Wilkinson 2000, unpublished observations).

reader's interest images of the median nerve are provided (Figs 10.14 and 10.15).

Physical examination

The primary descriptors for setting up the physical examination for carpal tunnel syndrome are slow, gentle and detailed. This is because it will be necessary to sense small and subtle changes in physical function and sensory responses. The nerve is palpated extensively along its course, the need for which may extend far proximally up the upper limb. Palpation and testing for Tinel's and Kingery's signs should also be performed as far distally as the motor branch of the median nerve in the hand (Fig. 10.16) as it passes into the muscles of the thenar eminence. With deft technique, the median nerve can often be palpated immediately proximal to the transverse carpal ligament, once the tendons are displaced manually. Frequently, swelling in and around the

nerve and in the tunnel can be palpated and this may also extend distally to the motor branch (Fig. 10.16) and Guyon's canal. In relation to neurodynamic testing, the MNT1 is the technique of choice. It is performed in accordance with the system set out in the chapter on standard neurodynamic testing (Ch 7).

Mechanical interface

Testing of the mechanical interface involves putting the interfacing structures through their paces to establish whether they are involved in producing neurodynamic changes. Hence, active and passive movements of all carpal and related joints are performed. Watson's test is also pertinent, along with specific tests for interface opening and closing. Clearly, apart from searching for physical changes such as swelling, thickening, tenderness and stiffness, reproduction of symptoms is a key aspect through Phalen's and other tests.

Opening – horizontal flexion – opener
Horizontal flexion as an opening movement is performed with the patient positioned in supine with the elbow flexed to approximately 90° so the patient's

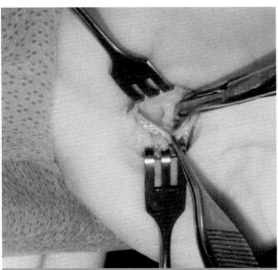

Figure 10.16   Motor branch of the median nerve as it passes into the muscles of the thenar eminence. It can be easily palpated and illustrates the importance of moving the innervated tissues (i.e. muscles) in mobilization of the nerve in cases of carpal tunnel syndrome.

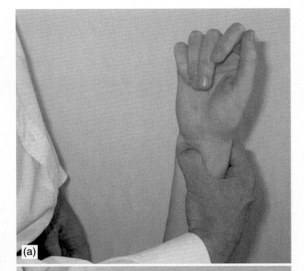

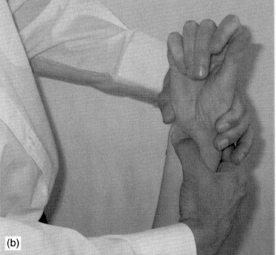

Figure 10.17   Technique of horizontal flexion. (a) Position of the therapist's proximal hand. (b) Technique of horizontal flexion.

forearm and hand point almost vertically. The therapist's hands approach the patient's wrist from different directions. The therapist's proximal hand gently clasps the patient's distal forearm radially so that the therapist's thumb is located on the ventral surface of the patient's forearm between, and parallel to, the patient's radius and ulna. This is so that the end of the therapist's thumb reaches up to the patient's distal palmar crease. No pressure is exerted by the thumb over the carpal tunnel during the test movement. The therapist's distal hand then passes dorsally around the patient's wrist, so that ventral pressure is applied on the radial side by the therapist's fingers and ulnarly by the therapist's thumb. The wrist and forearm are stabilized by the therapist's proximal hand. This manoeuvre makes the carpal bones and first and fifth metacarpals form an arch with the concave surface being on the ventral aspect of the wrist. When performed gently, it is likely that the ensuing movements produce reduced tension in the transverse carpal ligament and reduce pressure on the median nerve. This can be performed as a static or dynamic opener (Fig. 10.17).

Closing – horizontal extension – dynamic closer
In the performance of horizontal extension, the therapist's hands approach the patient's wrist from the dorsal aspect. Each hand creates a gentle pincer action with the therapist's index fingers and thumbs around the medial and lateral aspects of the wrist complex and first and fifth metacarpals. The hand that holds the radial aspect grips the first metacarpal and scaphoid bones whilst the hand that grips the ulnar structures clasps the hamate, pisiform and

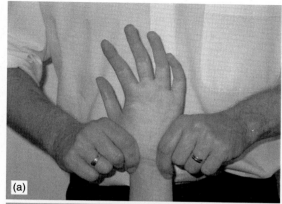

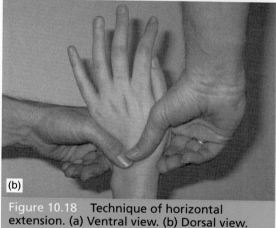

Figure 10.18 Technique of horizontal extension. (a) Ventral view. (b) Dorsal view.

fifth metacarpal bones. The movement is produced by the therapist levering gently over their thumbs as they apply a ventral pressure over the dorsum of the wrist and an outward wedging action of their index fingers. This movement produces an increase in tension in the transverse carpal ligament by angling the ulnar and radial structures posteriorly around the capitate (Fig. 10.18).

Neurodynamic testing

Levels 1 and 2

In neurodynamic testing, the level 1 testing for the median nerve at the wrist is limited and structural differentiation modified. The first movement is contralateral lateral flexion of the neck and the rest of the MNT1 is completed gradually to the first onset of symptoms. Contralateral lateral flexion is then released and, in the event that there is a genuine carpal tunnel syndrome, may well produce a change in the hand symptoms. Clearly, some movements may be omitted, such as wrist and finger extension if symptoms are likely to appear too early or too severely (Fig. 10.19).

At level 2, the standard MNT1 is performed whereas, at level 3, other component movements are added.

Level/type 3

Testing at level/type 3a involves performance of the MNT1, with contralateral lateral flexion and possibly scapular depression. Level/type 3b testing is achieved by, still using the MNT1, starting the test with wrist and finger extension and completing the manoeuvre by adding the movements in proximal order. Level/type 3c testing utilizes the wrist joint as the mechanical interface. In doing so, horizontal extension is combined with the MNT1. This way, pressure is applied during the neurodynamic test. Alternatively, resisted active wrist and finger flexion can be combined with the MNT1. It must be remembered that, since symptoms due to carpal tunnel syndrome can be easily provoked, decisions on which level/type of testing to perform are based on the system of planning the examination set out in chapter 6 (Fig. 10.20).

Treatment

Mechanical interface

Treatment of carpal tunnel syndrome naturally revolves around the diagnostic category. However, in the case of interface dominant problems, treatment will focus on improving function of the wrist complex. This, if necessary, can be by way of improving stability through exercises and is effectively treatment of an excessive closing disorder. The other kind of excessive closing problem is that produced by a tunnel that is too small for the nerve and tendons. In this category of diagnosis, it will be necessary to reduce pressure on the median nerve by performing interface opening techniques (horizontal flexion), as mentioned above. This would apply to the level 1 problem. As the disorder improves to level 2, the closing techniques (horizontal extension) can be applied whereby mobilization of the transverse carpal ligament is the aim. It is improbable that normal force applied during mobilization of the ligament will produce a sudden increase in

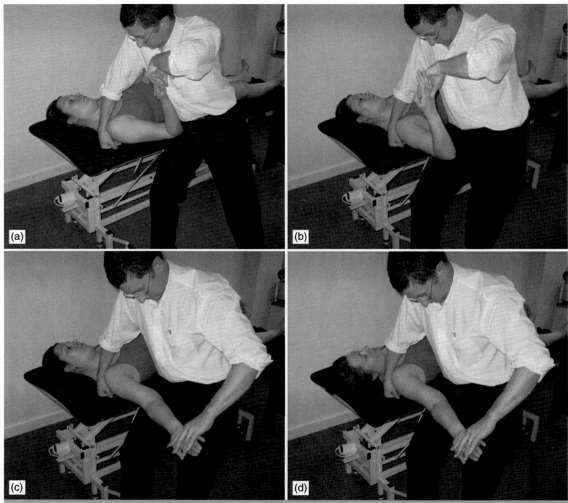

Figure 10.19 Performance of the MNT1 in physical examination of the patient with carpal tunnel syndrome at level 1. (a) Starting position. Note that the wrist and fingers are straight and the neck is in contralateral lateral flexion for modified structural differentiation. (b) Glenohumeral abduction. (c) Elbow extension. Note that the wrist and fingers remain straight so as not to stretch the median nerve at the wrist. (d) Modified structural differentiation in the form of release of contralateral lateral flexion.

its length. However, with repeated loading, it may be possible to achieve improvements in carpal tunnel pressures in two ways; subtle improvement of viscoelastic function of the ligament, thereby improving stresses on the median nerve and; by applying repeated pressure to the tunnel, thus milking it of excessive venous fluid, further reducing pressure in the area. This would improve its oxygenation by allowing new, fresh blood to enter the

tunnel. Hence, a valuable technique for the carpal tunnel problem is often the horizontal extension mobilization.

Neural component
Proximal sliding dysfunction

The essential ingredient of the proximal sliding dysfunction is that symptoms are evoked by proximal movement of the nerve in the carpal tunnel. In the

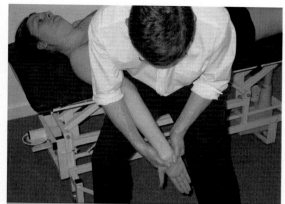

Figure 10.20 Median neurodynamic test 1 with horizontal extension of the wrist complex for assessment and treatment at level/type 3c.

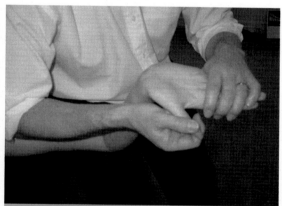

Figure 10.21 Distal slider of the median nerve at the wrist. Note that the elbow is flexed and tension is not applied from a proximal direction (position away/move away).

MNT1 position, increased symptoms with *release* of finger extension, flexing the fingers or cervical contralateral lateral flexion illustrate this dysfunction. The following slider techniques can be useful in such a scenario.

At first, the distal slider is performed to move the nerve away from the direction of the dysfunction. In the above illustration (Fig. 10.21) the technique is close to the end range. This may be tolerated by the patient who occupies level 1 but, if not, the technique can be varied by reducing the wrist and finger components. The patient can naturally perform this

actively as a home exercise. Progression of this mobilization to high level 1 is to add proximal components progressively, such as elbow extension and glenohumeral abduction but still mobilize in the distal direction with the use of finger extension movements (position towards/move away).

Position – the patient's upper limb is placed in the MNT1 position according to the patient's capabilities. The wrist and fingers are located in a straight position as if to make a paddle with the patient's hand. The neurodynamic technique is performed by positioning the elbow in more extension and mobilizing the fingers and thumb into extension, whilst the wrist joint remains stationary. The reason for holding it still is that, with movement of the wrist, the interfacing joint structures will tend to move with the nerve, which would then reduce the amount of longitudinal movement of the nerve relative to the joint structures. Prevention of wrist movement enables the nerve to slide relative to the neighbouring structures such as the transverse carpal ligament above and bones underneath. This will mean that the tendons will still slide longitudinally with the nerve somewhat, although their movement is greater in amplitude than the nerve as the fingers move. The ratio of tendon movement to nerve movement that we have observed informally tends to vary between approximately 5:1 and 20:1, however, formal measurement would be necessary to establish accurate values for this phenomenon.

At low level 2, the glenohumeral joint is gradually positioned toward 90° abduction and the nerve mobilization is reversed to it being performed in a proximal direction. Hence, in this position, the wrist and fingers are flexed whilst the elbow is extended during the mobilization (position towards/move towards).

At high level 2, the neurodynamic technique utilises scapular depression and/or contralateral lateral flexion of the neck as positional elements and the wrist and finger flexion and elbow extension movements are repeated. It is important to make the thumb move into the palm of the hand under the fingers so that the motor branch of the nerve is mobilized effectively (Figs 10.22 and 10.23).

Distal sliding dysfunction
In the MNT1 position, the distal sliding dysfunction displays itself as an increase in symptoms with finger

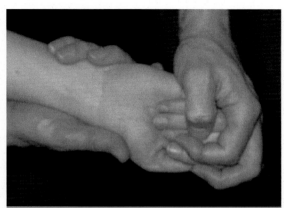

Figure 10.22   Hand positions and movement of the thumb and fingers during the proximal slider of the median nerve at the wrist. Note that the thumb leads the fingers into the palm during flexion so as to successfully mobilise the motor branch of the median nerve.

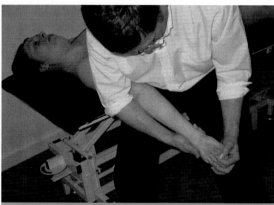

Figure 10.23   Technique of proximal sliding of the median nerve at the wrist using the MNT1 at high level 2.

extension movements and a decrease in symptoms with movements that produce proximal migration of the nerve. Hence, cervical contralateral lateral flexion will produce a reduction in hand symptoms in the MNT1 position.

The preparation for the distal sliding dysfunction with the MNT1 is the same as for the level 2 proximal sliding dysfunction above. Effectively, the progressions are reversed so that the principles of position and move away and towards are fulfilled. At

low levels of the distal sliding dysfunction, however, the clinician will modify the technique according to the patient's needs.

Sliding of the nerve on the adjacent tendons
What is interesting about the dynamics of the median nerve at the wrist is that the slider of the nerve in the direction of finger movement (e.g. extension) produces movement of the nerve *with* the tendons in this direction. In this situation, not as much sliding of the nerve relative to the tendons takes place as could be the case with other combinations of movements. What turns out to be the best slider of the nerve in the opposite direction of the tendons is in fact the tensioner of the nerve. This is because extension of the fingers produces distal movement of the tendons and, simultaneously, the nerve is pulled proximally by a proximal movement such as contralateral lateral flexion of the neck. Hence, all other things being equal and when the wrist joint stays still, the neural tensioner produces proximal movement of the nerve at the wrist whilst the tendons move distally with the fingers. I therefore advocate an element of gentle tensioners at some stage of carpal tunnel syndrome rehabilitation to make sure that all the sliding possibilities of the nerve have been optimized.

Tension dysfunction
The tension dysfunction is exhibited by the patient's symptoms being evoked when tension is applied to the nerves from both ends of the tract. Hence, in the MNT1 position, contralateral lateral flexion of the cervical spine and wrist and finger extension will be symptomatic and release of either of these movements will reduce symptoms. As mentioned earlier in this book, tensioners at level 1 are often unsuccessful but may be attempted and are similar to those for the median nerve at the elbow. Generally, sliders in both distal and proximal directions as large amplitude techniques are good for level 1 carpal tunnel syndromes with a significant sensitivity to tension.

At level 2, the tensioner can be introduced. It is performed as a wide amplitude movement, but at first it must not evoke symptoms. For instance, the patient is positioned for the MNT1 and, with no lateral flexion or wrist and finger extension and the arm is abducted to between 45° and 90°. The mobilizations consist of elbow and finger extension in an elbow position that is satisfactory for the patient. As the problem improves, wrist extension may be added as high level 2 treatment.

At level 3a, the movements of contralateral lateral flexion of the neck and/or scapular depression are added and the wrist, finger and thumb movements are repeated. The level/type 3b sequence can be to mobilize elbow extension after arriving gently toward the end of a comfortable range of the distal-to-proximal sequence of the MNT1. The level/type 3c treatment is also to mobilize elbow extension with additional interface treatment, for instance, performing horizontal extension. This technique is described under level/type 3c testing.

References

Akalin E, Peker O, Senocak O, Tamci S, Gulbahar S, Cakmur R, Oncel S 2002 Treatment of carpal tunnel syndrome with nerve and tendon gliding exercises. American Journal of Physical Medicine and Rehabilitation 81(2): 108–113

Coppieters M, Stappaerts K, Janssens K 2002 Reliability of detecting 'onset of pain'; and 'submaximal pain' during neural provocation testing of the upper quadrant. Physiotherapy Research International 7(3): 146–156

Coveney B, Trott P, Grimmer K, Bell A, Hall R, Shacklock M 1997 The upper limb tension test in a group of subjects with a clinical presentation of carpal tunnel syndrome. In: Proceedings of the Manipulative Physiotherapists' Association of Australia, Melbourne: 31–33

Grant R, Forrester C, Hides J 1995 Screen based keyboard operation: the adverse effects on the neural system. Australian Journal of Physiotherapy 41: 99–107

Kenneally M, Rubenach H, Elvey R 1988 The upper limb tension test: the SLR of the arm. In: Grant R (ed) Physical Therapy of the Cervical and Thoracic Spine, Churchill Livingstone, New York

McLellan D, Swash M 1976 Longitudinal sliding of the median nerve during movements of the upper limb. Journal of Neurology, Neurosurgery and Psychiatry 39: 556–570

Rozmaryn L, Dovelle S, Rothman E, Gorman K, Olvey K, Bartko J 1998 Nerve and tendon gliding exercises and the conservative management of carpal tunnel syndrome. Journal of Hand Therapy 11: 171–179

Selvaratnam P, Cook S, Matyas T 1997 Transmission of mechanical stimulation to the median nerve at the wrist during the upper limb tension test. In: Proceedings of the Manipulative Physiotherapists' Association of Australia, Melbourne: 182–188

Selvaratnam P, Matyas T, Glasgow E 1994 Non-invasive discrimination of brachial plexus involvement in upper limb pain. Spine 19: 26–33

Lumbar spine

11

Diagnosis and treatment – lumbar spine and radiculopathy, mid-lumbar disorders

Specific dysfunctions – mechanical interface (opening closing), neural sliding and tension dysfunctions, level/type 3c combination dysfunctions

Progression of physical examination and treatment through the levels

Off-loaders sliders and tensioners, openers and closers

Combined muscle, joint and neural treatments

PHYSICAL EXAMINATION AT LEVELS 1 AND 3

Slump test

Level 1

Neurodynamic sequencing

Recapitulating, the neurodynamic sequencing variations in the slump test for level 1 are designed to prevent physical stresses from rising unduly so that the patient's symptoms are not provoked.

Stage 1 – if the patient can sit without provocation of symptoms, they adopt the starting position as for the standard slump test. However, if they can not sit comfortably in this position, they are encouraged to alter their position so as to become comfortable. If this is successful, the appropriate neurodynamic movements, *except* lumbar and thoracic flexion are added to this position. The effect is to protect the painful interface whilst, at the same time, test the neural tissues in their inner range of motion. Consequently, the whole slump test is not completed, but sufficient information on the potential role of neuropathodynamics is gained. If the patient can not sit comfortably at level 1, then the slump test is not performed unless it will actually reveal useful information without undue provocation. Instead, the straight leg raise and passive neck flexion are performed as the means of obtaining information on the patient's neurodynamics.

Stage 2 – neck flexion is performed by the patient whilst the therapist supports the patient's forehead with their hand and prevents too rapid a descent of the head. The movement is taken to the first onset of symptoms only. If lumbar symptoms occur, the neck is then returned to the neutral position. When neck flexion produces an increase in the lumbar symptoms and they are the patient's clinical pain, the test is deemed to be an overt abnormal response (for classification of responses, see Chapter 5).

Stage 3 – dorsiflexion may then be performed passively by the therapist and this is followed by passive knee extension to the first onset of symptoms. As soon as lumbar symptoms occur, the dorsiflexion is released to ascertain if it produces an effect on (reduces) the lumbar symptoms. If the answer is yes, then the test is deemed to be abnormal. The value in the above sequences of movement is that they do not provoke the patient's symptoms yet the necessary information on neurodynamics has been obtained (Fig. 11.1).

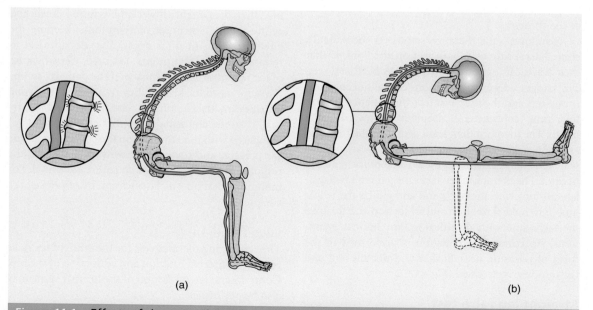

(a)   (b)

Figure 11.1   Effects of slump test biased to: (a) Musculoskeletal structures – the structures of the spinal canal are compressed with lumbar flexion during the standard slump test. (b) Neural tissues – removal of lumbar flexion during the slump test producing a bias of forces to the neural structures, thus exerting a protective effect on the musculoskeletal system.

Table 11.1 Types of dysfunction implicated by abnormal responses to the slump test	
Movement	**Dysfunction**
Neck flexion	Cephalad
Knee extension/dorsiflexion	Caudad
Neck flexion and knee extension	Tension

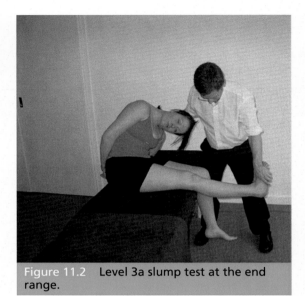

Figure 11.2   Level 3a slump test at the end range.

Diagnosis of dysfunctions

When neck flexion only is abnormal, the diagnosis of a cephalad sliding dysfunction is made and when knee extension alone is abnormal a caudad dysfunction may exist. In the case of both neck flexion and knee extension being abnormal when performed at the same time, a tension dysfunction is implicated, as summarized in Table 11.1.

The level 2 slump test is simply the standard one described in Chapter 7.

Level 3

Type 3a neurodynamically sensitized

The level/type 3a (neurodynamically sensitized) position for the slump test for the lumbar spine incorporates the additional sensitizing manoeuvres of medial rotation and adduction of the hip, dorsiflexion of the ankle and contralateral lateral flexion of the spine.

Technique – the therapist stands on the patient's contralateral side with both feet on the floor so that their reach can extend to the patient's head and feet. The patient adopts the position for the full standard slump test and the therapist tells the patient to droop their near (contralateral) shoulder downward to the plinth. The therapist then leans gently on the shoulder and upper trapezius region with their near forearm whilst the hand extends to the far side of the patient's occiput. The therapist then takes the patient's far (ipsilateral) foot with the free hand and guides the whole limb into medial rotation and adduction and finalizes the technique with dorsiflexion. For lumbar symptoms, structural differentiation is performed in the form of releasing neck flexion and dorsiflexion and the response is classified (Fig. 11.2).

Straight leg raise test

Level 1

Testing the lumbar spine with the straight leg raise test at level 1 is quite simple and should be performed

gently, slowly and carefully with close attention being paid to the patient's symptoms. This is particularly important on account of the problem being at level 1 and rather sensitive.

Technique – the patient in supine with a straight knee, if possible. Passive dorsiflexion is performed first, then the patient's lower limb is raised slowly and gently to the first onset of symptoms, keeping the knee straight. At this point, the dorsiflexion is released and the symptoms observed. Classification of the response is the next step. If the patient's symptoms are reproduced, and they reduce with releasing dorsiflexion, the response is classified as overt abnormal. If subtle abnormalities (physical or subjective) compared with the same test on the contralateral side are present, and they change with dorsiflexion, the response is then deemed to be covert abnormal. For more information on classification of responses, see Chapter 5.

Level/type 3a

The sensitizing manoeuvres for the straight leg raise consist of internal rotation and adduction of the hip. Contralateral lateral flexion of the lumbar spine may also be performed.

Technique – the straight leg is raised to the first point of symptoms, then internal rotation and adduction are performed. If contralateral lateral flexion is included in the test the movement is

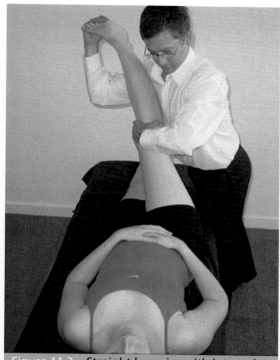

Figure 11.3   Straight leg raise with internal rotation and adduction of the hip (level/type 3a, sensitized neurodynamically).

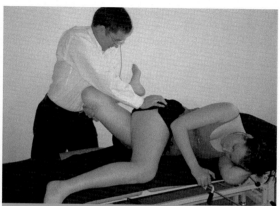

Figure 11.4   The level 3a femoral slump test which includes contralateral lateral flexion of the lumbar spine by applying cephalad pressure on the patient's trochanter and ilium.

performed as the first one to set the test up and prevent extraneous movement occurring. Dorsiflexion is added at the end of the manoeuvre for the purposes of differentiation (Fig. 11.3).

Prone knee bend

Level 1

The technique for the prone knee bend for level 1 is modified somewhat from the standard test because, by definition, the differentiation part must not increase symptoms. Hence, the first movement is to stabilize the pelvis, or even roll it slightly into a posterior rotated position by applying pressure on the sacrum in this direction. The knee is then flexed to the first onset of lumbar symptoms, if they actually occur. At this point, the pelvis is let to roll back into the anterior rotated position whilst the knee position is held stationary. This final manoeuvre is likely to reduce neural tension and release the nerves but it increases lumbar extension. Hence, if the

symptoms reduce with the release of posterior rotation, there may be a neural component to the test response.

Level 3

A level 3a technique for the L2–3/femoral component of the nervous system is simply to add contralateral lateral flexion to the prone knee bend prior to performance of the test. The same applies to the femoral slump test (Fig. 11.4).

TREATMENT

Mechanical interface

Reduced closing dysfunction
Introduction
Even though the following treatment techniques act through the musculoskeletal system, they are a magnificent illustration of neurodynamics in action. This is because, in the early low levels, treatment affects mainly the pathophysiological mechanisms in and around the nerve root and, as the problem progresses to higher levels, the dominant mechanism is pathomechanical in nature, which the treatment attacks specifically then too. The following is a good example of mechanics and physiology of the

nervous system interacting and treatment being tailor-made to affect each relevant component.

One of the more important aspects of the reduced closing dysfunction is that it is usually caused by a space-occupying lesion such as a disc bulge, swollen posterior intervertebral joint or stenotic changes. It may also be a result of inflammatory changes in or around the neural structures, causing them to become hypersensitive. The neural tissues themselves can be swollen and under pressure from dilated veins in the intervertebral foramen and rest of the radicular canal. These vascular changes therefore become part of the mechanical dysfunction through altered pressure dynamics. Hence, usually the best treatment in these circumstances is to open up the interface so as to reduce pressure. This is likely to improve intraneural venous return and capillary blood flow and produce a reduction in sensitivity and pressure in the area. The reason for not advocating a closing technique at level 1 is that it is likely to compress an already sensitive and potentially hypoxic neural structure. Generally therefore, I advocate opening techniques in the early stages of a reduced closing lumbar dysfunction. As the problem settles, techniques that improve the pathodynamics related to the motion segment can be applied, such as closing techniques and other forms of mobilization. As will be seen, an inadvertent result of this approach is that, in the early stages, treatment for the reduced closing dysfunction ends up being similar to that for the reduced opening category.

Level 1
Progressions 1, 2, 3 and 4 – static opener
The 'static opener' at level 1 of the reduced closing dysfunction is one of the most important and useful techniques for the patient with sciatica and distal neurological symptoms because, when performed well, it is so often effective.

Position – contralateral side lying (painful side uppermost) the hips and knees are flexed to 90° or higher and the patient is moved to the edge of the plinth so that their knees protrude a hand's breadth over the side of the bed. If the patient can not flex their hips and knees sufficiently, it is permissible to raise them only as high as is comfortable. This flexion manoeuvre is designed to open up the spinal canal and radicular canals. It does this by allowing the legs and feet to drape over the edge of the plinth and

therefore also produce contralateral lateral flexion of the lumbar spine on the symptomatic side. The result is that pressure is taken off the nerve roots. Nevertheless, a sudden rush of blood through the nerve root as pressure is removed can be painful. So, if the manoeuvre produces too much opening and is provocative, one of the patient's feet can be placed back on the plinth. A partial reversal of the lateral flexion therefore occurs. If this position is still painful, then the other foot can also be placed back on the plinth, which reduces the lateral flexion even further. At this point, much of the lateral flexion will have been removed, so it is then advisable to place a bolster in the form of a rolled up towel or other such object under the patient's waist to add a small amount of localized lateral flexion without producing symptoms. At the other end of the spectrum, in some patients, even their legs hanging off the side of the plinth is not sufficient to produce a good amount of lateral flexion. If this occurs, a bolster, as mentioned above, can again be used to increase the lateral flexion. In the general application of the technique, because problems at level 1 are somewhat irritable, the position adopted must be modified in small increments with careful reference to the patient's symptomatology.

During each of the applications of the 'opener', the therapist checks that the appropriate amount of lateral flexion has been achieved and monitors the effects of lateral flexion on the patient's symptoms. Once a comfortable position has been found, and this means one that reduces the patient's symptoms (particularly distal ones), the patient is asked to remain in this position for approximately one minute. This duration allows time for new blood to flow through the nerve root and improve nutrition. If this produces a small or moderate improvement, the position can be adopted twice more in the same session. If a dramatic improvement occurs, the technique is *not* repeated in the same session, and the patient is reassessed on another day. If symptoms develop whilst the patient is in this 'opened' position, the patient is instructed to return to a comfortable position until the symptoms settle. This treatment can still be repeated once or twice more to establish the consistency of the response, as long as the response is satisfactory. Reassessment is always performed after each application, particularly symptoms at rest, neurological symptoms and signs and optionally one neurodynamic test to the first change in symptoms only. The patient is not instructed to perform this technique as a home exercise at this stage because it is important to establish the long-term effect (at least 24 hours) of the treatment. The number of patients who improve with this treatment, particularly in relation to neurological signs and pain, is astounding. The patient most suited to this treatment is that in whom neurological symptoms, such as numbness and pins and needles, occur distally, and more so if they are present much of the time. In the patient who has severe pain near their spine and in the buttock, this treatment can be helpful but they are often quite sensitive to opening techniques so they are to be progressed cautiously and slowly. This technique is not appropriate for patients whose symptoms are provoked by opening techniques. However, to be sure this is the case, the therapist must perform the techniques carefully and correctly. If they are executed clumsily and without small incremental changes, the therapist will discard them hastily and the patient will miss an opportunity

to receive effective treatment. Mobilizations are not performed at this stage. However, if, at the second session, the patient reports an improvement, it is then advisable for them to use the 'static opener' as a home treatment, but as a position, not a mobilization.

In appointing each of the above positions to a scale of incremental steps, progression 1 is the patient lying on their side with a bolster under their waist with their hips and knees flexed comfortably. Progression 2 is with their lower or upper leg suspended over the side of the plinth whilst the other foot rests on the bed and the hips and knees flexed to 90° or more, if possible. Progression 3 is with both legs lying over the side of the plinth, producing lateral flexion. Progression 4 is as progression 3 but with an additional bolster under the patient's waist. In all progressions, the patient is asked to relax their trunk muscles so that they let their pelvis roll on the bed to allow lateral flexion. The patient's hands are placed according to the figures below. In more advanced cases, the therapist can hold the pelvis in a caudad direction (producing more contralateral lateral flexion) (Figs 11.5, 11.6, 11.7 and 11.8).

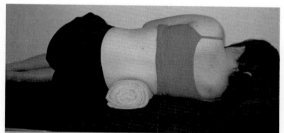

Figure 11.5   Progression 1 static opener for the level 1 lumbar reduced closing dysfunction.

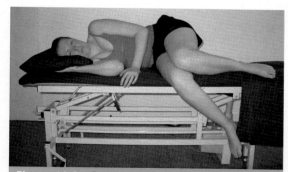

Figure 11.6   Progression 2 static opener for the level 1 lumbar reduced closing dysfunction. Either the upper or lower leg can be draped over the side of the plinth to produce increased contralateral lateral flexion.

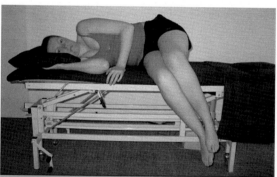

Figure 11.7   Progression 3 static opener for the level 1 lumbar reduced closing dysfunction.

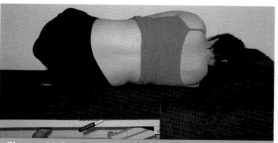

Figure 11.8   Amount of contralateral lateral flexion obtained with the progression 3 opener.

Dosage – as the patient becomes able to perform this opener at home, they may administer it approximately several times per day. It is not normally a case of the-longer-the-better and, in the early stages, holding the position for longer times increases the risk of reactive hyperaemia in the nerve roots and consequent reperfusion pain. Hence, the patient is told not to increase the time without careful supervision from the therapist. The maximum time I advocate for this manoeuvre is 5–15 minutes but this is attained with the addition of small increments over at least several treatments.

Dynamic opener

Movement – the therapist stands facing, and leans over, the patient. The intention is to gently mobilize the patient's pelvis, alternating between opening and returning to the starting position. This means that the therapist's proximal hand holds the superolateral surface of the patient's ilium whilst the distal hand and forearm pass over the patient's buttock to cup over the ilium as well. With maximum contact area for patient comfort, the movement is produced by the therapist applying pressure in a caudad direction on the patient's ilium making the pelvis rock over the downward greater trochanter. It is imperative that the therapist does not push or lean on the patient heavily, as this will cause discomfort in the downward hip as it presses into the plinth. The therapist uses their whole body from the feet upward to generate the movement. The mobilization is performed slowly and gently as a reasonably wide amplitude movement.

This mobilization probably produces more opening than earlier and certainly mobilizes the motion segment. It also produces a pumping action around the nerve root, which may help nerve root blood flow.

Dosage – up to 10 mobilizations initially before reassessing. This sequence may be repeated several times in the same session (Fig. 11.9) and ultimately can reach 20 or 50 movements each time.

Level 2 – dynamic closer

Position – for the dynamic closer, the patient is positioned in contralateral side lying, with their hips and knees flexed to 90°, but this time with their legs on the bed. The mobilization is now changed to be in the closing direction. This is because the problem will have settled sufficiently to the point where it will now tolerate, and benefit from, mobilizations that are directed more specifically at the mechanical dysfunction in the interface, that is, reduced closing. Like the dynamic opener, it will produce a gentle pumping action but the peak pressure will be greater than in the case of the opener. This treatment is aimed at improving the closing mechanism around the intervertebral foramen through mobilization of the motion segment.

Movement – the therapist leans over the patient whilst placing their distal hand or forearm on the patient's buttock between the trochanter and ischial tuberosity. This is the key contact point at which the mobilization is initiated and controlled. The other hand palpates the segmental motion to verify that the movement produced by the mobilization is satisfactory. The mobilization is produced from the therapist's feet upwards in which the key contact point is used to rock the pelvis in a cephalad direction, therefore producing a closing movement at the motion segment and intervertebral foramen.

Dosage – the manoeuvre should not evoke significant symptoms and can be oscillated 10–20 times. It may be repeated several times in one session.

Progression 2 – dynamic end range closer
Position – contralateral side lying, hips and knees flexed to 90°. If sufficient flexion of these joints is not achieved, the lumbar spine will not follow with

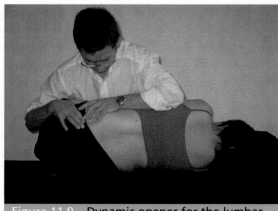

Figure 11.9   Dynamic opener for the lumbar spine.

lateral flexion correctly and, instead, lumbar flexion/extension will contaminate the procedure. Also, the patient will experience excessive pressure on their lower thigh as it is pressed too hard into the plinth. Then, facing cephalad, the therapist holds the patient's feet with their distal hand underneath the patient's lower foot and applies pressure to the posterior surface of the patient's greater trochanter with their proximal hand. The correct ipsilateral lateral flexion (closing) motion is achieved by the therapist moving the patient's feet around an axis that passes anteroposteriorly through the pelvis and moving the pelvis through application of pressure in a cephalad direction on the patient's buttock/greater trochanter. Care is taken to perform the movement correctly in the frontal plane by producing a slow rolling motion of the pelvis and legs.

Dosage – sometimes local lumbar symptoms occur with this mobilization but they should only be mild at most and should subside instantly. The technique may be oscillated 10–15 times and performed up to several times in one session (Fig. 11.10).

Reduced opening dysfunction

The dynamic openers for the reduced opening dysfunction are performed in a similar fashion to those for the reduced closing dysfunction. They are progressed gradually in the direction of opening and are effectively a standard lumbar mobilization for contralateral flexion.

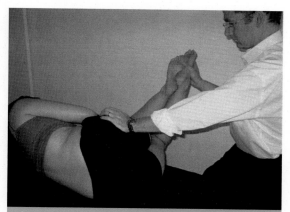

Figure 11.10   Dynamic closer for the lumbar spine.

Neural dysfunctions

Generalized two-ender sliders
Introduction

One of the more useful general neural techniques in relation to the lumbar spine is the two-ended slider because it is particularly effective in relieving pain. This slider is comparable to Maitland's grade III technique in which movement without much physical stress in the tissues is the key event. Hence, it can be used before and after mobilizations that evoke symptoms or approach the higher end of function. It can also be used to relieve persistent aches and hypersensitivities that are produced by inflammatory changes in or around the neural tissues. The two-ended slider is a general technique with wide application and moves the neural tissues in the lumbosacral region up and down in the spinal canal.

With all the two-ended sliders of the lumbar spine, amplitude of movement is a key factor. Generally, at the lower levels, small amplitudes are used, whereas, at the higher levels, larger amplitudes are the focus in order to facilitate sliding of the neural tissues with the aim of reducing sensitivity.

Position – side lying, painful side uppermost or if the problem is symmetrical the decision on which side should lay uppermost is arbitrary, hips and knees flexed to approximately 45°. The neck movements (both flexion and extension) are generally performed to a comfortable range and, if this is satisfactory, the movements may be progressed further into the range.

Movements – neck extension/bilateral knee extension then neck flexion/bilateral knee flexion. The neck movements are generally performed by the therapist whilst the patient moves their knees. Dorsiflexion is optional.

The two-ended sliders can also be performed in the sitting position if this is more convenient. A benefit is that the patient can perform them easily in this position as a home exercise (Fig. 11.11).

Cephalad/proximal sliding dysfunction
General points

The chief clinical features of this dysfunction are as follows. The patient usually strains their back during a lifting incident. The pain pattern often shows an inflammatory pattern with morning stiffness and aching. Even though the pain is often situated in the midline, it can be unilateral. The symptoms are reproduced by cephalad sliding of the neural structures in the lumbosacral region, that is, neck flexion, and are eased, or not affected, by straight leg raising. Lumbar flexion in standing can be painful and the pain increases with the addition of neck flexion. Interestingly, lumbar extension is often shows little in the way of abnormality. An essential aspect of treating this problem is to be familiar with the progressions of neurodynamic techniques from level 1 to 3 for this dysfunction.

Level 1

Position – the patient lies with their painful side uppermost with their neck in neutral and supported by a pillow. If this position does not ease the patient's symptoms sufficiently, the neck may be placed in some degree of extension. The hips and knees are flexed to approximately 45° in preparation for a knee extension mobilization (position away/move away).

Movement – ipsilateral knee extension. This should not reproduce the patient's symptoms (Figs 11.12 and 11.13).

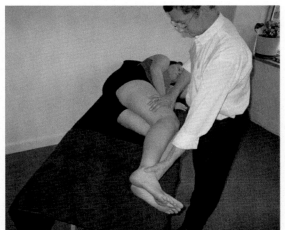

Figure 11.12   Starting position for the unilateral cephalad/proximal sliding dysfunction, painful side uppermost to reduce tension in the upper nerve roots.

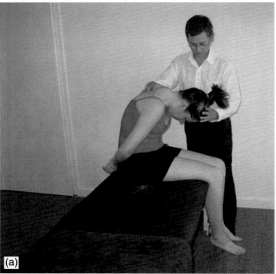

(a)

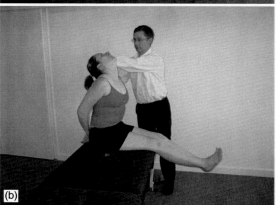

(b)

Figure 11.11   Two-ended slider for the lumbar nerve roots. (a) cephalad/proximal slider with neck flexion and knee flexion. (b) caudad/distal slider with neck extension and knee extension.

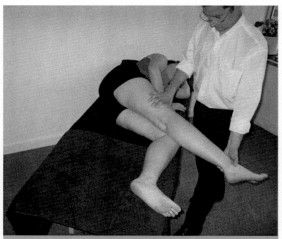

Figure 11.13   Caudad/distal slider at level 1 for the lumbosacral nerve roots, knee extension.

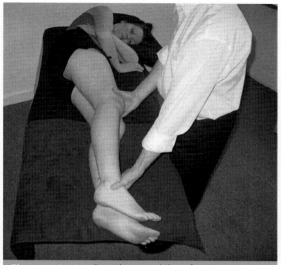

Figure 11.14   Starting position for the caudad/distal slider (level 2).

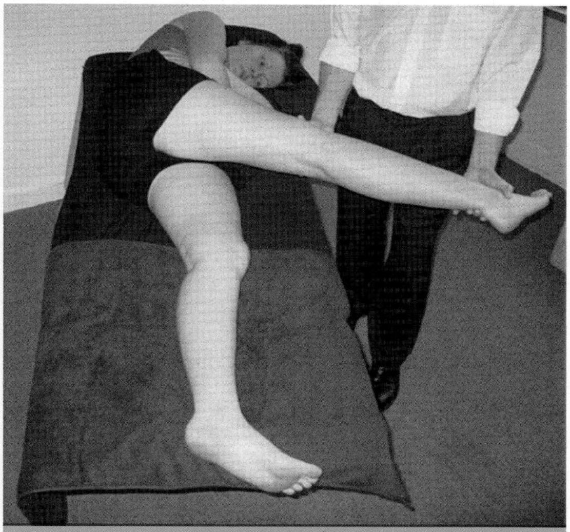

Figure 11.15   Movement for the progressed caudad/distal slider (level 2), unilateral straight leg raise.

The next progression is to position the patient's neck further into flexion and the leg movements, as above, are repeated (position towards/move away).

Level 2

At low level 2, the following progression applies.

Position – side lying, painful side uppermost, knees and hips straighter, neck flexed to a point immediately short of discomfort.

Movement – ipsilateral straight leg raise from the neutral position (Figs 11.14 and 11.15).
The subsequent progressions are as follows:

a. Position – as in the above progression, except the neck is positioned in neutral flexion/extension, ready for a passive neck flexion mobilization.

Movement – passive neck flexion is performed as far as comfortable into the available range. Some lumbar symptoms may be evoked. However, they should only be mild and should cease immediately after the technique is completed.

b. Position – sitting over the side of the bed.

Movement – neck and thoracic flexion to the end of the available range without provoking symptoms. This time, contralateral lateral flexion can be included in the mobilization (Fig. 11.16).

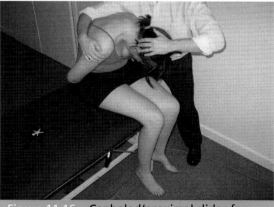

Figure 11.16   Cephalad/proximal slider for the lumbosacral neural structures.

In the event that the dysfunction is located in the midline, similar techniques are performed however they are made bilateral and symmetrical. Hence, the above techniques can be applied whilst in the supine position or still in side lying but with bilateral straight leg raise positioning and movements.

In addition, if the above techniques for a unilateral problem seem intrusive, they can be performed as bilateral techniques at lower levels because the contralateral nerve root will take some of the tension *off* the ipsilateral one.

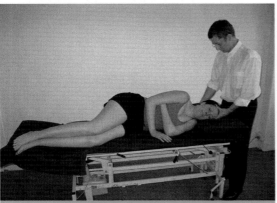

Figure 11.17   Starting position for treatment of the lumbar unilateral caudad/distal sliding dysfunction at low level 1. The mobilization is passive neck flexion to draw the lumbosacral neural contents cephalad in the spinal canal and proximal in the intervertebral foraminae (position away/move away).

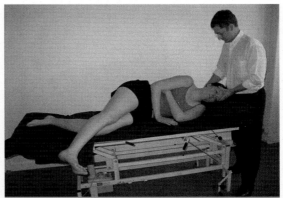

Figure 11.18   Mobilization for the caudad/distal sliding dysfunction at high level 1. The ipsilateral knee is positioned straighter than previously whilst passive neck flexion is mobilised (position toward/move away).

Caudad/distal sliding dysfunction

Clinical features

The symptoms of the caudad/distal neural sliding dysfunction are evoked by movements that produce sliding of the neural tissues in the lumbosacral region in a caudad direction. An example would be the straight leg raise reproducing the patient's symptoms whilst passive neck flexion does not. Performance of a neurodynamic movement can reduce the symptoms e.g. passive neck flexion *reduces* low back pain and permits more normal lower limb movement with the slump test. Sometimes, these patients say that they can bend over without back pain, as long as they have their neck flexed.

Level 1

Progression 1

Position – the patient lies with their painful side uppermost, the hips and knees at approximately 45° flexion and the neck in neutral flexion/extension. This position reduces the caudad tension in the ipsilateral neural elements and will assist in moving them away from the provoking (caudad) direction. The ipsilateral knee may need support in the form of a pillow so that it does not rest on the plinth and produce lumbar rotation. If the symptoms do not reduce sufficiently with this position, it is acceptable to flex both knees and reduce the amount of bilateral hip

flexion so as to reduce caudad tension even more (Fig. 11.17).

Progression 2

Position – side lying, painful side uppermost, the hips at approximately 45° flexion and the ipsilateral knee straight, although short of symptoms. This will draw the neural elements slightly caudad whilst the mobilization moves them in the cephalad (easing) direction with passive neck flexion (position towards/move away) (Fig. 11.18).

Level 2

Progression 1

Position – side lying, painful side uppermost and the neck flexed to its comfortable limit (position away).

Movement – gentle ipsilateral straight leg raise to its maximum comfortable range (move toward) (Fig. 11.19).

Progression 2

Position – as in the above progression, except the neck is positioned in neutral flexion/extension.

Movement – ipsilateral straight leg raise.

Progression 3

Position – side lying, painful side uppermost, neck positioned in extension to permit increased caudad sliding (position toward).

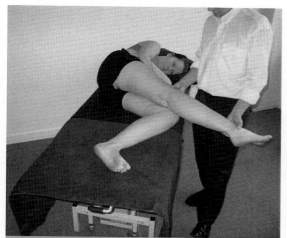

Figure 11.19   Mobilization for the caudad sliding dysfunction at level 2. The neck is positioned in flexion whilst passive knee extension is mobilized (position away/move toward).

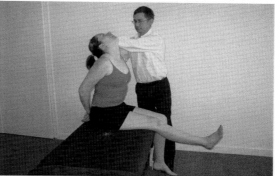

Figure 11.20   Mobilization for caudad slider of the lumbosacral nerve roots and sciatic nerve as progression 4 in the caudad/distal sliding dysfunction at level 2. Cervical and thoracic extension with knee extension with or without dorsiflexion.

Movement – unilateral straight leg raise (move toward). Some stretching symptoms may occur in the treated thigh with this procedure. However, these must cease when the technique is completed.

Progression 4
Position – seated on the plinth as for the slump test.

Movement – cervical and thoracic extension, knee extension with or without dorsiflexion. Care is taken to ensure that the neck and thoracic spines extend fully and are returned to the neutral position each time the movement occurs. The reason for stating this is that this technique often suffers from lack of amplitude (Fig. 11.20).

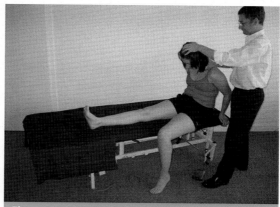

Figure 11.21   Starting position for progression 5 of the caudad sliding technique for the caudad/distal sliding dysfunction at the high end of level 2.

Progression 5
Position – ipsilateral long-sitting parallel with the plinth, short of symptoms.

Movement – neck and thoracic extension to the end of the available range combined with knee extension and dorsiflexion to optimize caudad sliding. The emphasis in terms of handling is through the therapist guiding the thoracic and cervical spines into extension, whilst, at the same time, making sure that the patient flexes over their hips (Figs 11.21 and 11.22).

In the event that the patient shows signs of a symmetrical sliding dysfunction, the following progressions can be executed as bilateral techniques through lower limb movements in a pattern similar to that of the above unilateral techniques. Such signs consist of midline lumbar pain and symmetrical restriction of limb and spinal movements.

Tension dysfunction
Clinical features
In the tension dysfunction, lumbar symptoms evoked by neurodynamic testing show a characteristic feature

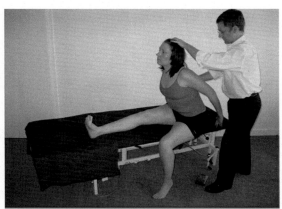

Figure 11.22   Mobilization for progression 5 of the caudad sliding technique for the caudad/distal sliding dysfunction at the high end of level 2, thoracic and cervical extension with hip flexion.

that differentiates them from the sliding dysfunction. The symptoms increase with performance of a neurodynamic movement in one direction and, with the addition of another movement from the opposite direction, the symptoms increase further. This is because tension in the nervous system increases when neurodynamic movements from opposite directions are performed. For instance, in the slump position, neck flexion reproduces the patient's low back pain, which increases further with the addition of knee extension/dorsiflexion.

Which end do I mobilize?
The true two-ended tensioner involves movement from both cephalad and caudad ends. However, this is sometimes impractical in those patients whose problem is quite irritable. Therefore, the over-riding condition placed on the following progressions related to the tension dysfunction is that the therapist decides which end to position and which to mobilize. The decision is quite arbitrary and is influenced by factors related to patient acceptance, therapist convenience and therapeutic efficacy.

Background and rationale for treatment
Just as it is in the cervical spine, so is using contralateral or bilateral neurodynamic tests a key principle in treatment of the neural tension dysfunction in the lumbar spine. As stated earlier, the mechanism of greatest benefit is that which produces a reduction in

tension in the treated side by the addition of a contralateral limb position or movement (see Chapter 2 on specific neurodynamics). The basic principles are as follows. Consistent with the progressional system 'position away/move away' advancing to 'position toward/move toward', addition of the contralateral neurodynamic test produces the effect of 'positioning or moving away' from the direction of the dysfunction because it reduces tension in the treated nerve roots. As the problem improves through the levels, the so-called assistance provided by applying the contralateral test reduces (position toward) and use of the ipsilateral test then progressively adds a small amount of tension in the neural tissues (move toward). Hence, what follows in a set of progressions that applies these principles at level 1.

At level 2, and to start with, the use of gravity takes place, in which the ipsilateral limb is placed uppermost so that the neural elements undergo a reduction in tension, to which tension movements are applied (position away/move toward). As the patient improves, they are then taken more into the tension movements (position toward/move toward).

Level 1
Progression 1
The patient is positioned in the generic off-loader for the lumbosacral nerve roots and sciatic nerve. The patient may apply this at home as frequently as they are capable (Fig. 11.23).

Progression 2
The next progression is to, in the position for progression 1, gently perform dorsiflexion or knee extension on the contralateral side (position away/move away). This should not produce an increase in symptoms. If it does, the technique should be ceased and other treatment applied. Incidentally, in view of the fact that neural tension dysfunctions at level 1 tend to be quite sensitive, it is recommended that musculoskeletal treatments in addition to neurodynamic techniques are performed, whenever appropriate.

Progression 3
Position – this mobilization is executed in the same general position as progression 2 except the knee is extended with ankle dorsiflexion.

Subsequent progressions include the addition of contralateral hip flexion. The overall result of the

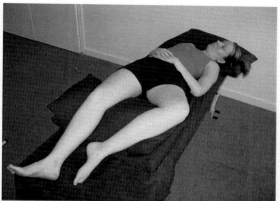

Figure 11.23   Generic off-loader for the left lumbosacral nerve roots and sciatic nerve, ipsilateral lateral flexion, hip flexion/abduction/external rotation, knee flexion, ankle plantarflexion.

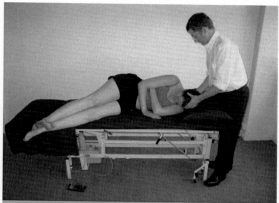

Figure 11.24   Progression 1 mobilization for the tension dysfunction affecting the lumbosacral nerve roots at low level 2. Active dorsiflexion and passive neck flexion are performed.

above is building of the contralateral straight leg raise in small increments.

Level 2
Progression 1
Position – the patient lies with their painful side uppermost with their neck in neutral and supported. Both hips and knees are flexed to a point short of symptoms in preparation for a mobilization involving dorsiflexion of the ankle. The reason both limbs are positioned as such is to decrease tension in the treated side. As mentioned, the patient lies on their contralateral side because this reduces tension in the treated nerve root.

Movement – active dorsiflexion of the ipsilateral ankle and passive neck flexion to a comfortable range. However, if necessary, it is possible to move one end, depending on the patient's symptomatology. This technique should not reproduce the patient's symptoms (Fig. 11.24).

Progression 2
Position – as in the above progression, except the straight leg raise angle of the contralateral (downward) lower limb is reduced. This will add a degree of tension to the treated nerve root.

Movement – passive neck flexion and active knee extension with some dorsiflexion are performed as far as comfortable into the available range. Lumbar

symptoms at this stage do not always occur. However, if they do, they should only be mild and should cease immediately after the technique is completed.

Progression 3
Position – as above, except the neck is placed in maximum comfortable flexion.

Movement – ipsilateral straight leg raise (without dorsiflexion) to mild to moderate resistance and mild symptoms.

Progression 4
Position – *ipsilateral* side lying (change to painful side down). This sensitizes the leg raise for the lower side (as described in Chapter 2).

Movement – ipsilateral straight leg raise, as in progression 3. Dorsiflexion can also be added to advance the technique further.

Progression 5
Position – seated as for the slump test.

Movement – neck flexion and knee extension. A subsequent progression would be to add active or passive dorsiflexion (Figs 11.25 and 11.26).

Level 3a
Progression 1
Position – sitting over the side of the plinth in the slump position.

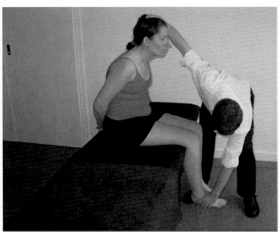

Figure 11.25   Starting position for the tensioner for the neural tension dysfunction in the lumbar spine at high level 2.

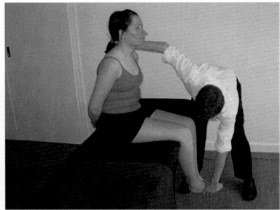

Figure 11.27   Starting position for the level/type 3a tensioner.

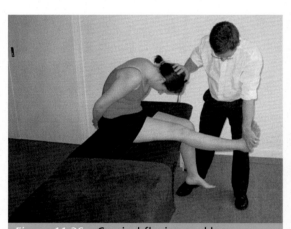

Figure 11.26   Cervical flexion and knee extension (with or without dorsiflexion) as the tensioner for the neural tension dysfunction in the lumbar spine at high level 2. Note that the hand that controls the head movement does not apply over-pressure. Instead it simply guides the neck movement.

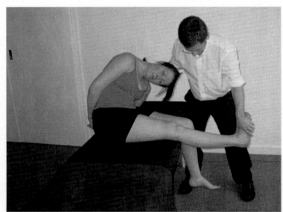

Figure 11.28   Movements of the level/type 3a tensioner. Flexion and contralateral lateral flexion of the spine, internal rotation and adduction of the hip and knee extension with optional dorsiflexion.

Movement – neck flexion and ipsilateral knee extension to the end comfortable available. This time, contralateral lateral flexion of the spine, internal rotation and adduction of the hip and knee extension are performed. No overpressure is given. Instead, the therapist uses their hands to help guide the movement, feel for resistance and muscular behaviour patterns and teach the patient how to control

the movement themself. The techniques of level 3 can produce some degree of resistance and muscular stretch symptoms. However, they must cease when the technique is completed.

Dosage – several mobilizations are performed. A pause is also given between each mobilization. The each set of mobilizations may be repeated several times per treatment session, however, I do not recommend more than this (Figs 11.27 and 11.28).

The technique can be progressed further by performing it in long sitting (Figs 11.29 and 11.30).

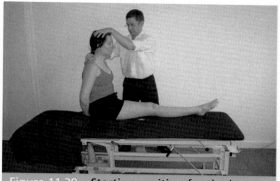

Figure 11.29   Starting position for the long sitting slump test (level/type 3a).

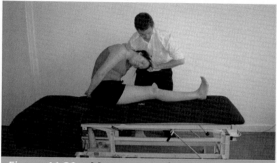

Figure 11.30   Movements of the long sitting slump test (level/type 3a).

Introduction to the complex dysfunctions

Because neuropathodynamic events usually come from the mechanical interface, I have dealt with conditions in which both components are affected with respect to the interface dysfunction categories. What then follows are progressions that are designed to treat both components simultaneously. As a consequence, this naturally places these dysfunctions in the level/type 3c bracket. This format is preferable, especially for the practitioner who is not particularly familiar with neurodynamics because it encourages the clinician to work through the single dysfunctions first before attempting to treat them as complex ones.

Level/type 3c – reduced closing with distal sliding dysfunction

Position – the patient is positioned on their contralateral side (painful side uppermost), the hips and knees are flexed to 90° and supported on a pillow.

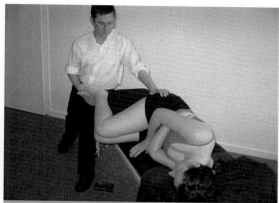

Figure 11.31   Starting position of the technique for the lumbar reduced closing dysfunction with distal sliding dysfunction.

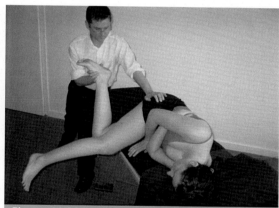

Figure 11.32   Technique for the lumbar reduced closing dysfunction with distal sliding dysfunction. Ipsilateral lateral flexion with active knee extension.

Movement – the closing manoeuvre, is performed whilst the patient performs knee extension actively. The next progression would be to add active dorsiflexion.

Dosage – 5–10 oscillations, can be repeated up to several times in one session (Figs 11.31 and 11.32).

Level/type 3c – reduced closing with proximal sliding dysfunction
Level 3c – multistructural
Progression 1
Position – the patient is positioned on their contralateral side (painful side uppermost), the hips and

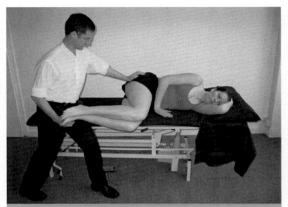

Figure 11.33 Starting position of the mobilization for the reduced closing dysfunction with proximal sliding dysfunction.

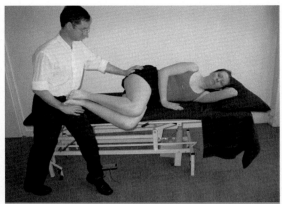

Figure 11.35 Starting position of the technique for the lumbar spine reduced closing dysfunction with tension dysfunction.

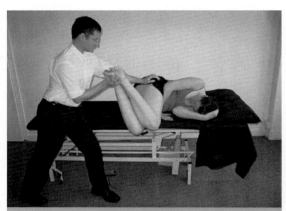

Figure 11.34 Technique for the reduced closing dysfunction with proximal sliding dysfunction. Ipsilateral lateral flexion with cervical flexion.

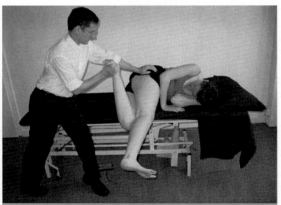

Figure 11.36 Technique for the lumbar spine reduced closing dysfunction with tension dysfunction. Closer with tensioner – ipsilateral lateral flexion with cervical flexion and knee extension with or without dorsiflexion.

knees are flexed to 90° with their thoracic spine in flexion and their neck in neutral supported by their own hand.

Movement – the closing manoeuvre of the reduced closing dysfunction is performed whilst the patient performs neck flexion actively, guided and supported by their hand. The patient will need to slide comfortably on the plinth. This mobilization sometimes evokes symptoms but, as usual, they should only be mild and should always subside instantly. The patient must relax their lumbar spine during this technique (Figs 11.33 and 11.34).

Reduced closing with tension dysfunction

Level 3c – multistructural

Progression 1

Position – the patient is positioned as for the previous technique.

Movement – a closing manoeuvre is performed whilst the patient performs neck flexion and ipsilateral knee extension actively (Figs 11.35 and 11.36).

Reduced opening with distal sliding dysfunction

Level 3c – multistructural

Position – the patient is positioned on their contralateral side (painful side uppermost), the hips and knees are flexed to 90° and their legs over the side of the bed.

Movement – contralateral lateral flexion (dynamic opener). This technique is performed in conjunction with knee extension as part of the straight leg raise and active dorsiflexion may be added. Frequently the lumbar muscles tighten during this mobilization. There may be a hyperactivity and protective dysfunction which can be treated with soft tissue techniques to the lumbar muscles during the mobilization. For instance, the muscles could be stretched manually whilst the patient relaxes them and performs knee extension as the therapist also mobilizes into the opened position.

Reduced opening with proximal sliding dysfunction

Level 3c – multistructural

Position – the patient is positioned on their contralateral side (painful side uppermost), the hips and knees are flexed to 90° and their legs over the side of the bed. Flexion of the thoracic spine is also performed. However, the neck is placed in neutral.

Movement – the opening manoeuvre for the reduced opening dysfunction is performed whilst the patient performs neck flexion.

Reduced opening with tension dysfunction

Level 3c – multistructural

Position – the patient is positioned on their contralateral side (painful side uppermost), the hips and knees are flexed to 90° with their thoracic spine in flexion and their neck in neutral supported by their own hands.

Movement – the opening manoeuvre, as before is performed whilst the patient performs neck flexion and knee extension actively.

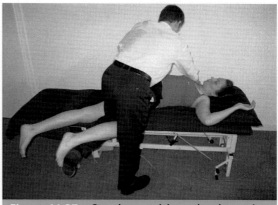

Figure 11.37 Starting position – lumbar spine rotation technique with neural mobilization.

Another technique that is commonly needed for the above dysfunction is that which involves lumbar rotation mobilizations and straight leg raise. The patient lies on their contralateral side and, whilst a lumbar rotation mobilization is performed, various components of the straight leg raise are also executed. The therapist holds the patient's lower limb between their lower legs whilst supporting the patient's lower leg with their caudad foot. This means that the therapist stands on one leg and rotates about this leg in the process of moving the patient's knee into extension. If hip flexion is performed, the therapist uses their pivot around the patient's hip joint in combination with pivoting around their grounded foot. This way different movements can be performed, knee extension or hip flexion, or a combination of both. The technique is rather unusual but, once perfected, can occupy a regular spot in the therapist's repertoire (Figs 11.37 and 11.38).

Muscle hyperactivity dysfunctions

Introduction

As mentioned in the chapter on general neuropathodynamics, dysfunction in the nerve root may produce physiological and behavioural changes in the innervated muscles. This following section introduces several key principles related to the treatment of the level 3c category of problem involving neural tension and muscle hyperactivity. The two types of disorders to consider in this context are the protective hyperactivity and the localized hyperactivity

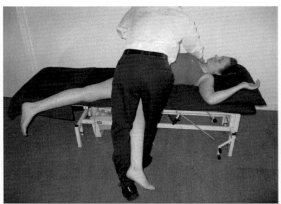

Figure 11.38   Lumbar spine rotation technique with neural mobilization – knee extension is produced as the therapist supports the patient's lower leg and ankle and rotates about their other leg.

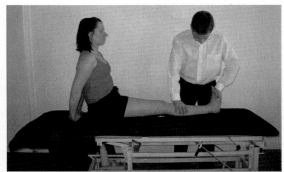

Figure 11.39   Lumbar spine protective hyperactivity dysfunction for the S1 nerve root, starting position – ipsilateral long sitting with full allowable dorsiflexion.

problems. In my experience, the protective hyperactivity dysfunction tends to act over a longer course of the neural structure. It therefore involves more muscles that are often biarticular. Such an example would be tight hamstring and calf muscles in response to pathodynamics in the S1 nerve root. These components often do not emerge until the nervous system is tested at level 3c such as stretching the hamstring and calf muscles during a long sitting slump test. In this situation, the muscles will not release very well and will be more painful when compared with those on the contralateral side. The other dysfunction (localized muscle hyperactivity – alias trigger point) tends to be more localized and offers the clinician a trigger point which can become accentuated in a neurodynamic position.

Protective hyperactivity dysfunction (e.g. S1 nerve root affecting the hamstrings and calf muscles)

Testing

Testing for the neural tension and protective hyperactivity dysfunction is performed using the straight leg raise and slump tests. At the end of each test, the muscle in question is elongated gently so that the therapist can ascertain its state of contraction in and out of the neurodynamic position. For instance, the calf muscles are passively elongated in isolation as a specific muscle test. The nervous system is then placed under tension and the same muscle test is repeated. In the

presence of the protective hyperactivity dysfunction, the muscles will become tighter when the limb is in the slump or straight leg raise position and this effect is greater than on the asymptomatic side.

1. Test 1 – nervous system off-loaded – the patient is positioned in ipsilateral long sitting, leaning backward on their hands to off-load the nervous system. The calf stretch test in the form of passive ankle dorsiflexion is performed in this position and the symptoms and physical behaviour, such as resistance and range of motion, are observed.
2. Test 2 – neurodynamic position – the patient then flexes their thoracic and lumbar spines and leans forward to the point of increased symptoms whilst the therapist holds the whole limb stationary. The calf stretch test is performed again and then once more with neck flexion. Normally, either forward leaning or neck flexion produces an increase in calf tension or posterior thigh discomfort but, when compared with the other side, the difference can be substantial and indicates an abnormal response (Fig. 11.39).

It should be emphasized that this technique is for level 3 patients with high expectations, such as athletes or people with only minor symptoms. Inclusion and exclusion criteria are covered in more detail in Chapter 6.

Treatment

The patient adopts the position for test 2 (spinal flexion), but stops immediately before the onset of symptoms. Facing the patient in a medial-to-lateral direction, the therapist grasps the limb so as to resist active plantarflexion and stabilize the rest of the limb. This position also gives the therapist the opportunity to easily control the patient's torso and head movements, if need be. The therapist's distal forearm then contacts the plantar surface of the patient's foot as the therapist's hand holds the calcaneum on its under surface. The therapist's proximal hand stabilizes the knee and the patient is instructed to press into the therapist's distal forearm, gently but firmly, with the ball of their foot. This is naturally a contraction of the calf muscles. The manoeuvre should be a resisted static one and may evoke some symptoms, but they should subside immediately afterwards. The contraction is held for a time between 5 and 15 seconds and, as the patient relaxes, the muscle is gently elongated by the therapist. This is essentially a contract-relax neurodynamic technique.

If the hamstrings were the focus of attention, the procedure would be modified somewhat. The therapist and patient would adopt a hamstring stretch position in supine and the muscles tested for symptoms and resistance patterns, as above, with and without dorsiflexion. A more dramatic change in the relevant parameters compared with the contralateral side indicates abnormality. Treatment would then be administered through contract-relax techniques in the straight leg raise position. Further sensitization could also be added by performing the procedure in the slump position and adding dorsiflexion if need be.

Localized muscle hyperactivity dysfunction (alias trigger point) (e.g. S1 nerve root)
Testing
Testing for this dysfunction involves placing the affected limb in the straight leg raise position and palpating the muscles innervated by the related nerve root, in this case, those in the S1 myotome. This technique can, and should at times, be performed along the whole length of the nerve and includes the gluteal muscles, piriformis, hamstrings, popliteus, calf muscles and muscles in the plantar aspect of the foot, if necessary. The technique is performed in the contralateral side lying position and should be compared with the same procedure on the other side. Sometimes, palpation reveals tender spots and localized muscle holding that become

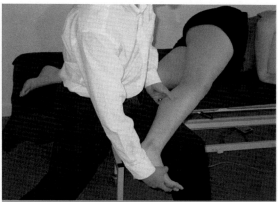

Figure 11.40   Localized muscle hyperactivity dysfunction located in the calf muscles. Both the muscle and neural elements are loaded gently whilst manual techniques are performed.

more noticeable in the straight leg raise position than in the off-loaded position. The neurodynamic movements to be added during the palpation are dorsiflexion and side lying slump.

Treatment
Treatment consists of performing local soft tissue manual techniques that are used by most therapists, such as trigger point therapy, soft tissue releases, contract-relax and connective tissue massage. In the event that a neurodynamic component exists, the techniques are performed in the neurodynamic position to maximize their effects. Clearly, these techniques can be applied to many areas of the body and are based on the above principles (Fig. 11.40).

MID-LUMBAR DISORDERS

Neurodynamic testing

Neurodynamic testing of the mid-lumbar region focuses on the prone knee bend. Sometimes, at level 1, the test can be used in its standard form, however, the variation is that knee flexion is only taken to the first onset of symptoms and usually does not advance as far into the range as with levels 2 and 3.

At level 1, sliders for the L2–4 nerve roots can be performed easily when the patient lies on their contralateral side and performs the neck and lower limb movements for the nerve root. For the proximal slider, neck flexion is combined with hip flexion and knee extension. The therapist takes the patient's thigh and knee to produce the limb movements and the patient performs the neck movements. The distal slider is produced by the therapist performing hip extension with knee flexion whilst the patient performs neck extension.

Tensioners are generally reserved for levels 2 and 3 and are created by forces being applied to both ends of the system, comprising the movements of neck flexion, hip extension and knee flexion and are sensitized with contralateral lateral flexion of the lumbar spine.

Level 3

As mentioned in specific neurodynamics, gravity assists in sensitizing spinal neurodynamic testing and the mid-lumbar region is no exception. Therefore, testing the femoral part of the nervous system at level 3 utilizes the femoral slump test in *ipsilateral* side lying.

In the femoral slump position, the test might be sensitized further by performing hip adduction and contralateral lateral flexion during the hip extension/knee flexion phase. The adduction movement with one of the therapist's arms and pressure applied to the pelvis with the other hand are what produce the contralateral lateral flexion movement (Fig. 11.41).

Interface and neural dysfunctions
Reduced opening and neural dysfunction

The mid-lumbar nerve roots and spine can be mobilized when the reduced opening interface problem interacts with a neural component. The patient lies on their contralateral side with their back near the edge of the plinth to allow the therapist good access to the patient's thigh and spine from a posterior direction. This is also so that their symptomatic limb can be placed into the knee bend position without the plinth preventing adduction of the hip. Hence, the limb may drape over the edge somewhat and this may warrant the patient being positioned diagonally on the plinth. With the contralateral (downward) limb in approximately 45° hip and knee flexion to prevent it being an obstruction, the ipsilateral limb is then placed in the hip extension/knee flexion (knee bend) position. Care

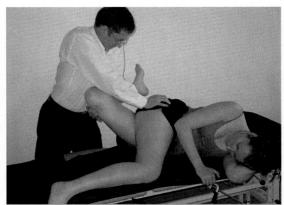

Figure 11.41   Lumbar spine femoral slump in painful side down – contralateral lateral flexion of the lumbar spine with hip extension/adduction and knee flexion.

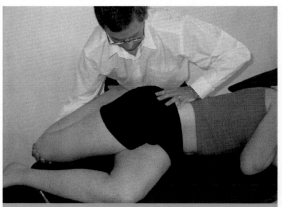

Figure 11.42   Femoral neurodynamic test in combination with opening of the lumbar spine (contralateral lateral flexion) for the mid-lumbar nerve root disorder (level/type 3c).

should be taken not to move the lumbar spine into too much extension due to the pulling action of the rectus femoris muscle with hip extension and it might be that this is what limits the amount of hip extension. Facing in a caudoanterior direction and in stride standing, the therapist holds the limb in this position with their far hand. With the other hand, the therapist mobilizes the lumbar spine into the open (contralateral lateral flexion) position by moving the patient's ipsilateral (upper) pelvis in a caudad direction. As with the opening dysfunctions of the lumbar spine, a bolster can be used to enhance the lateral flexion component of the mobilization (Fig. 11.42).

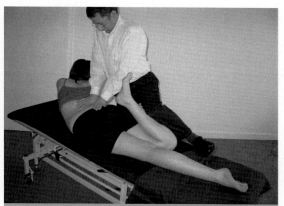

Figure 11.43   Femoral neural component to back pain. Mobilization of the mid-lumbar segments in the closed position with neural mobilization.

Reduced closing with neural dysfunction

For the reduced closing dysfunction with a tension or distal sliding dysfunction, the lumbar spine is placed in extension and ipsilateral lateral flexion. This is achieved by, in prone, the patient coming up onto their elbows and moving into ipsilateral lateral flexion. The prone knee bend is superimposed on this by the therapist leaning on the patient's leg (with their own leg) whilst the patient's knee is in flexion. The therapist then performs posteroanterior, or any other relevant, mobilizations at the appropriate level of the spine (Fig. 11.43).

Lower limb

12

Diagnosis and treatment – piriformis syndrome, knee pain, tarsal tunnel syndrome, peroneal and sural nerve disorders

Specific neuropathodynamics and clinical features of each problem

Specific dysfunctions – mechanical interface (opening closing), neural sliding and tension dysfunctions, level/type 3c combination dysfunctions

Progression of physical examination and treatment through the levels

Off-loaders sliders and tensioners, openers and closers

Combined muscle, joint and neural treatments

PIRIFORMIS SYNDROME

The piriformis syndrome as a cause of buttock and lower limb pain is usually overshadowed by the prospect of it being referred from the lumbar spine and pelvic joints. Unfortunately however, it can be a serious condition because of its potential to cause long term pain, scarring around the sciatic nerve and even paralysis in the more severe cases. In such cases, surgical decompression and external neurolysis can be indicated.

Several important features of the problem are worthy of mention.

Key points

1. The piriformis syndrome usually involves the peroneal portion of the sciatic nerve. This is either because the muscle is penetrated by this nerve in approximately 10–20% of cadavers, as the muscle forms two, or even three, heads. Also, in the event that the syndrome is not caused by the above anomaly, it is likely that the peroneal portion passes next to the adjacent tissues as the nerve emerges from under piriformis in its course out of the pelvis.
2. Pain may come from contraction of the muscle as its fibres and fascial edge are pressed onto the nerve. This implicates biomechanical and motor control approaches in treatment, as well as neurodynamic aspects.
3. Neuropathy can develop as the sliding actions of the nerve moving through the muscle during physical activity (e.g. running) cause friction irritation of the nerve and subsequent scarring. Scarring can also result from previous trauma to the region.
4. Severe compression can at times produce paralysis of the muscles in the field of the peroneal nerve, resulting in a foot drop.
5. The piriformis syndrome causes pain down the leg from the buttock to the anterolateral leg area and it is easy to see why this syndrome could be mistaken for an L5 radiculopathy.

In relation to the biomechanics of the piriformis muscle, I am informed that, below

70° of hip flexion, it produces lateral rotation of the hip joint and, above 70°, it becomes a medial rotator. Therefore, its dynamic interactions with the sciatic nerve will vary according to the angle of hip flexion and this will in turn influence neurodynamic testing, especially when it comes to examination at level 3, as reflected below.

Physical examination and diagnosis

Introduction

One of the key aspects of diagnosis of the piriformis syndrome is neurological examination. The key facets to test are sensation along the anterolateral aspect of the leg and dorsum of the foot, strength of dorsiflexion and the tibial and peroneal neurodynamic tests. The reason for mentioning the tibial component is that, clinically, I have observed that, in addition to plantarflexion/inversion, dorsiflexion can affect the symptoms in the buttock with neurodynamic testing. This could be related to a low division of the sciatic nerve into its tibial and peroneal branches, enabling dorsiflexion to act on the sciatic nerve in the region of piriformis.

The other aspects to weigh up are the preponderance of signs to palpation of the muscles in the buttock, especially piriformis. Frequently, pressure applied to this muscle reproduces local and referred pain along the line of the peroneal nerve from the buttock and more distally. Occasionally, pins and needles in the dorsum of the foot can also occur and, frequently, a trigger point in the muscle is evident.

In terms of neurodynamic testing, the standard straight leg raise can be abnormal but it is sometimes not as abnormal as the peroneal neurodynamic test. Besides, a problem is that, at level 3, the standard tests are often useless in detecting neuropathodynamics and do not address the complex array of factors that are relevant to the problem. The dynamic interactions between the mechanical interface (piriformis and gemellae) and the peroneal portion of the sciatic nerve are at issue here in which these interactions are not accounted for in level 1 or level 2 testing. As mentioned above, the piriformis syndrome can be mistaken for an L5 radiculopathy because it appears more prominently in the clinician's mind and is easier to diagnose. Another reason for missing the piriformis syndrome is that good neurodynamic tests, especially at higher levels, have until now not been available. Hence, new modified forms of testing are proposed below in order to detect the higher level of dysfunction that can exist in people such as athletes, and is often missed.

Levels 1, 2 and 3a

One of the key aspects of physical examination of the piriformis syndrome at level 1 is to test the interface structures separately from the neural ones. Therefore, along with palpation, active contraction and passive stretch of the muscle above and below 60°–70° of hip flexion are essential. This establishes the balance of the problem in terms of interface versus neural. More provocation with interface (piriformis muscle) testing than neural will lead the therapist toward treatment of the muscle as opposed to the nerve and vice versa. Naturally, in this case when the interface signs dominate the clinical picture, any muscle techniques known to the practitioner can be applied.

Coincidentally, neurodynamic testing at level 1 is the same as in level 2 and simply requires performance of the peroneal neurodynamic test (see Chapter 7) to the first onset of symptoms and differentiation with release of plantarflexion/inversion, for buttock pain. At level 1, it is simply performed more gently. Level 3a testing (neurodynamically sensitized) is the same as for level 3a in the slump and straight leg raise tests with their relevant sensitizing manoeuvres and plantar flexion/inversion.

Level 3b – neurodynamic sequencing

Physical examination at level 3b through modification of the neurodynamic sequence obliges the therapist to move the nerve from the hip first, then from other more remote sites. The test therefore starts with hip flexion, followed by knee extension, then plantarflexion/inversion. A hindrance with this technique is that, sometimes, because such a large amount of hip flexion is permitted before the knee extension is introduced, the hamstrings are pretensioned excessively. This prevents the knee extending much and renders the test useless because the sciatic nerve can not be tensioned sufficiently. Therefore, an alternative is to lower the hip flexion

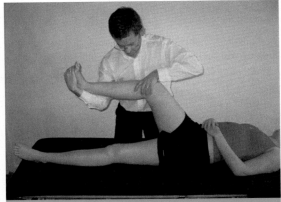

Figure 12.1   The piriformis neurodynamic test below 70° hip flexion at level/type 3b, stage 1 – starting position. Even though the foot is in neutral, it is supported so as to easily introduce plantarflexion/inversion later in the test.

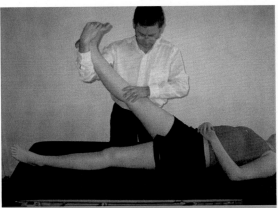

Figure 12.2   The piriformis neurodynamic test below 70° hip flexion at level/type 3b, stage 2 – knee extension.

enough to gain more knee extension. Plantarflexion/ inversion or dorsiflexion is then added and used for the purpose of differentiation (Figs 12.1, 12.2, 12.3 and 12.4).

Piriformis neurodynamic test

As mentioned, the piriformis neurodynamic test at level/type 3c is performed differently above and below 70° of hip flexion.

Exactly the same sequence of distal movements is used in executing the test above 70° of hip flexion.

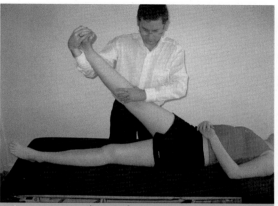

Figure 12.3 The piriformis neurodynamic test below 70° hip flexion at level/type 3b, stage 3 – internal rotation of the hip joint.

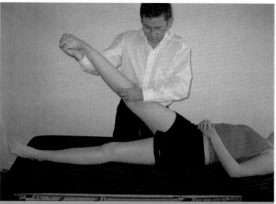

Figure 12.4 The piriformis neurodynamic test below 70° hip flexion at level/type 3b, stage 4 – plantarflexion/inversion of the ankle and foot.

Level/type 3c

At level/type 3c, the standard peroneal neurodynamic test is combined with testing of the mechanical interface in a rather complex fashion that accounts for the changes in function of the piriformis muscle below and above 70°.

In a modified peroneal neurodynamic test, the therapist's preparation is as for the standard test, but the sequence is different. As the lower limb is raised from the plinth, the hip is first positioned in full available internal rotation and the foot in plantarflexion/inversion (Figs 12.3 and 12.4). The entire lower limb is then raised from the plinth as in the straight leg raise whilst the therapist maintains full internal rotation and plantarflexion/inversion. The maintenance of internal rotation is crucial, because the reason for taking maximum advantage of the internal rotation is that the intent is to stretch the piriformis muscle onto the peroneal part of the sciatic nerve. This is in order to test as best possible the dynamic interactions between the two structures. The internal rotation is maintained maximally until approximately 70° of hip flexion is reached. At this point, the limb rotation is reversed into full external rotation and the straight leg raise component is taken further toward the end range, if permissible. The technique takes into account the change in interactions between the muscle and nerve throughout the whole range of straight leg raise, particularly at the transitional angle of 60°–70° hip flexion (Fig. 12.5).

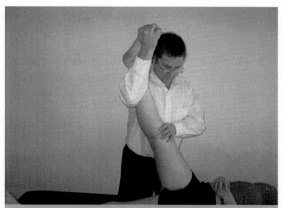

Figure 12.5 Modified piriformis neurodynamic test above 70° of hip flexion. External rotation of the hip joint is substituted for internal rotation (level/type 3c).

At any point in the testing procedure, the patient can resist the rotation as a means of applying pressure to the sciatic nerve with contraction of the piriformis. For instance, below 70° of hip flexion, the patient would actively produce external rotation (whilst the limb is positioned in internal rotation). When the limb is positioned above 70°, the patient would produce internal rotation (whilst the limb is positioned in external rotation).

Level 3c – piriformis slump test

In addition to the straight leg raise, the slump test can be modified to investigate the role of the piriformis

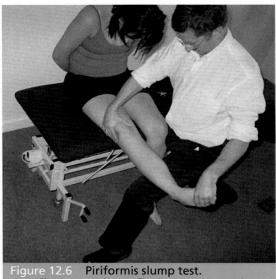

Figure 12.6   Piriformis slump test. Dorsiflexion or plantarflexion can be used.

syndrome in patients with buttock and lower limb symptoms. Since, in the slump position, the hips are flexed above 60°–70°, external rotation as a means of stretching the piriformis muscle onto the sciatic nerve is again utilized. In the slump position with the neck flexed, the patient's hip joint is brought into full external rotation, then the knee is extended and foot movements performed. The key is to keep the external rotation maximal at all times. Dorsiflexion or plantarflexion/inversion can be applied. In some people, their buttock pain is more easily reproduced by this test than with the standard slump test. The pain can, at times, also be differentiated with neck and foot movements (Fig. 12.6).

Neurodynamic treatment of the piriformis syndrome

Mechanical interface

Level 1

Treatment of the piriformis syndrome depends on its kind and severity. Cases with severe neurological changes should be evaluated medically, whereas the disorder in which mechanical dysfunction is the prime component will need conservative neurodynamic and musculoskeletal treatment such as what can be offered by the therapist. Of course, all relevant modalities other than neurodynamic ones can be used in the treatment of this syndrome.

Treatment at all levels is aimed at releasing pressure between the piriformis muscle and the sciatic nerve. This can be in the form of muscle release techniques, trigger point therapy, myofascial release and deep connective tissue massage, with which the reader will be familiar. Motor control techniques and biomechanical adjustments through orthotics and lumbopelvic stability treatments can also be of value, especially in the athlete or other persons in whom repetitive activities are a factor.

Progression 1 – static opener

The patient is positioned so as to off-load pressure and tension from the nervous system in the piriformis region. Therefore, the patient will be placed in an open position as far as the interface is concerned, also incorporating a low neural tension position.

Position – supine, a pillow under the knees to provide knee flexion, hips externally rotated (releases tension from the piriformis muscle and compression of the nerve). The ankle is relaxed comfortably. In the acute severe pain situation, this can be offered as a rest position as opposed to performing mobilizations, if movement is likely to provoke symptoms.

Progression 2 – dynamic opener

Position – as in progression 1. This time a mobilization is performed.

Movement – passive external rotation, performed at a slow speed and large amplitude, without producing symptoms. This is similar to Maitland's shaft rotations for hip pain and can be quite effective.

Dosage – up to 10–20 oscillations per mobilization, then reassess gently. Up to five repetitions of the same set of mobilizations can be performed in the same session. However, this is not obligatory.

Level 2

Progression 1 – closer mobilization
Position – as for level 1.

Movement – passive internal rotation of the hip joint is performed by the therapist, then it can be carried out as a home exercise by the patient. Even though this is a closer at the time of performing the manoeuvre, it is designed to produce an opening effect as the muscle releases and should take the pressure off the peroneal nerve. This mobilization is performed as a gentle manual oscillation.

Progression 2 – closer muscle release
Position – supine.

Movement – passive stretch of the piriformis muscle in which the hip is taken into flexion, adduction and external rotation. In addition, contract-relax techniques are carried out in which resisted internal rotation of the hip joint is performed.

Neural
Level 1
Progression 1 – off-loader as a position
The off-loader position for the neural dysfunction category at level 1 is the same as that for the lumbosacral nerve roots because they are continuous with one another (see lumbar spine).

Progression 2 – two-ended slider
Position – side lying, the painful side uppermost with the patient's body located in a slightly diagonal alignment relative to the plinth. The patient should be close enough to the edge so that their ipsilateral leg can move freely over the edge of the plinth. The ipsilateral hip is placed into flexion (below 70°) and external rotation so as to reduce tension and pressure in the buttock region. The thoracic spine is flexed whilst the neck is placed in neutral flexion/extension. The patient's symptomatic foot can at times drape over the edge of the plinth and pillows are sometimes needed to support the symptomatic limb in some degree of abduction (Fig. 12.7).

Movement – at first the therapist holds the patient's hip into external rotation and helps them learn the performance of the combined movements of knee extension/plantarflexion. Once this is accomplished, the therapist then performs passive neck flexion/extension as the patient performs the knee and foot movements which are sequenced as follows:

1. Proximal slider – neck flexion/knee flexion and the foot moves to the neutral position.
2. Distal slider – neck extension/knee extension and plantarflexion/inversion.

The same can be performed for the tibial nerve whereby dorsiflexion substitutes plantarflexion/inversion.

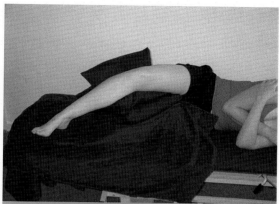

Figure 12.7   Off-loader and starting position (below 70° hip flexion) for the the two-ended slider for the piriformis syndrome involving the sciatic nerve.

Level 2
Position – as for level 1.

Movement – this time the sequence of movements is such that tension can be applied to the peroneal part of the sciatic nerve, namely neck flexion with knee extension and plantarflexion/inversion. The hip may be flexed above 70°, however, this will mean that it must be placed gently in internal rotation so as not to apply pressure to the nerve at this stage.

Level/type 3a – neurodynamically sensitized
The level/type 3a, two-ended tensioner for the piriformis syndrome is the same as that for the level/type 3a slump test for the lumbar spine. The end range is approached and the mobilization enters some degree of resistance, and symptoms can be evoked. However, the evoked responses should subside instantly. The problem with this technique is that it is not very refined in terms of attacking the causative mechanisms in which interactions of the nerve with the mechanical interface are a key problem. However, if a tension dysfunction exists, this may be the treatment of choice.

Level/type 3b – neurodynamic sequencing
The treatment technique for level 3b is the same as for the physical examination at this level. However, the mobilization can be taken into resistance and moderate symptoms, whilst the patient relaxes the buttock muscles in an attempt to increase range of

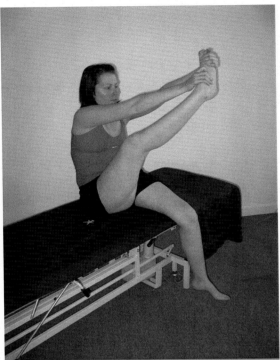

Figure 12.8 Self neurodynamic mobilization for the piriformis syndrome. Hip flexion/external rotation, knee extension and plantarflexion/inversion are the key movements.

simultaneous muscle lengthening and further neurodynamic movement in the direction of the manoeuvre.

Self neurodynamic mobilization

This exercise is designed for the athletic individual who has a mild piriformis syndrome at level/type 3c. The patient sits in the slump position. Then they bring their lower limb into full hip flexion/external rotation, knee extension and foot plantarflexion/inversion whilst, with their hands, holding their leg at as far distal a point as possible. The mobilization consists of knee flexion/extension. In the kinaesthetically aware, this action can be combined with contraction of piriformis (active internal rotation) in which the patient resists the movement by pushing into external rotation with their hands. They then move the limb passively into external rotation when they cease the contraction. If the patient cannot perform the contract-relax technique, they can simply lean on their ipsilateral buttock as a means of applying further pressure to the area (Fig. 12.8).

SCIATIC NERVE IN THE THIGH (E.G. HAMSTRING STRAIN)

Introduction

The main neuropathodynamic events in operation with problems affecting the sciatic nerve in the thigh will vary according to a number of factors. These are the location of the problem and the causative mechanisms. For instance, the problem of a hamstring strain with bleeding starts off in the mechanical interface and may initially produce a neural sliding dysfunction without causing much of a tension dysfunction. However, over time, as inflammation spreads into the nerve, an intrinsic pathology could develop (e.g. localized neuritis) and alter viscoelastic behaviour, thereby causing an additional secondary tension dysfunction. It is important to detect such changes from one domain to the other which necessitates a good understanding of the specific neuropathodynamics and detailed manual examination.

Dysfunction or pathology in the sciatic nerve in the thigh is not usually high on the clinician's list of possible diagnoses. However, the nerve at this site can be affected by a range of pathologies and pathodynamics. For instance, after trauma to the thigh,

motion and reduce hypersensitivity to the movement. It may also be performed as a wide amplitude movement out of the symptomatic position to allow symptoms to settle.

Level/type 3c – mechanical interface and neural

This technique is described earlier under examination with straight leg raise test at level/type 3c and combines interface and neural functions. At the outset, the lower limb is taken into full available range of internal rotation, then the peroneal neurodynamic test performed. Below 70° of hip flexion, the patient actively externally rotates their hip joint, which the therapist resists. Above 70°, the rotation component is reversed in which a resisted contraction of internal rotation is performed and the release is taken into external rotation. When the contraction is released, the muscle and nerve are treated with scar tissue can develop around the nerve and cause it to become compressed. In the more severe cases, this can need surgical intervention, even though one would think that the skilled therapist may at times be capable of dealing with the problem conservatively, given early intervention. In addition, tumours in the form of sarcoma, which are obviously sinister in nature, can appear in and around the hamstring muscles. This kind of problem has the potential to produce pathodynamics in the sciatic nerve, which highlights the point that patients with problems in this area that do not improve within normal time frames should be promptly referred for medical management. Hamstring injury is also a prime cause of pathodynamics in the sciatic nerve and, because of its specific relevance, is the focus of the following section.

Neurodynamic testing

Introduction

With respect to neurodynamics, the principal things to assess in the patient with hamstring injury naturally relate to investigation of the causative mechanisms. These consist of history in order to localize the reason for, and nature of, the onset of the problem; provoking and easing factors; understanding the pathological mechanisms (such as neuritis and movement dysfunction); investigations such as neurological examination, MRI and ultrasound and of course a thorough physical examination of the specific neurodynamics.

A key question is whether bleeding, swelling and bruising are observed after the injury. In severe cases, scarring from bleeding around the sciatic nerve from the hamstrings may significantly restrict the excursion of the nerve.

Clinical case

A young man appeared at my clinic early in the week following a weekend football match at which he injured himself. He reported experiencing only isolated pain in the posterior aspect of his thigh, which was provoked by walking, straightening his back and leaning to his contralateral side. His

lumbar spine listed ipsilaterally and manual correction of the list reproduced his posterior thigh pain. I thought the problem was located in his low back until I saw severe bruising in his posterior thigh. He experienced no back pain but was finding it increasingly difficult to stop leaning toward his painful side and to stretch out his leg to walk. In addition to the lumbar list, his protective deformity also consisted of a small amount of hip flexion and external rotation and knee flexion and even plantarflexion of his foot. In the standing position, passive knee extension also reproduced his hamstring pain and increased his lumbar ipsilateral list. It became clear that the purpose of the list was to reduce proximal sliding and tension in the sciatic nerve at the level of the thigh because the nerve may have become hypersensitive due to neuritis. Scar tissue may also have started to appear. This was an easy case to recognize, however, it is much more common for hamstring problems that affect the sciatic nerve to be subtle and covert, only to be missed with standard neurodynamic testing. The following illustrates some techniques for assessment and treatment of the hamstring/sciatic nerve problem.

Level 1

When investigating the possibility of sciatic nerve involvement in hamstring injuries at level 1, the following techniques should be used, especially in the acute situation. This is because they can assist in the early determination of specific neurodynamic dysfunctions. For instance, pain with proximal sliding will require different treatment from pain with distal sliding or a tension dysfunction. As follows, the straight leg raise and slump tests are utilized on a general level to ascertain whether neuropathodynamic changes exist.

Straight leg raise

At level 1, dorsiflexion of the foot is performed first so that, at the first onset of symptoms, this movement is released and a change in symptoms may indicate a neural component to the problem. This aspect is advanced later and, as will be seen, responses to specific manoeuvres can yield quite different information that naturally resolves to provide different treatment.

Slump test

In addition to the straight leg raise test, a modified slump test for level 1 can also be executed. Dorsiflexion and spinal flexion movements are performed first and knee extension is taken to the first onset of symptoms. One by one, neck flexion is released and returned and dorsiflexion is released.

Hence, the sequence of movements is as follows:

1. Starting position – slump sitting, flexion of the whole spine (including neck flexion) whilst keeping the sacrum in a vertical position.
2. Dorsiflexion.
3. Knee extension to the first onset of symptoms. If the calf muscles are too tight to permit sufficient knee extension, dorsiflexion may be released a little.
4. Release neck flexion and monitor changes in symptoms, return neck into flexion and/or:
5. Release dorsiflexion, monitor changes in symptoms.

Level 2

The standard straight leg raise and slump tests are applied for level 2, as presented in Chapter 7, and similar diagnostic manoeuvres as in level 1 are applied. The main differences are that the ranges of motion reached are mostly likely greater in level 2 than in level 1 and the differentiating movements are, for examination purposes, allowed to evoke mild symptoms.

Levels/types 3a and b slump tests

The level 3a (neurodynamically sensitized) examination for hamstring/sciatic nerve problems is as for the level 3a for the lumbar spine neural tension dysfunction.

The level 3b technique is possibly biased toward the proximal and middle portions of the hamstrings and sciatic nerve.

Position – the patient sits as for the standard slump test.

Movement – the patient flexes their hip as far as they can in a self-assisted manner whilst the knee

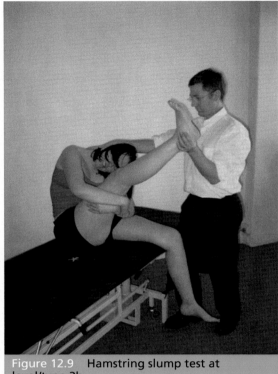

Figure 12.9   Hamstring slump test at level/type 3b.

stays flexed. At this point, the patient stabilizes their thigh with their forearms (cuddling their thigh), followed by moving their neck into flexion. The therapist moves the patient into contralateral lateral flexion of the whole spine and the patient completes the manoeuvre by performing knee extension and dorsiflexion actively. Structural differentiation is achieved with dorsiflexion and cervical flexion. I call this the 'hamstring slump test' (Fig. 12.9).

Level 3c – hamstring palpation with neurodynamic testing

The aim of this technique is to apply pressure to the sciatic nerve in the thigh during movement and elongation of the hamstrings and therefore deals with the dynamic interactions between the two components. In this position sliders and tensioners can be performed to offer the opportunity to apply pressure to the sciatic nerve and hamstrings simultaneously whilst they also move (Fig. 12.10).

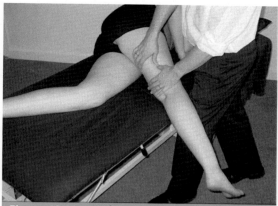

Figure 12.10   Technique of testing and treatment of sciatic nerve component to hamstring injury.

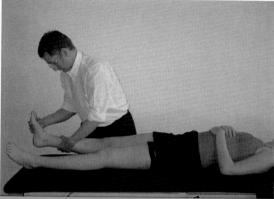

Figure 12.11   Starting position for sliders of the sciatic nerve related to hamstring injury.

Treatment

Treatment of the mechanical interface for the sciatic nerve in the thigh is essentially therapy for the hamstrings and associated soft tissue and will be well known to the practitioner. Therefore, this subject is omitted. What follows instead is a group of techniques for the sciatic nerve at levels 1, 2 and 3a, b and c with respect to hamstring strain that exhibits a neural component.

Proximal and distal sliding dysfunctions
Level 1

The two-ended slider can be used for the sliding dysfunction in either direction at level 1.

Position – supine lying.
The patient can perform the foot movements actively.

Movement – 1. Proximal slider – the therapist performs a straight leg raise without producing symptoms whilst, at the same time, plantarflexion is applied. 2. Distal slider – during the phase in which the leg is lowered, the foot is dorsiflexed. Clearly, at level 1, symptoms should not be provoked with the treatment (Figs 12.11, 12.12 and 12.13).

Level 2

Position – ipsilateral long sitting with the foot in a relaxed position.

Movement – 1. Distal slider – with the help of the therapist, the patient performs ipsilateral lateral

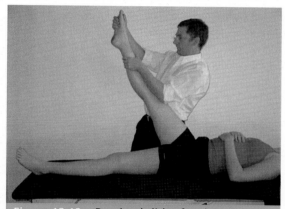

Figure 12.12   Proximal slider for the sciatic nerve related to hamstring injury, plantarflexion and straight leg raise.

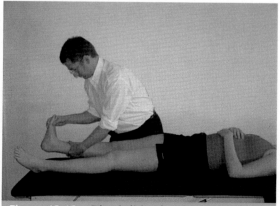

Figure 12.13   Distal slider for the sciatic nerve related to hamstring injury, dorsiflexion with lowering of the straight leg raise.

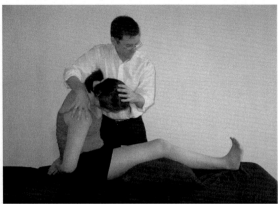

Figure 12.14 Distal slider of the sciatic nerve for hamstring injury at level 2, ipsilateral lateral flexion/dorsiflexion.

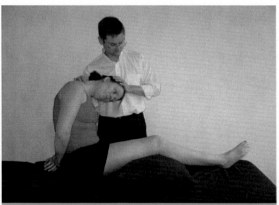

Figure 12.15 Proximal slider of the sciatic nerve for hamstring injury at level 2, contralateral lateral flexion/plantarflexion.

flexion of the whole spine (active assisted) and, at the same time, dorsiflexion of the foot. 2. Proximal slider – again, with the therapist helping to move the patient's spine, this time into contralateral lateral flexion and the patient performs plantarflexion of the foot (Figs 12.14 and 12.15).

Tension dysfunction

Level 1

The tension dysfunction is often a sensitive issue because treatment with tensioners can provoke. Often sliders are good at this level to decrease neural sensitivity. However, if the decision is to approach the tension component at level 1, gentle inner range one-ended tensioners in the form of dorsiflexion of the foot and internal rotation of the hip can be used. The patient is also shown the neurodynamic off-loaded position for the sciatic nerve (same as lumbar spine) which they can use at home to help their acute pain.

Level 2

The level 2 progression 1 mobilization is to perform gentle knee extension without reproducing symptoms whilst the patient is positioned in supine lying and the knee supported in approximately 45°–90° flexion. The progression 2 technique is the same as progression 1 except dorsiflexion is added. This can in turn be advanced to progression 3 in which the patient sits as for the slump test in which gentle active neck flexion, coupled with passive knee extension, is performed. If this technique is not extensive enough for the patient, dorsiflexion can be added.

Level/type 3a

The treatment progressions at level/type 3a for the tension dysfunction in hamstring injury are similar to those of the lumbar spine neural tension dysfunction.

Level/type 3b

The technique for treatment of the sciatic nerve problem at level/type 3b is as for the examination at this level. It is likely that, if the patient needs this treatment, it will evoke some symptoms and refined technique will be important. Range of motion without symptoms is a goal and dorsiflexion and spinal movements will be key elements. It will be necessary to maintain dorsiflexion carefully because the tendency with this manoeuvre is for the therapist and patient to neglect this movement and therefore reduce the effectiveness of the mobilization. I also recommend that contract-relax techniques also be applied to the hamstrings as a means of treating both the muscular and neural components (this effectively changes the technique to level 3c).

Level/type 3c

This technique is the same as for level 3c neurodynamic testing and involves palpation of the hamstrings adjacent to the sciatic nerve and making sure that pressure is applied toward the nerve itself. This necessitates that the therapist be familiar with palpation of the nerve. Treatment consists of deep massage in conjunction with other soft tissue techniques and neurodynamic movements in the form of active dorsiflexion. The patient can also perform a resisted static contraction of the hamstrings by pushing their hip into extension and their knee into flexion against the therapist's body. This way, many aspects of the dynamic interactions between the muscle (interface) and neural tissue can be treated. Finally, these techniques could massage the nerve and improve its blood flow to yield a reduction in inflammatory changes in the nerve and reduce its sensitivity to movement.

KNEE AND THIGH PAIN

Introduction

The contribution of the nervous system to anterior knee and thigh problems usually revolves around the femoral and saphenous nerves. The neurodynamic tests for these nerves are generally not very sensitive for minor neuropathodynamics and can even be quite normal in the presence of what would be suspected to be a significant neural problem. For instance, lateral femoral cutaneous neuropathy (meralgia paraesthetica) often shows a normal neurodynamic test for the nerve. What also happens is that the tests tend to show covert abnormal responses or solely tightness in the myofascial tissues to produce slight restrictions in range of motion of the knee and hip.

Clinical case

A patient was recently referred to our sports injury clinic for treatment of her meralgia paraesthetica. Even though she had all the localizing symptoms of the problem (and reduced sensation in the lateral thigh), palpation of the nerve was only slightly tender but symmetrical and the lateral femoral cutaneous neurodynamic test was tighter than on the contralateral side, and

differentiation was negative. The main difference between the symptomatic and asymptomatic sides was that her rectus femoris muscle was tight, such that, when she extended her hip with a flexed knee whilst on her hands and knees, her pelvis rotated into the anterior position much earlier than on the asymptomatic side. Her range of hip extension was less than what occurred contralaterally and her gluteal muscles were weak. This was a case of the neurodynamic tests exhibiting poor sensitivity and specificity, even though there was clear symptomatic evidence of a neural problem. Treatment focused on motor control for the lumbopelvic and knee regions, with excellent results. The therapeutic effect probably operated through improvement of mechanical stresses on the nerve via changing the behaviour of the mechanical interface.

The above means that, frequently, the neurodynamic tests for the knee and thigh must be taken to their end range to be of value and this is because of their relative lack of sensitivity. However, this is not to deny that some clinical problems in this region will need small range techniques when in the irritated state. Such cases could exist in particularly mobile people whose movement is sufficient to pass mechanical stresses to the nerves. However, if the person of average or limited mobility presents with markedly abnormal neurodynamic tests for the femoral region, one should suspect local pathology in the nerve or in the tissue adjacent to it. Nevertheless, the progressions that are possible for the femoral part of the nervous system are as follows and can be useful in patients with coexisting musculoskeletal and myofascial dysfunction in and around the knee and thigh.

Femoral nerve (groin, thigh and knee pain)

The prone knee bend and femoral slump tests are the techniques of choice in examination for neural contribution to thigh and knee pain, unless the problem focuses in the medial knee. In which case,

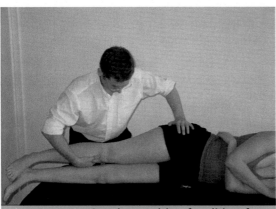

Figure 12.16   Starting position for sliders for the femoral nerve in the thigh.

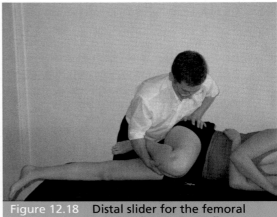

Figure 12.18   Distal slider for the femoral nerve in the thigh, hip flexion/knee flexion.

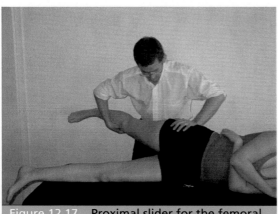

Figure 12.17   Proximal slider for the femoral nerve in the thigh, hip extension/knee extension.

the saphenous neurodynamic test may also be used. The progressions for treatment of the femoral nerve consist of the following.

Sliders and tensioners

The proximal slider is executed with the performance of hip extension (elongating the mechanical interface at the hip and therefore drawing the nerve proximally) and extension of the knee which lets the nerve pass proximally away from the knee (Figs 12.16, 12.17 and 12.18).

The tensioner is achieved by performance of femoral slump test, described in the chapter on standard neurodynamic testing (see Chapter 7) and is

sensitized at level/type 3a by performing it on the downward side and raising the treated thigh into adduction to produce contralateral lateral flexion of the lumbar spine in addition to the other spinal movements of the test.

The level/type 3b treatment can be to perform the femoral slump using a sequence that starts at the hip joint first. The level 3c testing and treatment for thigh and knee pain is to perform contract-relax techniques to the rectus femoris muscle and/or hip flexors in the neurodynamic position for the femoral nerve. This entails use of the modified Thomas test or side lying slump tests.

Because the femoral nerve relates anatomically to the inguinal region, it can be useful to apply the above techniques to groin pain and even perform manual soft tissue techniques in the neurodynamic position, such as in the side lying slump test.

Patellofemoral joint and neural dysfunction

A technique that is often useful in patients with a tight component to the femoral part of their nervous system as well as a tight rectus femoris muscle and lateral knee structures is the following. It is ranked at level 3c as a treatment to the innervated tissues of the femoral nerve and may influence the neural component to the problem.

The patient adopts a contralateral side lying position as if the therapist plans to mobilize their patellofemoral joint into a medial direction whilst

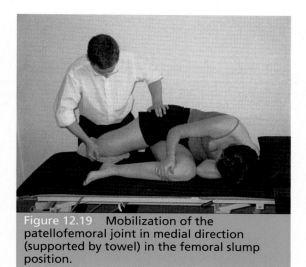

Figure 12.19 Mobilization of the patellofemoral joint in medial direction (supported by towel) in the femoral slump position.

the knee is in whatever degree of flexion is chosen. This is influenced by the location in the range of motion at which the joint dysfunction is located. Hip extension and the spinal movements for the femoral slump test are then added (Fig. 12.19).

PERONEAL NERVE

Introduction

The peroneal nerve and its distal extensions (superficial and deep branches) in the foot can become symptomatic in a range of disorders. Some of these include pressurization by ganglia that protrude from the adjacent joint (e.g. superior tibiofibular), compression from compartment syndrome, impact injury, stretch injury at sport or following fracture dislocation and the wearing of tight straps with high-heeled shoes. Also, altered biomechanics in the foot may produce altered mechanical stresses in the nerve. Damage due to sprained ankle can occur as high as the common peroneal nerve at the posterior aspect of the knee where haematomas can develop after traction injury caused by the sprain. Compromise can also occur as far distally as the superficial peroneal nerve. Inflammation then develops and the nerve may incur hypersensitivity, reduced mobility and, in some cases, reduced conduction (Kleinrensink 1997). The clinical correlates may include pain with movement (particularly plantarflexion/inversion),

tenderness and aching, dysaesthetic symptoms, tenderness and, in cases in which reduced conduction occurs, loss of sensation. In more recalcitrant cases, severe mechanical allodynia related to central sensitization may be a prominent feature. Loss of muscle power due to paralysis is not nearly as common as the other symptoms, however, this should still be kept in mind when treating such cases.

The area under consideration is along the anterolateral surface of the leg, extending distally, over the ankle, to the dorsum of the foot. Hence, symptoms in any of these areas may warrant examination of the peroneal part of the nervous system. Clearly, the musculoskeletal structures in the region should be examined and treated thoroughly. However, in relation to the nervous system, the most important aspects of examination related to the nervous system are neurological examination, neurodynamic tests and palpation of the nerves in question and these must of course be married with the biomechanics of the disorder.

Neurodynamic testing

The technique of choice for problems affecting the peroneal nerves (common and superficial) is the standard peroneal neurodynamic test. At level 1, it is modified to be performed as a straight leg raise whilst the foot is relaxed as best possible and, if needed, supported by the therapist. At the height of the leg raise, if symptoms have not been evoked, the therapist passively moves the ankle into plantarflexion/inversion to the first onset of symptoms and, at this point, to differentiate neurodynamic mechanisms, lowers the limb by reducing the hip flexion angle a small amount, whilst holding the foot stationary on the leg. This completes the neurodynamic test and structural differentiation.

At level 2, the same manoeuvre generally is performed, except that it is in the standard neurodynamic sequence. That is, initially plantarflexion/inversion is performed to the first onset of symptoms, followed by the straight leg raise, with care being taken not to contaminate the test with uncontrolled internal rotation of the hip.

One could separate testing the peroneal nerve into levels 3a, b and c, however, clinically, it is worthwhile starting with a technique that combines the three and, if this shows something of value, separate tests can be performed. In addition to the movements of the standard test, the level 3a examination (neurodynamically sensitized) incorporates internal rotation of the hip and can even be performed as a slump test.

The level 3b test (sensitized by neurodynamic sequencing) for the peroneal nerve is the same as that for level 2, except plantarflexion/inversion is taken further into range, whereby some local symptoms are often evoked prior to performing the straight leg raise. It is imperative that the toes are included properly with this test to ensure that all the right movements for the nerve occur. This stronger movement is likely to produce a more sensitized test than standard testing.

The level 3c test for the peroneal nerve is simply the same as that for level 3a and b, except resisted active dorsiflexion/eversion is performed as a means of applying force to the nerve through the mechanical interface (tendons and bone) and innervated tissue. Clearly, it is necessary to link the nature of testing to the disorder in the mechanical interface, in terms of stability and stiffness. For instance, it would not be wise to load the superficial peroneal nerve forcefully with plantarflexion/inversion, knowing that it might increase the instability of a sprained ankle. Conversely, it may be necessary to perform a technique at level 3b or c in the case of a stiff joint that is not especially irritable.

Treatment

Level 1

Treatment at level 1 for the peroneal nerve consists of proximal and distal sliders. This is to relieve pain, restore movement to the nerve, stimulate healing through alteration of intraneural blood flow and moulding of the connective tissues in the nerve and reduce its sensitivity.

Sliders

Proximal

Position – the patient lies supine whilst the therapist holds the patient's limb in approximately 45° hip flexion and sufficient knee flexion so that the leg can be held horizontal. Facing slightly distally, the therapist achieves this by placing the medial aspect of their near arm around the medial and/or posterior aspects of the patient's leg (almost using their armpit to grip the leg). The other hand holds the patient's

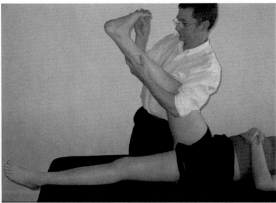

Figure 12.20   Proximal slider of the peroneal nerve, from the hip being flexed to approximately 45°, the knee is extended and the foot is moved into dorsiflexion/eversion.

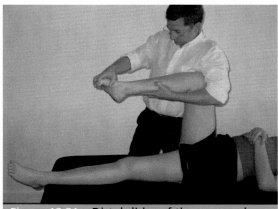

Figure 12.21   Distal slider of the peroneal nerve, plantarflexion/inversion with knee flexion.

foot under its plantar surface by the therapist placing their hand under the forefoot with the fingers spreading to the toes. The therapist's thumb then passes around the medial surface of the foot toward the dorsum of the forefoot, taking a firm but comfortable hold (Figs 12.20 and 12.21).

The distal slider incorporates the movements of knee flexion and plantarflexion/inversion (Fig. 12.21).

Level 2

Tensioners

The tensioner technique is simply the patient adopting an ipsilateral long sitting position and leaning forward over their hip at same time as performing plantarflexion/inversion. The therapist stabilizes the patient's knee in extension, if tolerated easily by the patient, and guides the foot into plantarflexion/ inversion so as to ensure that correct movement occurs.

Level 3

The technique for level 3a is as for the previous technique (level 2 progression 2 tensioner), except internal rotation of the hip and contralateral lateral flexion with the slump test are added.

Treatment at level 3b consists of the manoeuvre starting with plantarflexion/inversion first while the patient is in supine with their knees flexed comfortably. The knee is then extended and the remainder of the long sitting slump test is completed by the patient with execution of hip flexion, lumbar flexion and cervical flexion, in that order. It is crucial that the foot and knee positions have been stabilized properly during addition of the slump component.

The level 3c progression is as for level 3a except the foot is actively dorsiflexed against the therapist and contract-relax releases are performed at the end range of the technique. If by chance, the joint is found to be stiff in conjunction with housing a peroneal nerve problem, another way of executing treatment at this level is to perform joint mobilizations and neurodynamic techniques. For instance, in the slump position with plantarflexion/inversion, the ankle, or any of the foot joints can be mobilized into the stiff direction.

POSTERIOR TIBIAL NERVE – ALIAS HEEL PAIN AND PLANTAR FASCIITIS

Introduction

Dysfunction in the posterior tibial nerve as a contributor to ankle and heel pain and plantar fasciitis is completely underestimated and neglected and is, in my opinion, common. It is the carpal tunnel syndrome of the lower limb and does not select a particular age group because I have seen it occur in the young athlete, middle-aged and the elderly. Causes can be pressure from anomalous tendons and muscles, neurilemmomas, Schwannomas, tendonitis and tenosynovitis, ganglia, diabetes, overuse with a pronated foot and trauma. The area of symptoms is usually in the medial ankle region and spreads along the medial aspect of the foot and/or heel to the plantar aspect of the foot. It can produce pain and dysaesthesias and weakness of the muscles in the plantar aspect of the foot because it ultimately feeds the plantar and digital nerves. It is also for this reason that forefoot and toe movements are included in neurodynamic testing in evaluation of this problem. This painful and potentially disabling lesion can respond superbly to treatment. For a case history of neurodynamic treatment and clinical reasoning of a clear case of posterior tibial neuropathy causing heel pain and plantar fasciitis, see Shacklock (1995).

The posterior tibial nerve can become compressed or irritated at the posterior tarsal tunnel, located on the medial aspect of the ankle. The key aspects in diagnosis of this problem are palpation of the nerve and its surrounding tissues and specific neurodynamic and neurological testing. On occasions, patients with this problem show neurological changes in the form of numbness in the field of medial calcaneal nerve (supplying the medial and plantar aspect of the heel). With palpation, they also exhibit swelling and tenderness of the nerve and its surrounding tissues and this often extends along the course of the nerve, through the abductor hallucis muscle, and into the plantar aspect of the foot. A lesion in the nerve can produce obvious signs of neurogenic inflammation in the heel and plantar fascia (e.g. swelling and pain on compression), which should always be an indication that a neural component ought to be investigated. The mechanisms for this phenomenon are presented in the chapter on general neuropathodynamics (see Chapter 3). The distal symptoms in the foot can often be reproduced by applying pressure over the nerve at, and adjacent, the tunnel and even proximal and distal sliding dysfunctions can be detected with specific neurodynamic testing. Foot biomechanics should also be accounted for because excessive pronation increases stress in the nerve (Daniels et al 1998).

Mechanical interface testing and treatment

The reason for including the mechanical interface in examination of the posterior tibial nerve dysfunction is that it has a critical role to play. Specific passive physiological and accessory movements of the joints of the ankle and foot should be examined thoroughly. Imbalance in function, such as, stiffness or hypermobility should be interpreted in terms of their possible effects on the nerve. For instance, a stiff joint with a reduced closing dysfunction may not produce sufficient closing to facilitate normal nerve nutrition and movement. This may need mobilization of the joint in conjunction with a neurodynamic technique. Alternatively, an excessive closing dysfunction will need treatment that reduces closing on the nerve. This could require biomechanical intervention such as taping, orthotics or gait analysis and re-education and exercises with the aim of normalizing the mechanical events in and around the nerve.

The key physiological movements in relation to opening and closing of the interface revolve around plantarflexion/inversion (opener) and dorsiflexion/eversion (closer).

Neurodynamic testing

Levels 1, 2 and 3
Neurodynamic testing for the posterior tibial nerve disorder involves performing the standard tibial neurodynamic test and its variations. The order of movements at level 1 is to perform the standard straight leg raise to the point of symptoms in the foot and localize their site. Effectively, at this point, the necessary structural differentiation has been performed with hip flexion and it is not necessary to perform dorsiflexion/eversion, unless symptoms have not been evoked. In this case, at the top of the straight leg raise, the foot is taken into dorsiflexion/eversion to the first onset of symptoms and the limb is then lowered slowly, keeping the position of the foot on the leg stationary. If the symptoms change, a neurodynamic mechanism may be implicated.

Level 2 testing consists of the standard tibial neurodynamic test. The straight leg raise is again used to perform the differentiation by raising and lowering it to ascertain if this component movement produces a change in symptoms that were initially evoked by the dorsiflexion/eversion.

Level/type 3a testing (progression 1) is to perform the standard tibial neurodynamic test with the addition of internal rotation and adduction of the hip. A further progression (progression 2) would be the long sitting slump test in which the patient flexes

over their limb and the therapist performs the passive dorsiflexion/eversion. In the supine position, testing at level/type 3b is performed by the therapist performing the foot movements first. This is then followed by the rest of the tibial neurodynamic test in proximal order. The therapist performs internal hip rotation and the patient executes the hip flexion moving into a sitting position followed by spinal flexion and contralateral lateral flexion of the spine. Level/type 3c testing entails the long sitting slump in which the foot is dorsiflexed and everted by the therapist and the patient superimposes the slump with its sensitizing movements. The duet is then completed by performance of a resisted contraction of plantarflexion/inversion and great toe flexion/abduction to apply loading to the nerve through the mechanical interface. Clearly similarities exist between testing and treatment of the posterior tibial nerve and the other nerves. The main difference is that the foot movements vary according to the local anatomy and biomechanics.

Sliding and tension dysfunctions
Proximal sliding of the posterior tibial nerve is tested in the following way. With the patient in supine, the leg is supported so that the hip is in approximately 45° flexion and the leg horizontal. The foot is held so that the therapist's fingers can control the ankle, forefoot and toes. To achieve this, the therapist will later have to stabilize the calcaneum with their proximal hand.

Dorsiflexion/eversion of the ankle and forefoot and dorsiflexion of the toes are the first movements and these should be taken as far as practicable into the range. Knee extension is the next movement and is taken to a change in symptoms. Whilst stabilizing the ankle joint and the rest of the limb, release of dorsiflexion of the forefoot and toes is the final movement because this event releases distally directed natural tension from the digital nerves and allows the tibial part to displace further in a proximal direction. If the symptoms increase, a proximal sliding dysfunction is implicated (Figs 12.22 and 12.23).

In testing for a distal sliding dysfunction, again the hip is flexed to approximately 45° and the leg held horizontal as the starting position. This is to release proximal tension and allow distal sliding. The foot and toes are moved into dorsiflexion/eversion and the toes into dorsiflexion to move the

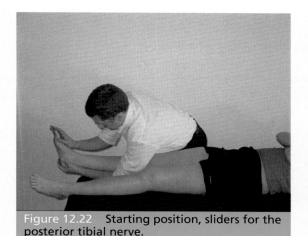

Figure 12.22   Starting position, sliders for the posterior tibial nerve.

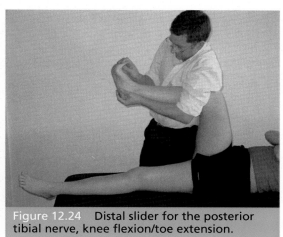

Figure 12.24   Distal slider for the posterior tibial nerve, knee flexion/toe extension.

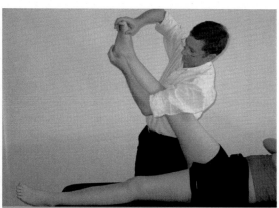

Figure 12.23   Proximal slider for the posterior tibial nerve, straight leg raise combined with flexion of the toes.

nerve distally in its tunnel. This movement must sometimes be relatively strong because, if not, it is often not sufficient to evoke symptoms. If symptoms are present with this movement, knee extension is used to produce proximal movement in the nerve whilst the toes, foot and ankle are held stationary. If the symptoms decrease with knee extension, a distal sliding dysfunction may be implicated. However, if at this point in the symptomatic range, further toe extension produces a reduction in symptoms (which sometimes happens), toe flexion produces an increase in symptoms, a proximal sliding dysfunction may be the problem (Fig. 12.24).

Clinical case – proximal sliding dysfunction of the posterior tibial nerve

A case in point is a young athlete who experienced pain in her heel and plantar fascia area. Plantar fasciitis was diagnosed and had been treated with local electrical modalities, deep frictions, taping for foot alignment and orthotics, corticosteroid injections and joint mobilizations. Even though a small improvement had occurred in the following several months, she remained unable to run without burning pain developing toward the end of her run, which would at times be severe and last until the next day. In the tibial neurodynamic test position with full toe extension, release of toe extension *increased* her pain. Palpation of the posterior and medial calcaneal nerves revealed local swelling and tenderness in the region of the nerve and posterior tarsal tunnel, particularly at its distal end and reproduced the symptoms in her heel and foot. This, coupled with the fact that there was reduced sensation to light touch in her first and second toes, is strong evidence of posterior tarsal tunnel syndrome masquerading as plantar fasciitis. Since the dynamics suggested a proximal sliding dysfunction, I believe that the problem was at the distal end of the tarsal tunnel as the nerve moved proximally against its fascial edge during daily movements. Palpation at this site was exquisitely tender, providing further support for the presence of this problem.

The tension dysfunction is tested by performing the tibial neurodynamic test and examining the effect of dorsiflexion of the toes and hip flexion. If, at the top of the straight raise to the first onset of symptoms, the performance of dorsiflexion of the ankle, foot and toes increases the symptoms, and reduction of the hip flexion angle reduces them, a tension dysfunction may be present.

Treatment

The proximal and distal sliders for the posterior tibial nerve consist of the tests for their respective dysfunctions, as above.

At low levels, treatment of the distal sliding dysfunction is achieved by moving the nerve in a *proximal* direction with the use of toe flexion with the knee moving from a flexed to extended position. As the patient progresses through to higher levels, they will need a change in treatment to a distal slider, as presented in Figures 12.22 to 12.24. The same principles apply for the proximal slider except the progressions are applied in the reverse order.

Tension dysfunctions (level 2 and higher) are treated with the use of the standard tibial neurodynamic test and movement of the foot and hip simultaneously as a wide amplitude movement to prevent provocation of symptoms.

Nerve massage

The notion of massaging a nerve is particularly interesting because it seems unusual to massage nerves. In my experience with posterior tarsal tunnel syndrome, massage of the nerve and its surrounding tissues can be very effective. The technique is performed by the therapist locating the nerve and massaging directly on it, as well as on the interfacing soft tissues and even the tissues innervated by the nerve. The massage passes along the course of the nerve distally into the foot and proximally into the calf. Focusing the treatment immediately proximal and distal to the tunnel is also performed so as to move

fluid in the nerve away from the tunnel and improve intraneural fluid pressures and blood flow. The movements are made with the thumb or fingers and consist of small circular and longitudinal motions. The technique is basically a combination of gentle deep friction and effleurage in which swelling in the nerve and environs is removed from the area. The changes in swelling in the nerve are often remarkably palpable following treatment. Furthermore, the most striking reassessment findings often evident immediately after the massage can be a reduction in sensitivity of the nerve to palpation, improvements in neurodynamic testing and even improvements in neurological findings. The technique can be performed in problems at all levels.

SURAL NERVE

Introduction

Disorders of the sural nerve cause pain anywhere along the distal posterolateral calf region, posterolateral ankle and dorsolateral edge of the foot to the lateral two toes. As with all neuropathies, this one has the potential to produce the gamut of neuropathic symptoms in addition to aches and pains that will masquerade as a problem in the nearby musculoskeletal tissues. It can be affected by sprained ankle, particularly when the mechanism of injury is related to severe adduction of the calcaneum or dorsiflexion/inversion of the ankle. Naturally, this is because the nerve passes around the dorsolateral surface of the ankle posterior to the lateral malleolus. The sural nerve may also cause pain in the region of, and coexist with stiffness in the joints that surround, the cuboid bone. Clearly, biomechanics in the lower limb and ensuring that the local joints and muscles function optimally are important aspects of assessment and treatment of this problem.

Neurodynamic testing

Neurodynamic testing at level 1 is similar in principle to that for the peroneal and tibial nerves. Naturally, the sural neurodynamic test is used and the specific foot movements of dorsiflexion/inversion are employed to detect the presence of distal and proximal sliding and tension dysfunctions in the same way as the posterior tibial nerve. If symptoms occur in the field of the nerve, palpation of the nerve can confirm the diagnosis.

At level 2, the standard sural neurodynamic test is used, whereby the foot movements of dorsiflexion/ inversion are performed to the first onset of symptoms, followed by the leg raise. The second progression at level 2 would be to perform the test in long sitting whilst the therapist positions and stabilizes the knee in extension and the foot in dorsiflexion/ inversion. At level/type 3a, the test is combined with the long sitting slump test, internal rotation of the hip and contralateral lateral flexion of the spine is added. The level/type 3b test involves performance of the sural neurodynamic test, starting with the foot movements whilst the patient is in the supine position and following with the remaining movements in proximal order (internal rotation of the hip, hip flexion whilst moving into the long sitting position and contralateral lateral flexion of the spine). The final progression (level/type 3c) is to perform the test for level/type 3b except add resisted contraction of plantarflexion/eversion of the foot. This activates the peronei and will apply increased pressure to the nerve and offer information on minimal dysfunction in the nerve. The reader should bear in mind that the sural neurodynamic test is highly sensitive when compared with the tibial neurodynamic test, especially to movements from a remote location such as the hip. This reactivity is characterized by the sudden onset of symptoms in the foot with only small changes in range of motion at the end of the movement. It will therefore be necessary to perform movements of the remote sites slowly and carefully.

Treatment

At level 1, treatment for the sural nerve dysfunction is best executed with sliders that do not evoke symptoms at first and move away from the specific dysfunction. The sliders for the nerve are as follows and they are applied and progressed in the same way as in the posterior tibial nerve (Figs 12.25, 12.26 and 12.27).

At level 2, the first progression is much the same as that for the peroneal and tibial nerves but the difference is that the foot movements revolve around dorsiflexion/inversion. In level 2, tensioners are applied in which the straight leg raise is combined with dorsiflexion/inversion in the supine position and is the standard sural neurodynamic

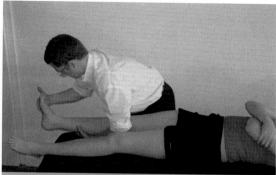

Figure 12.25   Starting position for the slider for the sural nerve.

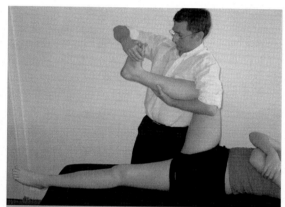

Figure 12.26   Distal slider for the sural nerve, knee flexion with dorsiflexion/inversion of the ankle.

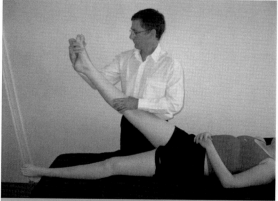

Figure 12.27   Proximal slider for the sural nerve, knee extension with plantarflexion/ eversion.

test. Progression 2 is the same test in long sitting with more potential for performance of hip flexion and fixation of the knee in extension or foot dorsiflexion/inversion by the therapist.

The level/type 3a progression is the long sitting slump test for the sural nerve with internal rotation of the hip, hip flexion and contralateral lateral flexion. The progression for level/type 3b is the same as for level/type 3a except the sequence of movements starts at the foot and finishes with the spinal movements.

The level/type 3c progression is as for level/type 3b except a resisted active plantarflexion/eversion is performed.

Another useful technique at level 3c is the joint mobilization whilst the sural nerve is in a neurodynamic position. It may be used in cases of stiffness in the joints on the lateral aspect of the foot or those that involve inversion. For instance mobilization of the calcanoecuboid joint can be performed in the long sitting sural slump position.

References

Daniels T, Lau J, Hearn T 1998 The effects of foot position and load on tibial nerve tension. Foot and Ankle International 19(2): 73–78

Kleinrensink G 1997 Influence of posture and motion on peripheral nerve tension. Inversion trauma as a cause of lowered motor conduction velocity of the peroneal nerve.

A prospective longitudinal study. Chapter 7, PhD Thesis, Erasmus University, Rotterdam

Shacklock M 1995 Clinical applications of neurodynamics. Moving in on Pain. Butterworth Heinemann, Sydney: 123–131

Glossary

Adverse mechanical tension
Ankle – dorsiflexion, eversion, dorsiflexion/inversion, plantarflexion/inversion
Axillary neurodynamic test
Biopsychosocial model of pain
Carcinoma
Carpal tunnel syndrome
Central pain mechanisms
Cervical spine
Clinical cases/examples
Clinical neurodynamics
Clinical reasoning
Closers – dynamic, static
Closing mechanisms
Compression
Continuum
Contraindications
Convergence
Covert abnormal response
Diagnosis
Diagnostic efficacy
Elbow – extension, flexion, supination, pronation
Endoneurium
Epineurium
Examination – planning, method, level/type zero, 1, 2, 3a, b, c, d
Excessive closing dysfunction
Excessive opening dysfunction
Excursion/sliding
Femoral slump test
Filum terminale
General neurodynamics
Glenohumeral – external rotation, internal rotation, horizontal extension
Glenohumeral abduction
Gravity – neurobiomechanics, clinical application
Headache
Hip – flexion, medial rotation, adduction, extension
Hypermobility
Inflammation dysfunction – increased, reduced
Innervated tissue – definition, dysfunctions, diagnosis
Intervertebral foramen
Intraneural blood flow
Kingery's sign
Knee – extension, flexion
Lateral flexion – contralateral, ipsilateral
Lateral glide – contralateral, ipsilateral
List – ipsilateral, contralateral

Localized muscle hyperactivity dysfunction
Lumbar spine
Mechanical dysfunction
Mechanical interface – definition, dysfunctions, reduced closing, excessive closing, reduced opening, excesssive opening
Mechanical irritation
Mechanosensitivity – normal, abnormal, clinical correlates
Median neurodynamic test 1
Median neurodynamic test 2
Mesoneurium
Metabolic disorders
Motor control dysfunctions
Movement diagram
Muscle hypoactivity dysfunction
Muscle imbalance dysfunction
Nerve bending
Nerve instability
Nerves – median, radial, ulnar, brachial plexus, axilliary, sciatic, tibial, sural, peroneal, saphenous, lateral femoral cutaneous, obturator
Neural container
Neural sliding dysfunction – definition, diagnosis, treatment
Neural stretching
Neural tension
Neural tension dysfunction
Neurodynamic sequencing
Neurodynamic tests – standard, median 1, median 2, radial, ulnar, axilliary, obturator, lateral femoral cutaneous, tibial, sural, peroneal, straight leg raise, slump, contralateral, bilateral, classification of responses, diagnosis with, method
Neurodynamics – general, specific
Neurogenic inflammation
Neurogenic pain – definition
Neurological examination
Neuropathodynamics – general, specific, classification
Non-organic signs
Openers – dynamic, static
Opening mechanisms
Overt abnormal response
Passive neck flexion
Pathoanatomical dysfunction – neural, mechanical interface, definition, mechanical interface, neural
Pathophysiological dysfunction – neural, mechanical interface, definition
Perineurium

Peroneal neurodynamic test
Phalen's test
Physiology
Piriformis neurodynamic test
Prone knee bend test
Primary mechanical functions
Provocative testing
Radial neurodynamic test
Radiculopathy – cervical, lumbar
Reduced closing dysfunction
Reduced opening dysfunction
Relationships between neuropathodynamics and
    clinical problems – optimal/desirable, suboptimal/
    undesirable, normal, abnormal, relevant, irrelevant
Scapular depression – neurobiomechanics, effect
    on symptoms
Sciatica
Sensitization
Sliders – cephalad, caudad, proximal, distal
Specific dysfunctions – diagnosis, treatment
Spinal canal

Standard testing
Stenosis
Straight leg raise
Strain
Stress
Structural differentiation
Sural neurodynamic test
Syndromes – thoracic outlet, pronator, supinator,
    carpal tunnel, hamstring strain, lumbar, cervical
    nerve root, radiculopathy, piriformis, knee pain,
    thigh, treatment pain, groin pain
Tension gradient
Tensioners
Tibial neurodynamic test
Tourniquet effect
Trigger point
Ulnar neurodynamic test
Upper cervical slump test
Viscoelasticity
Wrist – flexion, extension, neurobiomechanics

Index

Note: page numbers in *italics* refer to figures.

A

Abnormal, 51, 52
Abnormal neurodynamic response,
    101–103
  covert (CAR), 101–103
  irrelevant, 103
  overt (OAR), 101
  relationship to clinical problem,
    103–104
  relevant, 103
  subclinical, 103–104
Active movements
  in closing dysfunction, 80–81, 82
  in inflammation dysfunction, 95
  in mechanical interface
    dysfunction, 79
  in tension dysfunction, 89–90
Allodynia, 64, 79
Ankle, 44–45
  dorsiflexion, 44
  dorsiflexion/inversion, 45
  eversion, 44
  plantarflexion/inversion, 45
  sprains, 45, 88, 230, 235
Anomalous neurodynamic response,
  104
Antalgic movements, 115
Anti-tensioners *see* Offloaders
Atypical (but normal)
    neurodynamic response, 104
Axillary neurodynamic test (ANT),
  130–131

B

Back pain, low
  caudad/distal sliding dysfunction,
    205
  non-organic contribution, 39
  tension dysfunction, 206–207
  see also Lumbar spine
Back strain, 202–203
Bending, nerve, 8, *9*

Bilateral neurodynamic tests, 38–39,
  114
Bilateral straight leg raise (BSLR)
    test, 135–137
  common problems, 137
  median neurodynamic test 1 and,
    38–39
  normal response, 136
  structural differentiation, 136, *136*
  technique, 135–136, *136*
Biomechanics, nervous system, 14
Biopsychosocial model of pain,
  98–99
Blood flow, intraneural *see*
    Intraneural blood flow
Brachial plexus
  lateral neck flexion and, 40
  shoulder movements and, 40
  in thoracic outlet syndrome,
    176–177
  tumour, *61*
Buttock pain, 218

C

C nociceptive fibres, 62
  peripheral nerves, 18
  role in inflammation, 18, 69, 70
Calcitonin gene-related peptide
    (CGRP), 18
  in inflammation, 18, 62, 69
  vasodilator effect, 16
Calf muscles, in S1 radiculopathy,
  213–214
Calf stretch test, 213
Capsaicin, 18
Carpal tunnel syndrome, 187–194
  mechanical interface testing,
    188–190
  muscle hyperactivity after release,
    68
  nerve clicking, 90
  neurodynamic testing, 190
  opening dysfunction, 54–55

  pathophysiological dysfunction, 92
  physical examination, 188–190
  provocative testing, 42, 43
  sliding dysfunction, 60
  treatment, 190–194
    mechanical interface, 190–191
    neural component, 191–194
Central nervous system, nociceptive
    innervation, 18
Central pain mechanisms, 98
Cervical radiculopathy, 160–169
  mechanical interface, 160
  physical examination, 160–164,
    164
  treatment, 164–169
    combination dysfunctions,
      168–169
    mechanical interface
      dysfunctions, 164–166
    neural dysfunctions, 166–168
    tension dysfunctions, *167*,
      167–168, *168*
Cervical slump test, 160–162
  level 1 and 2, 160–161
  level 3, 161–162, *162*
  see also Upper cervical slump test
Cervical spine, 39–40, 159–174
  flexion *see* Neck flexion
  lateral flexion, 39–40
Clicking, nerve, 90
Clinical neurodynamics, defined, 2
Closers, 154
  carpal tunnel syndrome, 190–191
  cervical radiculopathy, 165–166
  dynamic, 154
  lumbar radiculopathy, 201–202,
    202
  piriformis syndrome, 221–222
  pronator tunnel syndrome, 181
  static, 154
Closing, 10
  dysfunctions, 52–54
    diagnosis, 80–82, *86*
    excessive *see* Excessive closing
      dysfunctions

Closing (*contd*)
   reduced *see* Reduced closing
      dysfunctions
   mechanisms, 11–12
Compression, 7, *7*
   closing and, 12
   intraneural blood flow and, 17
   see also Pressure, elevated
Connective tissues, nervous system,
   3–4
Contralateral movements, clinical
   application, 38
Contralateral neurodynamic tests,
   37–38, *38*, 114
Convergence, 5, 7–8, *9*
   spinal neural tissues, 33–34, *35*
Covert abnormal response (CAR),
   101–103
Cubital tunnel syndrome, 41, 82

D

De Quervain's disease, 10, *10*, 131
Deformity, protective
   in closing dysfunctions, 80
   in hamstring injury, 224
   in mechanical interface
      dysfunctions, 79
   in opening dysfunctions, 83,
      85–86
Desirable, 51, 52
Diabetes, 15, 65
Diagnosis
   general points, 78
   importance of specificity, 12–13
   innervated tissue dysfunctions,
      92–95
   lateral flexion and, 36
   mechanical interface
      dysfunctions, 78–88
   neural dysfunctions, 88–92
   with neurodynamic tests,
      97–104
   specific dysfunctions, 77–95
   spinal flexion and extension and,
      35
Diagnostic categories, 50–52,
   99–104
Diagnostic efficacy, 99–100
Differentiation *see* Structural
   differentiation
Dorsal root ganglion,
   mechanosensitivity, 64

Dura
   sensory innervation, 18
   in spinal flexion, 32
Duration of testing (movement),
   21–22
Dysaesthesiae, 64, 85, 87, 89, 90

E

Egypt, ancient, xi
Elbow, 41–42
   extension, 41
   flexion, 41
   supination and pronation, 41–42
Endocrine diseases, 65
Endoneurial blood flow, 62
Epineurium, 7
Evoking symptoms
   during testing, 114
   during treatment, 158
Examination, physical *see* Physical
   examination
Excessive closing dysfunctions,
   53–54, *54*
   diagnosis, 82
   treatment, 155
Excessive opening dysfunctions, 56,
   56
   diagnosis, 85–86
   treatment, 155
Excursion, neural *see* Sliding, neural
Explanation to patient, before
   testing, 113–114
Extent of movement, 21

F

Femoral nerve
   neurodynamic tests, 228
   treatment, 228–229, *229*
Femoral slump test (FST), 148–150,
   150
   femoral nerve in thigh, 228–229
   lumbar radiculopathy, 198, *198*
   mid-lumbar disorders, 215, *215*
   patellofemoral joint, 229–230, *230*
   side lying, 149–150
   structural differentiation, 150
Fibroblasts, 63, 69
Filum terminale, 32
Finger flexion and extension, 43
Foot, 44–45

   dorsiflexion, 44
   dorsiflexion/inversion, 45
   eversion, 44
   plantarflexion/inversion, 45
Force
   general application, 20–21
   localization, 21
   viscoelasticity and, 15

G

General neurodynamics, 1–26
General neuropathodynamics,
   49–75
Glenohumeral joint
   abduction, 40–41
   external rotation, 41
   horizontal extension, 41
   internal rotation, 41
Gravity, spinal effects, 37, *37*
Groin pain, 228–229

H

Hamstring slump test, 225, *225*
Hamstring strain, 223–228
   neurodynamic testing, 224–225
   treatment, *226*, 226–228, *227*
Hamstrings
   palpation with neurodynamic
      testing, 225
   in S1 radiculopathy, 213–214
Headache (cervicogenic), 169–174
   mechanical interface, 170
   muscle testing, 174
   upper cervical slump test,
      170–173
Heel pain, 232–235
   inflammation dysfunction, 70–71
   sliding dysfunction, 89
Hip, 43–44
   adduction, 44
   extension, 44
   flexion, 43–44
      see also Straight leg raise
   medial rotation, 44
History
   closing dysfunctions, 80, 82
   inflammation dysfunction, 95
   mechanical interface
      dysfunctions, 78–79
   opening dysfunctions, 83, 85

pathoanatomical dysfunction, 87
pathophysiological dysfunction, 88
reduced neural sliding, 89
Horizontal extension technique,
    carpal tunnel syndrome,
    189–190, *190*, *192*
Horizontal flexion technique, carpal
    tunnel syndrome, 188–189,
    189, 190
Hyperalgesia, 64, 79
Hyperlordotic lumbar spine, 82, *83*
Hypermobility, neural, 61, 90

I

Inflammation, *16*, 18–19
    in mechanical irritation, 62–63
    neural triggers, 70
    neurogenic, 18, *19*, 69–70
    release of peptides stimulating,
        69, *69*
Inflammation dysfunction, 69–72
    diagnosis, 94–95
    increased, 70–71, 94–95
    reduced, 71–72, *72*, 95
Inflammatory response, assessment,
    19, 71–72, 95
Innervated tissues, 4
    dysfunctions, 50, 65–72
        diagnosis, 92–95
    movement, 8–10
    physiology and, 18–19
    testing, 23–24
Instability
    musculoskeletal, 54, 56, 82
    neural, 61, 90
International Association for the
    Study of Pain, 50
Intervertebral foramina
    closing and opening, 11, 12
    flexion and extension and, 33, *33*
    lateral flexion and lateral glide
        and, 35
    rotation and, 36
Intraneural blood flow, 15–18
    in clinical reasoning, 92
    compression and, 17
    elevated pressure and, 62, *62*
    practical relevance, 17–18
    regulation, 15–17
    tension and, 17
    tension and compression
        interactions, 17

Irrelevant (problems), 52
Irrelevant abnormal neurodynamic
    response, 103
Irritability, Maitland's concept, 108
Irritation, mechanical *see*
    Mechanical irritation

J

Joint
    movements, 7–8, *9*, 14
    opening and closing, 12

K

Kingery's sign, 188
Knee, 44
    extension, 44
    flexion, 44
    pain, 228–230
Knee-extension-in-sitting (KEIS)
    test, 39

L

Lateral femoral cutaneous
    neurodynamic test
    (LFCNT), 148, 228
Lateral femoral cutaneous
    neuropathy, 228
Lateral flexion, 35–36
Lateral glide, 35–36
List
    contralateral, 80
    ipsilateral, 83, 224
Localized examination (level 3b), 111
Localized muscle hyperactivity
    dysfunction, 68, 94
Lower limb/quarter, 217–237
    neurodynamic tests, 132–151
    pain, 218
    sensitizing movements, 98
    specific neurodynamics, 43–45
Lumbar radiculopathy, 196–215
    mid-lumbar region, 214–216
    physical examination, 196–198
    treatment, 198–215
    vs piriformis syndrome, 218–219
    see also S1 radiculopathy
Lumbar spine, 195–216
    caudad/distal sliding dysfunction,
        205–206

cephalad/proximal sliding
    dysfunction, 202–204
complex dysfunctions, *210*,
    210–212, *211*, *213*
hyperlordotic, 82, *83*
mechanical interface
    dysfunctions, 198–202
muscle hyperactivity
    dysfunctions, 212–214, *213*
neural dysfunctions, 202–209
physical examination, 196–198
reduced closing dysfunction,
    198–202
reduced opening dysfunction, 202
tension dysfunction, 206–209
see also Back pain, low
Lumbosacral nerve roots, hip
    movements and, *43*, 43–44
Lumbosacral trunk, hip flexion and,
    43, 43–44

M

Maitland, G, 10, 106, 108
Manual testing
    in closing dysfunctions, 81, 82
    in mechanical interface
        dysfunctions, 79–80
    in opening dysfunctions, 83–84,
        86
Massage, neurodynamic
    median nerve at elbow, 184, *185*
    posterior tibial nerve, 235
    supinator tunnel syndrome, 187
Mechanical changes
    nervous system responses, 14
    physiological effects, 15, *15*
    spread, 14
Mechanical dysfunction
    as cause of pain, 50
    interactions between different
        types, 51
    types, 51
Mechanical functions, primary, 4–7
Mechanical interface, 2–3
    compression by, 7
    movement, 10–12
    testing, 23
Mechanical interface dysfunctions,
    50, 52–59
    cervical spine, 164–166
    closing *see under* Closing
    defined, 52

Mechanical interface dysfunctions
      (*contd*)
   diagnosis, 78–88
   history, 78–79
   instability and, 56
   opening *see under* Opening
   pathoanatomical, 57–58
   pathophysiological, 59
   physical findings, 79–80
   radiological investigation, 79
   symptoms, 78
   treatment guidelines, 154–155
Mechanical irritation, 62–63, *63*
   pressure interactions, 63, *63*
Mechanosensitivity, 63–65
   chemical, 64–65
   clinical correlates, 65
   in clinical reasoning, 92
   defined, 64
   normal *vs* abnormal, 64
Medial calcaneal nerve, 232
Median nerve
   bleeding around, 58, *58*
   in carpal tunnel, *188*
   closing mechanisms, 11–12
   elbow movements and, 41–42
   finger movements and, 43
   lateral flexion and glide and, 36
   lateral neck flexion and, 40
   longitudinal sliding, 5
   massage at elbow, 184, *185*
   palpation, 188, *189*
   shoulder movements and, 40–41
   sliding dysfunction, 60
   transverse sliding, 6
   wrist movements and, 42
   see also Carpal tunnel syndrome
Median neurodynamic test, *xi*
Median neurodynamic test 1
      (MNT1), 118–121
   carpal tunnel syndrome, 188, 190,
      191, 192
   cervical nerve root tension
      dysfunction, 167–168, *168,*
      169
   cervical radiculopathy, 161,
      162–164, *164*
   cervicogenic headache, 171
   common problems, 120–121
   contralateral, 37
   diagnostic efficacy, 100
   indications, 119
   level/type 3, *164*

modified (supported), 121, *122*
   movements, 120, *120, 121*
   normal response, 121, *122*
   preparation, 119, *119*
   pronator tunnel syndrome,
      181–183, 184
   sequencing, 24
   thoracic outlet syndrome, *179,*
      179–180
   using movement diagram, 106
Median neurodynamic test 2
      (MNT2), 125–128
   cervical spine, 161
   common problems, 127–128, *128*
   indications, 125
   normal response, 128
   pronator tunnel syndrome, 183,
      183
   technique, 125–127, *126, 127*
Meralgia paraesthetica, 228
Mesoneurium, 6
Metabolic disorders, 65
Mid-lumbar disorders, 214–216
   interface and neural dysfunctions,
      215–216
   neurodynamic testing, 214–215
Motor control
   dysfunctions, 66–69, 92–94
   importance, 66
   neurodynamics and, 66
Movement
   duration, 21–22
   extent, 21
   feeling for changes, 106
   innervated tissues, 8–10
   joint, 7–8, *9,* 14
   mechanical interface, 10–12
   nervous system responses, 14–15
   neural *see* Neural movement
   resistance to, 21
   speed, 22
   see also Active movements
Movement diagram, 10, *11*
   application, 11, 106, 115
Multistructural examination
      (level 3c), 110, 111–112
Muscle
   as innervated tissue, 66
   as interface, 66
   nerve compression by, 12
Muscle hyperactivity dysfunction
   localized, 68, 94
   lumbar spine, 212–214, *213*

protective, 66–67, 92–93
Muscle hypoactivity dysfunction, 68,
   94
Muscle imbalance dysfunction, 68,
   93–94, *94*
Muscle release techniques, cervical
   radiculopathy, 169, *169*

N

Neck flexion
   neural effects, 33–34, *34*
   test, passive, 118
Nerve bending, 8, *9*
Nervi vasa nervorum, 16, 18
Nervous system, *3*
   as a continuum, 13–14
   general layout, 2–4
   links between mechanics and
      physiology, 15, *15*
   physiology *see* Physiology
   primary mechanical functions,
      4–7
   responses to movement, 14–15
   transmission of forces along, 13
Neural dysfunctions, 50, 59–65
   diagnosis, 88–92
   pathoanatomical, 61, *61*
   pathophysiological, 62–65
   sliding (excursion), 59–60, 88–89
   treatment guidelines, 156–158
Neural movement
   dynamics, 14–15
   intraneural blood flow during,
      16–17
   mechanisms, 7–13
Neural sliding *see* Sliding, neural
Neural stretching, 2, 23
Neural structures, 3–4
   testing, 23
Neural tension *see* Tension, neural
Neuroanatomy, xiii
Neurodynamic massage *see* Massage,
   neurodynamic
Neurodynamic sequencing, 19–25
   defined, 20
   importance, 24–25
   key facts, 20
   key variables, 20–24
   level 3b examination, 111
   origin of concept, 19–20
   personalizing, 24–25
   serial, 24

Neurodynamic tests, *25*, 25–26
  abnormal response *see* Abnormal
      neurodynamic response
  bilateral, 38–39, 114
  classification of responses,
      100–104, *102*
  in closing dysfunctions, 82
  contraindications, 107–108
  contralateral, 37–38, *38*, 114
  defined, 25
  diagnosis with, 97–104
  diagnostic efficacy, 99–100
  factors affecting accuracy, 24
  false positive, 88
  feeling for changes in movement,
      106
  general points on technique,
      113–116
  history, xi
  individual variability, 99
  in inflammation dysfunction, 95
  interpretation, 99–104
  levels *see under* Physical
      examination
  in mechanical interface
      dysfunctions, 80
  musculoskeletal response, 100
  in nerve hypermobility, 90
  neurodynamic response, 100–104
  normal response, 101
  in opening dysfunctions, 84, 86
  in pathoanatomical dysfunction,
      90–91
  in pathophysiological
      dysfunction, 88
  planning and extent, 106–113
  positive/negative distinction, 52,
      100
  sequence, 113
  sequencing *see* Neurodynamic
      sequencing
  in sliding dysfunction, 89
  standard, 113, 117–151
  in tension dysfunction, 90
  terminology, 25, 118
  use, 26
  see also Physical examination;
      specific tests
Neurodynamically sensitized
    examination (level 3a), 111
Neurodynamics
  clinical, defined, 2
  concept, 2

general, 1–26
  specific, 2, 31–45
Neurogenic inflammation, 18, *19*,
    69–70
Neurogenic pain, defined, 50
Neurological examination
  in inflammation dysfunction, 95
  in mechanical interface
      dysfunctions, 80
  in nerve hypermobility, 90
  in pathoanatomical dysfunction,
      91
  in piriformis syndrome, 218
Neuropathodynamics, 50–75
  classification of problems, 50–52
  clinical problems and, 51–52,
      103–104
  general, 49–75
  neurodynamic testing and, 98–99
  specific, 50
  see also Abnormal neurodynamic
      response
Neuropeptides, 69, *69*
  see also Calcitonin gene-related
      peptide; Substance P
Nociceptors
  in central nervous system, 18
  intraneural blood flow regulation,
      16
  in mechanical irritation, 62
  in peripheral nerves, 18
Noradrenaline (norepinephrine), 72
Normal, 51, 52
Normal neurodynamic response,
    101
Nucleus pulposus, protrusion, 59
Numbness, 85

O

Obturator neurodynamic test
    (ONT), 150–151, *151*
Oedema, neural, 16, *16*
  elevated pressure and, 62, *62*
  in mechanical irritation, 63
Offloaders (anti-tensioners), 158
  cervical radiculopathy, 167, *167*
  lumbar radiculopathy, 207–208,
      208
  piriformis syndrome, 222, *222*
  pronator syndrome, 183–184
  supinator tunnel syndrome, 185,
      187, *187*

Openers, 154
  carpal tunnel syndrome, 190–191
  dynamic, 154
    cervical radiculopathy, 165,
        165, 166
    lumbar radiculopathy, 201, *201*
    piriformis syndrome, 221
    pronator tunnel syndrome, 181
    supinator tunnel syndrome, 185
    thoracic outlet syndrome, 178
  static, 154
    cervical radiculopathy,
        164–165, *165*
    lumbar radiculopathy,
        199–201, *200*
    piriformis syndrome, 221
    pronator tunnel syndrome, 181
    supinator tunnel syndrome,
        185
    thoracic outlet syndrome, 178
Opening, 10
  dysfunctions, 54–56
    diagnosis, 83–86
    excessive *see* Excessive opening
        dysfunctions
    reduced *see* Reduced opening
        dysfunctions
  mechanisms, 12
Optimal, 51, 52
Overpressure, in slump test, 143, *143*
Overt abnormal response (OAR),
    101

P

Pain
  biopsychosocial model, 98–99
  central mechanisms, 98
  latent, 108
  neurodynamic testing and, 107,
      108
  neurogenic, defined, 50
  in pathophysiological
      dysfunction, 87–88
  peripheral mechanisms, 4
  receptors in nervous system, 18
  slider techniques, 156
Painful arcs, 78
Palpation
  in closing dysfunctions, 82
  in inflammation dysfunction, 95
  in mechanical interface
      dysfunctions, 80

Palpation (*contd*)
  in nerve hypermobility, 90
  in opening dysfunctions, 84, 86
  in pathoanatomical dysfunction, 91
  in sliding dysfunction, 89
  in tension dysfunction, 90
Paraesthesiae, 87, 89, 90
Paralysis, 69
Passive movements, in tension dysfunction, 89–90
Passive neck flexion test, 118
Patellofemoral joint, 229–230, *230*
Pathoanatomical dysfunction, 57–58
  clinical examples, 57–58, 91
  defined, 57
  diagnosis, 86–87, 90–91
  mechanical interface, 57
  neural, 61, *61*
Pathophysiological dysfunction, 59
  definition, 59
  diagnosis, 87–88, 91–92
  mechanical interface, 59
  neural, 62–65
Perilunate instability, 82
Perineurium, 5
Peripheral nerves
  inflammation and, 18–19
  nociceptive innervation, 18
Peripheral neuropathies, classification, 50
Peroneal nerve, 230–232
  neurodynamic testing, 230–231
  in piriformis syndrome, 218
  tensioning movements, 45
  treatment, *231*, 231–232
  see also Superficial peroneal nerve
Peroneal neurodynamic test (PNT), *139*, 139–140
  in peroneal nerve problems, 230–231
  in piriformis syndrome, 219
Phalen's test, 7, 11–12, 188
Physical examination, 105–116
  in closing dysfunctions, 80–81, 82
  feeling for changes in movement, 106
  general points on technique, 113–116
  in inflammation dysfunction, 95
  level 0 (none), 107–108
  level 1 (limited), 108–109
  level 2 (standard), 109–110, 113

level 3, 110–113
    type 3a, 111
    type 3b, 111
    type 3c, 111–112
    type 3d, 112–113
  in mechanical interface dysfunctions, 79–80
  in motor control dysfunctions, 93
  nerve hypermobility, 90
  in opening dysfunctions, 83–84, 85–86
  in pathoanatomical dysfunction, 90–91
  in pathophysiological dysfunction, 88
  planning and extent, 106–113
  in sliding dysfunction, 89
  in tension dysfunction, 89–90
  see also Neurodynamic tests
Physiology, 15–19
  events, 15–18
  innervated tissues and, 18–19
  links with mechanics, 15, *15*
  see also Pathophysiological dysfunction
Piriformis neurodynamic test, 219, *219*, *220*
  modified, 220, *220*
Piriformis slump test, 220–221, *221*
Piriformis syndrome, 45, 218–223
  physical examination/diagnosis, 218–221
    level 1, 2 and 3a, 219
    level 3b, 219, *219*, *220*
    level 3c, 220–221
  sliding dysfunction, 89
  treatment, 221–223
Plantar fasciitis, 232–235
Posterior interosseous nerve
  compression, 12
  elbow pronation and supination, 42
  neurodynamic massage, 187
Posterior tibial nerve, 232–235
  mechanical interface testing and treatment, 232–233
  neurodynamic testing, 233–235
  tensioning movements, 44
  treatment, 235
Posture
  cervical radiculopathy and, 160
  in closing dysfunctions, 80, 82

head, cervicogenic headache and, 169–170
  in opening dysfunctions, 83, 85–86
Pressure, elevated
  causes, 62
  in clinical reasoning, 92
  interaction with mechanical irritation, 63
  neural effects, 62, *62*
  see also Compression
Pronator tunnel syndrome, 180–184
  mechanical interface, 181
  neural component, 181–184
Prone knee bend (PKB), 44, 145–147
  common problems, 147
  lumbar radiculopathy, 198
  mid-lumbar disorders, 214
  normal response, 147
  sensitizing movements, 44, 147
  structural differentiation, 146
  technique, 146, *147*
Protective muscle hyperactivity dysfunction, 66–67
  clinical example, 93, *93*
  diagnosis, 92–93
Provocative testing, 114
  carpal tunnel syndrome, 42, 43
Provoking symptoms, during treatment, 157–158

R

Radial nerve
  glenohumeral internal rotation and, 41
  lateral neck flexion and, 40
Radial neurodynamic test (RNT), 128–130, *129*, *130*
  history, *xii*
  supinator tunnel syndrome, 185–187, *186*
Radial sensory neurodynamic test (RSNT), 10, *10*, 131–132, *132*
Radiculopathy *see* Cervical radiculopathy; Lumbar radiculopathy
Radiological investigation, 79, 80
Red blood cells, 69
Reduced closing dysfunctions, 53, *53*
  cervical spine
    diagnosis, 164, *164*
    treatment, 164–166, *165*, 169

clinical example, 81
diagnosis, 80–81
lumbar spine, 198–202
    causes, 199
    level 1, 199–201, *200*
    level 2, *201*, 201–202
    level 3, 202, *202*
    mid-lumbar region, 216, *216*
    thoracic outlet syndrome,
        178–179, 180
    treatment, 154–155
        level 1, 154–155
        level 1 *vs* level 2, 155
        level 2, 155
Reduced opening dysfunctions,
    54–56, *55*
    case example, 84–85
    cervical spine
        diagnosis, 163, *164*
        treatment, 166, 168–169, *169*
    diagnosis, 83–85
    lumbar spine, 202
    mid-lumbar region, 215, *215*
    treatment, 155
Relevance, 51, 52
Relevant abnormal neurodynamic
    response, 103
Resistance to movement, 21
Rib
    first, 176, 177
    mobilization, 178, *179*, 180

S

S1 radiculopathy, 68
    muscle hyperactivity dysfunction,
        213, 213–214
    pathophysiological dysfunction,
        92
    trigger points, 214
Saphenous neurodynamic test
    (SAPHNT), 147–148, *148*,
    228
Sarcoma, muscle, 224
Scalene muscles, 177
Scapular depression, 40
Scarring, neural, 60, 63
Sciatic nerve
    hip movements and, 43, 44
    knee extension and, 44
    spinal lateral flexion and glide
        and, 36

in thigh, 223–228
    neurodynamic testing, 224–225
    treatment, *226*, 226–228, *227*
Sciatica, 199
Self neurodynamic mobilization,
    piriformis syndrome, 223,
    223
Sensation, loss of, 87
Sensitivity, diagnostic test, 99
Sensitization, 110
    contralateral lateral flexion and,
        36
    level 3a testing, 111
    level 3b testing, 110, 111
    level 3c testing, 110, 111–112
    level 3d testing, 110, 112–113
Sensitizing movements, 98
Sequencing *see* Neurodynamic
    sequencing
Shoulder, 40–41
    pain, 176–180
    see also Glenohumeral joint
Sliders, 14, 22, 156
    carpal tunnel syndrome, 191–193,
        192, *193*
    caudad, 156, 158
    cephalad, 158
    cervical radiculopathy, 166, *166*,
        167
    cervicogenic headache, 170–171,
        171
    defined, 22
    femoral nerve, 229, *229*
    lumbar spine, 202–206, *203*, *204*,
        206
    mid-lumbar disorders, 214–215
    one-ended, 156
    peroneal nerve, 231, *231*
    piriformis syndrome, 222, *222*
    posterior tibial nerve, *234*, 235
    pronator tunnel syndrome,
        181–183, *182*, *183*
    sciatic nerve in thigh, *226*,
        226–227, *227*
    supinator tunnel syndrome,
        185–186, *186*, *187*
    sural nerve, 236, *236*
    technique and dosage, 156
    thoracic outlet syndrome, 180,
        180
    two-ended, 156
    uses, 22, 156
Sliding, neural, 5–6

interfascicular, 6
longitudinal, 5, *6*
spinal neural tissues, 33–34
transverse, 6, *6*
Sliding dysfunctions, 59–60
    carpal tunnel syndrome, 191–193
    diagnosis, 88–89
    lumbar spine, 202–206
    posterior tibial nerve, 233–234
    pronator tunnel syndrome,
        181–183
    sciatic nerve in thigh, 226–227
    supinator tunnel syndrome,
        185–186
    thoracic outlet syndrome, 179
    treatment, 156, 158
SLR *see* Straight leg raise
Slump test, 8–10, 141–145
    common problems, 145
    diagnosis of dysfunctions, 197
    hamstring, 225, *225*
    indications, 141
    level 1, 196, *196*
    level 3a, 197, *197*
    long sitting, 209, *210*, 232, 233,
        237
    lumbar radiculopathy, 196–197,
        197
    non-organic back pain and, 39
    normal response, 144–145
    piriformis, 220–221, *221*
    structural differentiation, 144, *145*
    technique, 141–144, *143*, *144*
    see also Cervical slump test;
        Femoral slump test
Specific neurodynamics, 2, 31–45
Specific neuropathodynamics, 50
Specificity, diagnostic test, 99–100
Speed of movement, 22
Spinal canal, 32–33
    length change during flexion,
        32, *32*
    opening during flexion, 33
Spinal cord
    effect of gravity, 37, *37*
    during spinal flexion, 33, *34*
    during spinal rotation, 36
    tethering, 14, 59–60
Spinal nerve roots
    closing mechanisms, 11
    contralateral neurodynamic tests
        and, 37–38
    hip flexion and, *43*, 43–44

Spinal nerve roots (*contd*)
  opening dysfunction, 54
  see also Cervical radiculopathy;
    Lumbar radiculopathy
Spine, 32–39
  bilateral neurodynamic
    techniques, 38–39
  contralateral neurodynamic tests,
    37–38
  effect of gravity, 37
  flexion and extension, 32–35
  lateral flexion and lateral glide,
    35–36
  radiological investigations, 79
  rotation, 36–37
  sequencing, 24
Straight leg raise (SLR) test, 43–44,
    132–135
  ankle dorsiflexion and, 44
  bilateral *see* Bilateral straight leg
    raise (BSLR) test
  biomechanics, 14
  common problems, 134–135
  effect of gravity, 37
  effects on neural tissues, *43*, 43–44
  hamstring injury, 224–225
  indications, 133
  level 1, 197
  level/type 3a, 197–198, *198*
  lumbar radiculopathy, 197–198,
    198
  mechanical interface, 43
  neural sliding, 5, 33
  non-organic back pain and, 39
  normal response, 135, *135*
  sensitizing movements, 44, 133,
    134
  sequencing, 24, 25
  structural differentiation,
    133–134, *134*
  technique, 133, *134*
Strain, spinal neural tissues, 33, *34*
Stretch, pain and, 18
Stretching, nerve, 2, 23
Structural differentiation, 13–14, 115
  contralateral lateral flexion and,
    36
  modified, 108–109
  movements, 98
  negative, 100
  positive, 100–101
Subclinical neurodynamic response,
    103–104

Suboptimal, 51, 52
Substance P, 18
  in inflammation, 18, 62, 69
  vasodilator effect, 16
Superficial peroneal nerve, 230
  impaired sliding, 88
  transverse sliding, 6
Supinator muscle, 42
Supinator tunnel syndrome,
    184–187
  mechanical interface, 185
  neural component, 185–187
Sural nerve, 235–237
  neurodynamic testing, 235–236
  tensioning movements, 45
  treatment, *236*, 236–237
Sural neurodynamic test (SNT), *140*,
    140–141, *142*, 235–236
Sympathetic nervous system, 16, 72
Symptoms
  closing dysfunctions, 80, 82
  inflammation dysfunction, 94–95
  mechanical interface
    dysfunctions, 78
  nerve hypermobility, 90
  opening dysfunctions, 83, 85
  pathoanatomical dysfunction, 87,
    90
  pathophysiological dysfunction,
    87–88
  reduced neural sliding, 88–89
  tension dysfunction, 89

T

Tarsal tunnel syndrome, 232
  nerve massage, 235
  sliding dysfunction, 60, 234–235
Tension, neural, 2
  dynamics, 14–15
  generation, 5, *5*
  intraneural blood flow and, 17
  lateral spinal flexion and, 35, *36*
  spinal flexion and, 33, *34*
  transmission along system, 13
Tension dysfunctions, 60–61, *61*
  carpal tunnel syndrome,
    193–194
  cervical spine, 167–169
  diagnosis, 83, 89–90
  lumbar spine, 206–209
  posterior tibial nerve, 235

pronator tunnel syndrome,
    183–184
  sciatic nerve in thigh, 227–228
  supinator tunnel syndrome,
    186–187
  thoracic outlet syndrome, 180
  treatment, 157, 158
Tensioners, 14, 22–23, 157
  carpal tunnel syndrome, 193–194
  cervical radiculopathy, 167–168,
    168, *169*
  cervicogenic headache, 171
  defined, 22
  femoral nerve, 229
  lumbar radiculopathy, 207,
    208–209, *209*
  mid-lumbar disorders, 215
  one-ended, 157
  peroneal nerve, 231–232
  piriformis syndrome, 222
  pronator tunnel syndrome,
    183–184, *184*
  sciatic nerve in thigh, 227
  sural nerve, 236–237
  technique and dosage, 157
  thoracic outlet syndrome, 179
  two-ended, 157
  uses, 22–23, 157
Tethered median nerve stress test, 43
Thigh pain, 228–230
Thixotropy, 64–65
Thoracic outlet syndrome, 176–180
  clinical features, 177–178
  interface closing dysfunction,
    178–179
  mechanical interface dynamics,
    177
  mechanical interface evaluation,
    178
  neurodynamics, 179–180
  neuropathodynamics, 176–177
  physical examination and
    treatment, 178–180
  problems in diagnosis and
    treatment, 176
Three part system, 2–4, *3*
Tibial nerve, posterior *see* Posterior
    tibial nerve
Tibial neurodynamic test (TNT),
    137–138
  in posterior tibial nerve
    dysfunction, 233, 235
  technique, *137*, 137–138, *138*

Tinel's test, 188
Tissues, innervated *see* Innervated
    tissues
Tourniquet effect, 62, *62*
Trapezius muscle, imbalance
    dysfunction, 93–94, *94*
Trauma, past history, 79, 83, 160
Treatment, 153–158
    contralateral movements, 38
    mechanical interface
        dysfunctions, 154–155
    neural dysfunctions, 156–158
    progression through levels,
        157–158
    spinal flexion and extension
        and, 35
Trigger points, 68
    diagnosis, 94
    lumbar radiculopathy, 213, 214

U

Ulnar nerve
    bending, 8

clicking, 90
closing mechanisms, 12
elbow flexion and, 41
impaired sliding, 88
instability, 61
lateral neck flexion and, 40
Ulnar neuritis, 87, 90
Ulnar neurodynamic test (UNT),
    xii, 121–125
    common problems, 123–124
    indications, 122
    normal response, 124–125, *125*
    sequencing aspects, 20, *20*
    technique, 122–123, *123*, *124*
    thoracic outlet syndrome, 180
Ultrasound scanning, 79
Upper cervical slump test (UCST),
    170–173
    level 1, 170–171
    level 2, 171
    level 3a, 171
    level 3b, 171–173, *172*, *173*
    level 3c, *173*, 173–174
Upper limb/quarter, 175–194
    neurodynamic tests, 118–132

occupational overuse, 60
sensitizing movements, 98
sliding dysfunction, 89
specific neurodynamics, 39–43

V

Vasoconstriction, 16
Vasodilation, 16
Viscoelasticity, 15

W

Watson's test, 188
White cells, 69
Wrist, 42–43
    flexion and extension, 42
    radial and ulnar deviation, 42–43

ELSEVIER CD-ROM LICENSE AGREEMENT

PLEASE READ THE FOLLOWING AGREEMENT CAREFULLY BEFORE USING THIS PRODUCT. THIS PRODUCT IS LICENSED UNDER THE TERMS CONTAINED IN THIS LICENCE AGREEMENT ("Agreement"). BY USING THIS PRODUCT, YOU, AN INDIVIDUAL OR ENTITY INCLUDING EMPLOYEES, AGENTS AND REPRESENTATIVES ("You" or "Your"), ACKNOWLEDGE THAT YOU HAVE READ THIS AGREEMENT, THAT YOU UNDERSTAND IT, AND THAT YOU AGREE TO BE BOUND BY THE TERMS AND CONDITIONS OF THIS AGREEMENT. ELSEVIER LIMITED ("Elsevier") EXPRESSLY DOES NOT AGREE TO LICENSE THIS PRODUCT TO YOU UNLESS YOU ASSENT TO THIS AGREEMENT. IF YOU DO NOT AGREE WITH ANY OF THE FOLLOWING TERMS, YOU MAY, WITHIN THIRTY (30) DAYS AFTER YOUR RECEIPT OF THIS PRODUCT RETURN THE UNUSED PRODUCT AND ALL ACCOMPANYING DOCUMENTATION TO ELSEVIER FOR A FULL REFUND.

DEFINITIONS As used in this Agreement, these terms shall have the following meanings:

"Proprietary Material" means the valuable and proprietary information content of this Product including without limitation all indexes and graphic materials and software used to access, index, search and retrieve the information content from this Product developed or licensed by Elsevier and/or its affiliates, suppliers and licensors.

"Product" means the copy of the Proprietary Material and any other material delivered on CD-ROM and any other human readable or machine-readable materials enclosed with this Agreement, including without limitation documentation relating to the same.

OWNERSHIP This Product has been supplied by and is proprietary to Elsevier and/or its affiliates, suppliers and licensors. The copyright in the Product belongs to Elsevier and/or its affiliates, suppliers and licensors and is protected by the copyright, trademark, trade secret and other intellectual property laws of the United Kingdom and international treaty provisions, including without limitation the Universal Copyright Convention and the Berne Copyright Convention. You have no ownership rights in this Product. Except as expressly set forth herein, no part of this Product, including without limitation the Proprietary Material, may be modified, copied or distributed in hardcopy or machine-readable form without prior written consent from Elsevier. All rights not expressly granted to You herein are expressly reserved. Any other use of this Product by any person or entity is strictly prohibited and a violation of this Agreement.

SCOPE OF RIGHTS LICENSED (PERMITTED USES) Elsevier is granting to You a limited, non-exclusive, non-transferable licence to use this Product in accordance with the terms of this Agreement. You may use or provide access to this Product on a single computer or terminal physically located at Your premises and in a secure network or move this Product to and use it on another single computer or terminal at the same location for personal use only, but under no circumstances may You use or provide access to any part or parts of this Product on more than one computer or terminal simultaneously.

You shall not (a) copy, download, or otherwise reproduce the Product or any part(s) thereof in any medium, including, without limitation, online transmissions, local area networks, wide area networks, intranets, extranets and the Internet, or in any way, in whole or in part, except for printing out or downloading nonsubstantial portions of the text and images in the Product for Your own personal use; (b) alter, modify, or adapt the Product or any part(s) thereof, including but not limited to decompiling, disassembling, reverse engineering, or creating derivative works, without the prior written approval of Elsevier; (c) sell, license or otherwise distribute to third parties the Product or any part(s) thereof; or (d) alter, remove, obscure or obstruct the display of any copyright, trademark or other proprietary notice on or in the Product or on any printout or download of portions of the Proprietary Materials.

RESTRICTIONS ON TRANSFER This Licence is personal to You, and neither Your rights hereunder nor the tangible embodiments of this Product, including without limitation the Proprietary Material, may be sold, assigned, transferred or sublicensed to any other person, including without limitation by operation of law, without the prior written consent of Elsevier. Any purported sale, assignment, transfer or sublicense without the prior written consent of Elsevier will be void and will automatically terminate the Licence granted hereunder.

TERM This Agreement will remain in effect until terminated pursuant to the terms of this Agreement. You may terminate this Agreement at any time by removing from Your system and destroying the Product and any copies of the Proprietary Material. Unauthorized copying of the Product, including without limitation, the

Proprietary Material and documentation, or otherwise failing to comply with the terms and conditions of this Agreement shall result in automatic termination of this licence and will make available to Elsevier legal remedies. Upon termination of this Agreement, the licence granted herein will terminate and You must immediately destroy the Product and all copies of the Product and of the Proprietary Material, together with any and all accompanying documentation. All provisions relating to proprietary rights shall survive termination of this Agreement.

LIMITED WARRANTY AND LIMITATION OF LIABILITY Elsevier warrants that the software embodied in this Product will perform in substantial compliance with the documentation supplied in this Product, unless the performance problems are the result of hardware failure or improper use. If You report a significant defect in performance in writing to Elsevier within ninety (90) calendar days of your having purchased the Product, and Elsevier is not able to correct same within sixty (60) days after its receipt of Your notification, You may return this Product, including all copies and documentation, to Elsevier and Elsevier will refund Your money. In order to apply for a refund on your purchased Product, please contact the return address on the invoice to obtain the refund request form ("Refund Request Form"), and either fax or mail your signed request and your proof of purchase to the address indicated on the Refund Request Form. Incomplete forms will not be processed. Defined terms in the Refund Request Form shall have the same meaning as in this Agreement.

YOU UNDERSTAND THAT, EXCEPT FOR THE LIMITED WARRANTY RECITED ABOVE, ELSEVIER, ITS AFFILIATES, LICENSORS, THIRD PARTY SUPPLIERS AND AGENTS (TOGETHER "THE SUPPLIERS") MAKE NO REPRESENTATIONS OR WARRANTIES, WITH RESPECT TO THE PRODUCT, INCLUDING, WITHOUT LIMITATION THE PROPRIETARY MATERIAL. ALL OTHER REPRESENTATIONS, WARRANTIES, CONDITIONS OR OTHER TERMS, WHETHER EXPRESS OR IMPLIED BY STATUTE OR COMMON LAW, ARE HEREBY EXCLUDED TO THE FULLEST EXTENT PERMITTED BY LAW.

IN PARTICULAR BUT WITHOUT LIMITATION TO THE FOREGOING NONE OF THE SUPPLIERS MAKE ANY REPRESENTATIONS OR WARRANTIES (WHETHER EXPRESS OR IMPLIED) REGARDING THE PERFORMANCE OF YOUR PAD, NETWORK OR COMPUTER SYSTEM WHEN USED IN CONJUNCTION WITH THE PRODUCT, NOR THAT THE PRODUCT WILL MEET YOUR REQUIREMENTS OR THAT ITS OPERATION WILL BE UNINTERRUPTED OR ERROR-FREE.

EXCEPT IN RESPECT OF DEATH OR PERSONAL INJURY CAUSED BY THE SUPPLIERS' NEGLIGENCE AND TO THE FULLEST EXTENT PERMITTED BY LAW, IN NO EVENT (AND REGARDLESS OF WHETHER SUCH DAMAGES ARE FORESEEABLE AND OF WHETHER SUCH LIABILITY IS BASED IN TORT, CONTRACT OR OTHERWISE) WILL ANY OF THE SUPPLIERS BE LIABLE TO YOU FOR ANY DAMAGES (INCLUDING, WITHOUT LIMITATION, ANY LOST PROFITS, LOST SAVINGS OR OTHER SPECIAL, INDIRECT, INCIDENTAL OR CONSEQUENTIAL DAMAGES ARISING OUT OF OR RESULTING FROM: (I) YOUR USE OF, OR INABILITY TO USE, THE PRODUCT; (II) DATA LOSS OR CORRUPTION; AND/OR (III) ERRORS OR OMISSIONS IN THE PROPRIETARY MATERIAL.

IF THE FOREGOING LIMITATION IS HELD TO BE UNENFORCEABLE, OUR MAXIMUM LIABILITY TO YOU IN RESPECT THEREOF SHALL NOT EXCEED THE AMOUNT OF THE LICENCE FEE PAID BY YOU FOR THE PRODUCT. THE REMEDIES AVAILABLE TO YOU AGAINST ELSEVIER AND THE LICENSORS OF MATERIALS INCLUDED IN THE PRODUCT ARE EXCLUSIVE.

If the information provided In the Product contains medical or health sciences information, it is intended for professional use within the medical field. Information about medical treatment or drug dosages is intended strictly for professional use, and because of rapid advances in the medical sciences, independent verification of diagnosis and drug dosages should be made. The provisions of this Agreement shall be severable, and in the event that any provision of this Agreement is found to be legally unenforceable, such unenforceability shall not prevent the enforcement or any other provision of this Agreement.

GOVERNING LAW This Agreement shall be governed by the laws of England and Wales. In any dispute arising out of this Agreement, you and Elsevier each consent to the exclusive personal jurisdiction and venue in the courts of England and Wales.

Minimum System Requirements

To function properly, the computer utilizing this CD should support at least an 800×600 pixels screen resolution, 256 colors, 64MB RAM and operate on the Windows 98, 2000, NT, ME or XP operating system or the MAC OS 9.1+ operating system. Additionally, before beginning, be sure the browser is JavaScript enabled, has cookies enabled and has the 'show images' checkbox enabled.

Technical Support

Technical support for this product is available between 7.30 a.m. and 7.00 p.m. CST, 8.00 a.m. and 1.00 a.m. UK, Monday through Friday.

Before calling, be sure that your computer meets the minimum system requirements to run this software.

Inside the United States and Canada, call 1-800-692-9010.

Inside the United Kingdom, call 00800-6929-0100.

Outside North America, call +1-314-872-8370.

You may also fax your questions to +1-314-997-5080,

or contact Technical Support through e-mail: technical.support@elsevier.com.

Printed in the United States
By Bookmasters